# Colitis: Diagnosis and Therapeutic Strategies

FALK SYMPOSIUM 147

# Colitis: Diagnosis and Therapeutic Strategies

### Edited by

**D.P. Jewell**
*The Radcliffe Infirmary*
*Oxford*
*United Kingdom*

**J.-F. Colombel**
*Claude Huriez Hospital*
*CHRU, Lille*
*France*

**A.S. Peña**
*Free University*
*Amsterdam*
*The Netherlands*

**A. Tromm**
*Evangelical Hospital*
*Hattingen*
*Germany*

**B.F. Warren**
*John Radcliffe Hospital*
*Oxford*
*United Kingdom*

*Proceedings of the Falk Symposium 147 held in Birmingham, UK,*
*May 6–7, 2005*

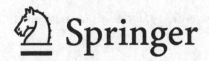 Springer

Library of Congress Cataloging-in-Publication Data is available.

ISBN-10 1-4020-4315-5
ISBN-13 978-14020-4315-4

---

Published by Springer,
PO Box 17, 3300 AA Dordrecht, The Netherlands

Sold and distributed in North, Central and South America
by Springer,
101 Philip Drive, Norwell, MA 02061 USA

In all other countries, sold and distributed
by Springer,
PO Box 322, 3300 AH Dordrecht, The Netherlands

*Printed on acid-free paper*

Printed and bound in Great Britain by MPG Books Limited, Bodmin, Cornwall.

# Contents

## SECTION VI: IMMUNOMODULATORY THERAPY
### Chair: SPL Travis, A Tromm

## SECTION VII: CANCER AND IBD
### Chair: S Prantera, J Satsangi

## SECTION VIII: NEW THERAPEUTIC APPROACHES
### Chair: F Pallone, EF Stange

# List of principal contributors

**A Axon**
Department of Gastroenterology
The General Infirmary at Leeds
Great George Street
Leeds, LS1 3EX
UK

**S Bar-Meir**
Chaim Sheba Medical Center
Department of Gastroenterology
2 Sheba Road
52 621 Tel Hashomer
Israel

**J Bohr**
Division of Gastroenterology
Örebro University Hospital
SE-701 85 Örebro
Sweden

**J-F Colombel**
Department of Hepato-
  Gastroenterology
Hopital Claude Huriez
CHRU Lille
1 Place de Verdun
F-59037 Lille Cedex
France

**J Emmrich**
Klinikum der Universität Rostock
Gastroenterologie
Ernst-Heydemann-Str. 6
D-18057 Rostock
Germany

**F Fernández-Bañares**
Department of Gastroenterology
Hospital Universitari Mutua Terrassa
Plaza Dr Robert 5
E-08221 Terrassa, Barcelona
Spain

**A Forbes**
Department of Gastroenterology
University College Hospital
235 Euston Road
London, NW1 2BU
UK

**K Geboes**
Department of Pathology
University Hospital St. Rafael
Catholic University of Leuven
Minderbroederstraat 12
B-3000 Leuven
Belgium

**E Hertervig**
Department of Gastroenterology
Lund University Hospital
S-221 85 Lund
Sweden

**S Itzkowitz**
Mount Sinai School of Medicine
Gastrointestinal Division, Box 1069
One Gustave Levy Place
New York, NY 10029
USA

**DP Jewell**
The Radcliffe Infirmary
Oxfordshire Health Authority
Gastroenterology Unit
Nuffield Department of Medicine
Woodstock Road
Oxford, OX2 6HE
UK

**D Kelleher**
Department of Clinical Medicine
Trinity Centre, St James' Hospital
Dublin
Ireland

**R Kiesslich**
I. Med Klinik und Poliklinik
Johannes Gutenberg Universität
  Mainz
Langenbeckstr. 1
D-55131 Mainz
Germany

**EV Loftus Jr**
Division of Gastroenterology and
  Hepatology
Mayo Clinic College of Medicine
200 First Street, SW
Rochester, MN 55905
USA

**P Marteau**
Service d'Hepato-Gastroenterologie
Hopital Europeen Georges
  Pompidou
20 rue Leblanc
F-75908 Paris Cedex 15
France

**NJ Mortensen**
Department of Colorectal Surgery
John Radcliffe Hospital
Oxford
OX3 9DU
UK

**MF Neurath**
I. Department of Medicine
University of Mainz
Langenbeckstrasse 1
D-55131 Mainz
Germany

**TR Orchard**
St Mary's Hospital and Imperial
  College London
Department of Gastroenterology
Praed Street
London, W12 1NY
UK

**AS Peña**
Department of Gastroenterology
Department of Pathology
VU University Medical Center
PO Box 7057
NL-1007 MB Amsterdam
The Netherlands

**CSJ Probert**
Clinical Sciences at South Bristol
University of Bristol
Bristol Royal Infirmary
Bristol, BS2 8HW
UK

**JM Rhodes**
University of Liverpool
Gastroenterology Research Group
Duncan Building
PO Box 147
Liverpool, L69 3BX
UK

**J Schölmerich**
Klinik und Poliklinik für Innere
  Medizin I
Klinikum der Universität Regensburg
D-93042 Regensburg
Germany

**A Tromm**
Klinik fur Innere Medizin
Evangelisches Krankenhaus
  Hattingen
Akademisches Lehrkranenhaus
Bredenscheider Str. 54
D-45525 Hattingen
Germany

**GNJ Tytgat**
Academic Medical Center
Department of Gastroenterology and
  Hepatology
University of Amsterdam
Meibergdreef 9
1105 AZ Amsterdam
The Netherlands

**S Vermeire**
Department of Internal Medicine
Gastroenterology Unit
University Hospital Leuven
Herestraat 49
B-3000 Leuven
Belgium

**BF Warren**
John Radcliffe Hospital
University of Oxford
Department of Cellular Pathology
Headley Way Headington
Oxford, OX3 9DU
UK

**JV Weinstock**
Division of Gastroenterology/
  Hepatology
Tufts New England Medical Center
  (Box 223)
750 Washington Street
Boston, MA 02111
USA

# List of chairpersons

**J-F Colombel**
Department of Hepato-
  Gastroenterology
Hôpital Claude Huriez
CHRU Lille
1 Place de Verdun
F-59037 Lille Cedex
France

**A Forbes**
Department of Gastroenterology
University College Hospital
235 Euston Road
London NW1 2BU
UK

**K Geboes**
Catholic University of Leuven
University Hospital St. Rafael
Department of Pathology
Minderbroederstraat 12
B-3000 Leuven
Belgium

**S Ghosh**
Imperial College London
Hammersmith Hospital Campus
Department of Gastroenterology
Du Cane Road
London, W12 0NN
UK

**MA Kamm**
St. Mark's Hospital
Gastroenterology Unit
Colorectal Disorders
Watford Road
Harrow, HA1 3UJ
UK

**MRB Keighley**
Whaleborne Cottage
Tanworth Arden
West Midlands
B94 5AN
UK

**F Pallone**
Università di Roma
Cattedra di Gastroenterologia
Dipartimento di Medicina Interna
Via Di Tor Vergata 135
I-00133 Roma
Italy

**AS Peña**
Department of Gastroenterology
Department of Pathology
VU University Medical Center
PO Box 7057
NL-1007 MB Amsterdam
The Netherlands

**C Prantera**
Azienda Ospedaliera
S. Camilo Forlanini
Via Portuense 292
I-00149 Roma
Italy

**DB Sachar**
Mount Sinai School of Medicine
Division of Gastroenterology
Box 1069
One Gustave L. Levy Place
New York, NY 10029-6574
USA

**J Satsangi**
University of Edinburgh
Western General Hospital
Gastrointestinal Unit
Crewe Road
Edinburgh, EH4 2XU
UK

**E-F Stange**
Innere Medizin I
Robert-Bosch-Krankenhaus
Auerbachstr. 110
D-70376 Stuttgart
Germany

**SPL Travis**
John Radcliffe Hospital
University of Oxford
Headley Way, Headington
Oxford, OX3 9DU
UK

**A Tromm**
Klinik für Innere Medizin
Evangelisches Krankenhaus
 Hattingen
Akademisches Lehrkranenhaus
Bredenscheider Str. 54
D-45525 Hattingen
Germany

**C Tysk**
Örebro Medical Center Hospital
Department of Gastroenterology
SE-70185 Örebro
Sweden

**BF Warren**
John Radcliffe Hospital
University of Oxford
Department of Cellular Pathology
Headley Way, Headington
Oxford, OX3 9DU
UK

# Preface

The 147th Falk Symposium was held in May 2005 in Birmingham to mark the launch of Dr Falk Pharma UK. Thus, it seemed appropriate to provide mainly a clinical forum but with some basic science underpinning the advances in clinical diagnosis and management. Indeed, these advances have been truly remarkable over recent years, which have not only led to a more optimal use of existing therapies but have seen an explosion in new therapeutic strategies. Many of these have stemmed from an increased understanding of the mechanisms of intestinal inflammation and the interaction between host and the environment (especially the intestinal flora). Thus, after many years of hope and considerable investment of both time and money, the benefits of translational research are becoming apparent. Patients with ulcerative colitis and Crohn's disease are genuinely benefiting from the 'bench-to-bedside' approach.

In the splendid surroundings of the International Convention Centre in Birmingham, equally splendid reviews were given and enthusiastically discussed. This book is based on those reviews and the Organising Scientific Committee thanks all the Authors for their excellent contributions. We also thank Ms Silvia Maresch of the Falk Foundation for her outstanding organising abilities without which these Symposia and the extraction of manuscripts might never occur. Our thanks are also given to Mr Phil Johnstone of Springer Science and Business Media b.v. who ensures a high level of editing.

*D.P. Jewell, J-F. Colombel, A.S. Pena, A. Tromm and B.F. Warren*

# Section I
# Diagnosis

Chair: K. GEBOES and D. SACHAR

# 1
# Role of capsule endoscopy in Crohn's disease

S. BAR-MEIR

Capsule endoscopy (CE) is used with increased frequency in patients with Crohn's disease (CD). The number of publications on CE in CD in peer-reviewed journals is now about 20, and half of them have been published in the past year alone.

The sensitivity of CE in the diagnosis of CD has been shown to be the highest compared to other tests available. This was first shown by Costamagna et al.[1], who compared CE to small bowel follow-through (SBFT) in the evaluation of small bowel pathologies. Twenty patients underwent both examinations; CE identified CD in three patients and SBFT in 1. Herrerias et al.[2] studied 21 patients who were suspected of having CD, but with a negative work-up. All patients underwent CE and in 43% the diagnosis of CD was confirmed. The location of the disease was mainly in the terminal ileum but also in the jejunum and duodenum. The ability to identify Crohn's lesions in the proximal small intestine is far more frequent with CE. Similar findings were reported by Fireman et al.[3] who diagnosed CD in 12 of 17 patients suspected of having CD. These patients were followed for a mean of 6 years and failed to be diagnosed by any other diagnostic modality. Ileal intubation during colonoscopy was achieved only in six patients. In another study only patients in whom retrograde ileoscopy was performed were included. CE had a similar yield to ileoscopy and both were superior to SBFT in the terminal ileum. However, only CE proved to be of diagnostic value in the proximal small intestine. An impressive study came from Indianapolis[4], where three patients with significant findings of CD on CE underwent state-of-the-art enteroclysis. The radiologist, although being aware of the findings by CE, was unable to detect any pathology on enteroclysis. Thus the workers concluded that CE is the gold standard examination for the detection of small bowel ulcers and is better than the best enteroclysis available. Its incremental yield over other modalities such as computed tomography (CT) enterography, push enteroscopy and small bowel magnetic resonance imaging (MRI) ranges between 20% and 44%.

Our group analysed 78 patients suspected of having CD. In all the patients investigations had been negative. The aim of the study was to assess which symptom is most likely to be associated with CD on CE. Results showed that none of the 11 patients with only abdominal pain had a positive study, whereas in 42 patients with anaemia, and in nine patients with diarrhoea, 9.5% and 11%, respectively, had CD. Among patients with at least two symptoms, the likelihood of finding CD increased to 38% (6/16). The low yield of CE in patients with abdominal pain confirms our previous findings[5].

CE also has a role in patients with established inflammatory bowel disease (IBD). Mow et al.[6] used CE in 50 patients with IBD, the majority being patients with colitis or pouchitis and minority patients with CD. CE was diagnostic for CD in 20 patients and suspicious for small bowel CD in another 10 patients. As a result of the findings on CE, management was changed in half of the patients. Voderholzer et al.[7] compared the extent of disease in 41 patients with known CD using CT enterography and CE. A similar rate of terminal ileum involvement was seen by both techniques. CE, however, detected twice as many lesions in the proximal small intestine compared to CT enterography. Outcome was changed due to CE findings in 10 patients. Consequently, all of them improved clinically. In two patients the capsule was entrapped. In one patient it passed following corticosteroids administration, and in the second patient it was removed via an enteroscope.

There are several caveats while using CE in patients with suspected CD. The first is related to the fact that the ileocaecal valve is reached in only 70–80% of the examinations while the batteries are still active. In order to exclude CD of the small intestine it is essential to confirm that the entire small intestine was examined and that the ileocaecal valve was reached. Failure to reach the ileocaecal valve may result in a false-negative study.

The second caveat is related to the scoring system. At the present time there is no good scoring system to quantify the damage to the mucosa. A description such as 'erosions in the terminal ileum' is not good enough to describe the extent and severity of the disease. Lewis suggested a scoring system based on the localization of lesions within the small intestine, number, shape and distribution of the lesions and whether erythema, oedema, nodularity, ulceration or stenosis exists. The correlation between the Lewis scoring system and the CDAI is poor. Graham et al. developed a simpler scoring system based on the number and size of the lesions[8]. Such scoring systems may be of help in clinical trials when the therapeutic effect of a medication is being evaluated.

It is important to keep in mind that a small number of mucosal erosions and petechiae were seen in the small bowel in from 10% to 13.8% of the normal population[8,9]. Thus the diagnosis of CD should be reserved only for patients with significant and unequivocal findings.

Erosions and ulcers seen on CE may result from other causes/diseases such as the intake of non-steroidal anti-inflammatory drugs (NSAID), lymphoid hyperplasia, lymphoma, radiation enteritis, HIV with opportunistic infection, intestinal tuberculosis and Behçet's disease. Thus it is important to exclude the intake of NSAID prior to the final diagnosis of CD.

There has always been a concern regarding the capsule becoming impacted in the stenotic segment of the small bowel. An analysis of the data of 937 capsule studies made available by the company (Given imaging), suggested that in seven (0.75%) patients the capsule could not be excreted naturally[10]. Only in one patient did the capsule cause an acute obstruction. All these patients were operated on, and a stricture was identified and resected. In all patients the symptoms resolved following surgery. Six out of seven patients had a previous SBFT which was interpreted as normal. Thus, a prior SBFT was not enough to prevent capsule retention. The failure of SBFT to demonstrate strictures was shown very clearly by Kastin et al.[11]. They described a CD patient with a normal SBFT in whom the capsule became impacted. At surgery, 10 strictures were found, none of them seen on SBFT.

The rate of capsule retention in a meta-analysis of 240 patients with either established or suspected CD is 4.6%. This is higher than the rate of retention seen in the general population who undergo CE. A retained capsule can stay intact in the small bowel for almost 2 years without causing any symptoms.

A retained capsule which is within the reach of an endoscope can be removed endoscopically using a Roth basket or a snare. Administration of corticosteroids to a CD patient with a retained capsule may relieve the inflammation and allow the capsule to pass through. Capsule retention may be prevented by using the 'patency' capsule.

The 'patency' capsule is a capsule of a similar size to a regular capsule. It is composed of lactose with 10% of barium and is thus radio-opaque. Inside the capsule there is a thin radio-frequency tag which can be detected by a radio-frequency scanner. The capsule at one end has a timer plug which, after 40–50 h, will permit water penetration into the capsule and result in the disintegration of the capsule. When there is a patient at risk for capsule retention the patency capsule is administered first. On the second day the radio-frequency scanner is used to detect the capsule. By that time the majority of capsules are expected have been excreted. If the scanner does not detect the patency capsule inside the patient, a regular capsule can be given. Where the capsule is detected, the ingestion of a regular capsule may carry an increased risk for retention. It is expected that parts of the disintegrated patency capsule will pass through the stricture uneventfully.

Costamagna et al.[13] studied 63 patients with CD, 54 with known strictures. All ingested the patency capsule and 36 excreted the capsule intact. Fifteen of these patients then ingested a regular capsule and underwent an uneventful study. In the other 27 patients the capsule dissolved; 15 of them had abdominal pain at the time of the examination and one needed to be operated because of capsule impaction.

Similar findings were described by Boivin et al.[14], who administered the patency capsule to 12 patients with CD. In seven patients capsule excretion was uneventful, and four of them later also had an uneventful regular CE study. Four patients had significant abdominal pain from the patency capsule and an additional patient was operated because of impaction. Thus, the patency capsule may rarely cause an acute intestinal obstruction which will necessitate an emergency operation.

The majority of authors state that not only was the CE more sensitive in detecting CD, but the outcome in most of these patients was also improved. Goldfarb et al.[12] performed a cost-effective analysis and concluded that, in patients with suspected CD and a negative SBFT, CE is more cost-effective than enteroclysis. Furthermore, based on economic considerations, CE should become the first diagnostic test in patients suspected of CD.

In conclusion, CE seems to be the most sensitive test for the diagnosis of CD. The yield of CE is highest when more than one symptom exist. The study must be complete with visualization of the ileocaecal valve. The rate of capsule retention in CD patients is 5%. The retained capsule can be removed in most cases, and if such a patient is operated on, a significant pathology always exists with patient improvement after surgery. Obtaining a careful history for NSAID intake is crucial. The diagnosis of CD should be based on significant mucosal damage and one should refrain from diagnosing CD based on a few erosions only.

## References

1. Costamagna G, Shah SK, Riccioni ME et al. Prospective trial comparing small bowel radiographs and video capsule endoscopy for suspected small bowel disease. Gastroenterology. 2002;123:999–1005.
2. Herrerias JM, Caunedo A, Rodriguez-Tellez M, Pellicer F, Herrerias JM Jr. Capsule endoscopy in patients with suspected Crohn's disease and negative endoscopy. Endoscopy. 2003;35:564–8.
3. Fireman Z, Mahajna E, Broide E et al. Diagnosing small bowel Crohn's disease with wireless capsule endoscopy. Gut. 2003;52:390–2.
4. Liangpunsakul S, Chadalawada V, Rex DK, Maglinte D, Lappas J. Wireless capsule endoscopy detects small bowel ulcers in patients with normal results from state of the art enteroclysis. Am J Gastroenterol. 2003;98:1295–8.
5. Bardan E, Nadler M, Chowers Y, Fidder H, Bar-Meir S. Capsule endoscopy for the evaluation of patients with chronic abdominal pain. Endoscopy. 2003;35:688–9.
6. Mow WS, Lo SK, Targan SR et al. Initial experience with wireless capsule enteroscopy in the diagnosis and management of inflammatory bowel disease. Clin Gastroenterol Hepatol. 2004;2:31–40.
7. Voderholzer WA, Beinhoelzl J, Rogalla P et al. Small bowel involvement in Crohn's disease: a prospective comparison of wireless capsule endoscopy and computed tomography enteroclysis. Gut. 2005;54:369–73.
8. Graham DY, Opekun AR, Willingham FF, Qureshi WA. Visible small-intestinal mucosal injury in chronic NSAID users. Clin Gastroenterol Hepatol. 2005;3:55–9.
9. Goldstein JL, Eisen GM, Lewis B, Gralnek IM, Zlotnick S, Fort JG. Video capsule endoscopy to prospectively assess small bowel injury with celecoxib, naproxen plus omeprazole, and placebo. Clin Gastroenterol Hepatol. 2005;3:133–41.
10. Barkin JS, O'Loughlin C. Capsule endoscopy contraindications: complications and how to avoid their occurrence. Gastrointest Endosc Clin N Am. 2004;14:61–5.
11. Kastin DA, Buchman AL, Barrett T, Halverson A, Wallin A. Strictures from Crohn's disease diagnosed by video capsule endoscopy. J Clin Gastroenterol. 2004;38:346–9.
12. Goldfarb NI, Pizzi LT, Fuhr JP Jr et al. Diagnosing Crohn's disease: an economic analysis comparing wireless capsule endoscopy with traditional diagnostic procedures. Dis Manag. 2004;7:292–304.
13. Costamagna G, Spada C, Spera G et al. Evaluation of the Given patency system in the GI tract: results of a multicenter study. Gastrointest Endosc. 2004;59:A145.
14. Boivin MI, Voderholzer W, Loch H. The M2 patency capsule: the Berlin experience. Gastroenterology. 2004;126:A459.

# 2
# Endoscopy in Crohn's disease

## G. N. J. TYTGAT

## INTRODUCTION

An overview is given of the current role of colonoscopy in the diagnosis of Crohn's disease (CD). Particular attention will be given to the significance of aphthoid lesions as the earliest endoscopically detectable abnormality in CD. Other novel imaging modalities such as ultrasonography, magnetic resonance, spectroscopy etc. will not be considered. Experimental imaging technologies such as narrow-band imaging, fluorescence endoscopy, endocytoscopy, and laser confocal microscopy will also not be covered[1].

## INDICATIONS FOR ENDOSCOPY IN CROHN'S DISEASE (CD)

The indications for endoscopy in CD include: (1) the early diagnosis of and differentiation between CD and other inflammatory infectious diseases, particularly ulcerative colitis; (2) the initial and perioperative assessment of disease extent and presence of disease complications; (3) assessment of disease activity; (4) assessment of the efficacy of medical therapy; (5) assessment of postoperative disease recurrence; (6) balloon dilation of strictures.

## AETIOPATHOGENIC CONSIDERATIONS

In the acute phase of inflammatory bowel disease (IBD) the intestinal pathology of CD is similar to that of *Yersinia enterocolitica* or *Mycobacterium tuberculosis* and *Paratuberculosis*. An association of CD with mycobacteria has often been suggested; however, in spite of numerous studies, findings have failed to show any consistent association between mycobacterial infection and disease.

It is generally accepted that infectious agents gain entry to intestinal tissue, mainly via M-cell-rich mucosa of intestinal lymphoid aggregates, presumably also the earliest site of CD pathology. Yet bacteria are rarely observed in uninflamed CD mucosa.

# EARLY ENDOSCOPIC CHARACTERISTICS OF CD

## The aphthous or aphthoid lesion or erosion

Presumably the earliest endoscopic abnormalities in CD are tiny reddish spots which might evolve into typical aphthoid lesions[2-4]. Aphthoid lesions are flat or slightly depressed and are usually 2–3 mm but less than 5 mm in diameter, with a greyish or yellowish centre crater and surrounded by a red halo. Aphthoid lesions often occur in crops. The mucosa surrounding aphthoid lesions looks endoscopically normal with a non-disturbed vascular pattern. Occasionally the surrounding mucosa appears slightly opalescent with blurring of the microcirculation because of oedema.

Peyer's patches, in highest density in the terminal ileum and lymphoid follicles in the colon, are considered sites of early lesions[5]. They play a role in the selective uptake of luminal antigens. Perhaps the ability of the M cells to take up luminal antigens and to deliver them to the underlying lymphoid structures may be involved in the initiation of CD. A similar process may be considered to induce apthous lesions or lymphoid collections in the colon.

The aphthous lesions may then result from necrosis of M cells over Peyer's lymphoid follicles[4] or colonic lymphoid collections.

Subsequent inflammation in the follicle and lymphoid collections presumably leads to cytokine-mediated hyperaemia of the coronal capillary ring encircling the lymphoid collection responsible for the so-called red ring sign, which is occasionally quite conspicuous.

Surrounding the lymphoid collection there is often aberrant expression of major histocompatibility complex (MHC) class II antigens such as HLD: DR[6], relevant in antigen presentation.

Another hypothesis to explain the lymphoid cell accumulation relates to the observation that the induction of apoptosis in the mucosal T cell compartment is severely impaired. Because apoptosis of activated T cells is an important mechanism of peripheral immune tolerance, this finding may explain why the inflammatory reaction in IBD patients is resilient to resolution. Mucosal T cells proliferate more, express higher levels of IL-2 receptor $\alpha$, and are more cytotoxic in CD than in ulcerative colitis (UC). Production of IL-2, IFN-$\alpha$, IL-12 and IL-18 are elevated in CD but not in UC[7].

## Specificity of aphthoid lesions

Aphthoid lesions, thought to be quite characteristic for CD, do however lack specificity as they may develop in many other conditions such as early tuberculosis[8], the psychotrophic bacteria *Y. enterocolitica* and *Listeria monocytogenes*, shigellosis, salmonellosis, balantidiasis, diversion colitis, sodium phosphate colonic preparation, diverticulitis, and Behçet's disease[9,10]. Phosphate preparations have also been noted to induce rectosigmoid aphthous lesions, occurring in up to 5% of patients receiving such preparations[11].

## Small and medium-sized ulcers

As the disease progresses, smaller and larger ulcers develop. Whether such ulcers develop from those aphthous lesions, or whether they are the expression of a granulomatous vasculopathy, is still unknown. Certainly aphthous lesions and ulcers can coexist. The mucosa surrounding small and larger ulcers remains in principle intact, which constitutes a fundamental difference compared with the inflamed periulcerous mucosa in UC. Whatever the cause of CD, the latter has to explain the patchy discontinuous distribution of the ulcerous abnormalities. In active disease there is usually a spectrum of tissue defects, varying from very small well-delineated breaks to larger, irregularly shaped or serpiginous and ultimately deep excavating ulcers.

Particularly in the descending and sigmoid colon, ulcers tend to align and coalesce in a longitudinal fashion, causing the characteristic 'railroad-track' appearance. The anatomical substrate responsible for such longitudinal parallel alignment remains speculative. The interplay between railroad-tracking and superimposed transverse fissuring-type ulceration is considered to lead to the pathognomonic appearance of 'cobblestoning'. A similar 'bamboo'-like appearance may be seen in the stomach. The mucosa covering the 'cobblestones' is usually intact and not friable, but may reveal 'top-erythema' as a consequence of mucosal friction in a vigorously contracting tubular organ.

## Specificity of ulcerous defects

Despite rumours to the contrary, ulcers in CD are not entirely specific. Many conditions lead to patchy ulceration such as Behçet's disease, tuberculosis, amoebiasis, yersiniosis, cytomegalovirus and herpes infection, NSAID, etc. Only railroad tracking and cobblestoning appear almost pathognomonic for CD, although the latter has also been described in diverticulitis[12].

## SEVERE DISEASE

In severe disease, ulceration may involve almost the complete circumference of the affected segment, rendering the differential diagnosis with severe UC more difficult, if not impossible. Obvious inequality in the intensity of inflammation of the periulcerous mucosa should be thought of as suggestive for CD.

Strictures usually develop in areas of severe ulceration. Cobblestoning may be present at the mouth of such narrowed areas. Fistulas may develop between adjacent bowel loops or hollow organs. Intensive swelling of the surrounding mucosa may sometimes obscure the fistulous opening. Both stricture and fistula formation are rather characteristic for CD.

## HEALING PHASE

Healing leads to development of inflammatory pseudopolyps area scarring. In case of deep ulceration, thick whitish fibrous bands may dissect the mucosal lining and lead to diverticular-like outpouching of adjacent less-involved areas.

## ROLE OF ENDOSCOPY IN MONITORING MEDICAL THERAPY

If anti-inflammatory therapy is successful, this should lead to endoscopic regression of the inflammatory changes and healing of the ulcerous defects. It has been demonstrated that some 30% of patients treated with infliximab have complete mucosal healing after receiving three doses at 0, 2 and 6 weeks. Between 46% and 53% will have mucosal healing at week 52 after receiving maintenance therapy with infliximab every 8 weeks for the course of 1 year[13]. Patients who enter endoscopic remission are less likely to experience relapse, and have fewer disease-related complications than those with persistent mucosal ulceration. The latest endoscopic scoring system, the Simple Endoscopic Score for Crohn's Disease (SES-CD)[14], appears relatively easy to use but has to compete with other, less invasive surrogate markers and imaging procedures such as faecal calprotectin, magnetic resonance, ultrasound, capsule endoscopy, etc. (Table 1).

## WIRELESS CAPSULE ENDOSCOPY

Capsule endoscopy has attracted much interest in recent years. An increasingly explored indication is the possibility of small bowel CD[15–19]. Herrerias et al.[20] observed pathological findings for 43% of patients in whom there was a clinical suspicion of small bowel CD that could not be confirmed using traditional techniques, indicating that in these cases capsule endoscopy could be a valuable diagnostic tool.

## CONDITIONS MIMICKING CD

Many conditions may masquerade as CD; they include other inflammatory conditions, malignancies, drug-induced damage, endometriosis, radiation damage, pelvic inflammatory disease, diverticular disease, prolapse-associated wall damage, infectious diseases, ischaemic conditions, and a spectrum of miscellaneous pathologies. Particularly disturbing features in UC may mislead the endoscopist, such as rectal sparing, focal peri-appendiceal inflammation, patchiness both before and after therapy, stricturing, etc. Multiple biopsies from both normal and abnormal areas is sometimes but not always helpful in the differential diagnosis.

A high index of suspicion of confounding diseases, and a willingness to re-evaluate the diagnosis as time progresses, ultimately guarantee a high degree of diagnostic accuracy.

## ENDOSCOPIC ACTIVITY SCORES IN CD

The Crohn's Disease Endoscopic Index of Severity (CDEIS) was launched by French investigators in 1989[21]. At present the CDEIS to considered the gold standard for evaluation of endoscopic activity but the correlation with clinical

**Table 1**   Definitions of the Simple Endoscopic Score for Crohn's disease (SES-CD) variables

| Variable | SES-CD score | | | |
| --- | --- | --- | --- | --- |
| | *0* | *1* | *2* | *3* |
| Presence of ulcers | None | Aphthous ulcers ($\varnothing$ 0.1–0.5 cm) | Large ulcers ($\varnothing$ 0.5–2 cm) | Very large ulcers ($\varnothing$ 0.1–0.5 cm) |
| Ulcerated surface | None | <10% | 10–30% | >30% |
| Affected surface | Unaffected segment | <50% | 50–75% | >75% |
| Presence of narrowings | None | Single, can be passed | Multiple, can be passed | Cannot be passed |
| Number of affected segments | All variables = 0 | At least one variable $\geqslant$1 | | |

activity remains rather poor. The CDEIS, although reliable and reproducible, is rather time-consuming, and elaboration of the score requires analogue scale transformation.

More recently the SES-CD was proposed[14] (Table 1). The SES-CD is the sum of all variables – 1.4 × (number of affected segments).

## DISCUSSION

Pan-endoscopy, preferably before anti-inflammatory therapy, remains the key diagnostic modality for diagnosing CD in spite of major progress in pathogenesis, genetic and immunological characterization[21]. However, none of the characteristic endoscopic features in CD is truly pathognomonic except perhaps cobblestoning. A large number of disease entities may masquerade as CD. Therefore sequential information over a period of months or years should always be obtained.

Aphthoid lesions appear the earliest endoscopically detectable abnormality. The true aetiopathogenesis of aphthoid lesions is still elusive. Aphthoid lesions can occur in other conditions, particularly infectious disorders. Whether all aphthoid lesions have the same pathogenetic pathway remains unclear.

There is also uncertainty whether all small–large ulcers ultimately develop from aphthoid lesions, or whether the larger focal defects correspond to areas of vascular occlusion (due to granulomatous vasculitis?).

The role of endosocopy will remain substantial for several years to come in the overall diagnosis and differential diagnosis of CD[22]. Yet ultimately only detailed study of early phases of CD in multiple disciplines (microbiology, genetics, immunology, etc.) will allow discovery of the true cause of this still-enigmatic disease(s).

## References

1. Dekker E, Fockens P. New endoscopic tools for the IBD physician. Inflamm Bowel Dis. 2004;10:S7–S10.
2. Makiyama K, Bennett MK, Jewell DP. Endoscopic appearances of the rectal mucosa of patients with Crohn's disease visualized with a magnifying colonoscope. Gut. 1984;25:337–40.
3. Okada M, Maeda K, Yao T, Iwashita A, Nomiyama Y, Kitahara K. Minute lesions of the rectum and sigmoid colon in patients with Crohn's disease. Gastrointest Endosc. 1991;37: 319–24.
4. Rickert RR, Carter HW. The 'early' ulcerative lesion of Crohn's disease: correlative light- and scanning electron-microscopic studies. J Clin Gastroenterol. 1980;2:11–19.
5. Fujimura Y, Kamoi R, Iida M. Pathogenesis of aphthoid ulcers in Crohn's disease: correlative findings by magnifying colonoscopy, electron microscopy, and immuno-histochemistry. Gut. 1996;38:724–32.
6. Chiba M, Iizuka M, Horie Y, Ischii N, Iasamune O. Expression of HLA-DR antigens on colonic epithelium around lymph follicles. Dig Dis Sci. 1994;39:83–90.
7. Sturm A, Leite AZA, Danese S et al. Divergent cell cycle kinetics underlie the distinct functional capacity of mucosal T cells in Crohn's disease and ulcerative colitis. Gut. 2004; 53:1624–31.
8. Pettengell KE, Pirie D, Simjee AE. Colonoscopic features of early intestinal tuberculosis. Report of 11 cases. S Afr Med J. 1991;79:279–80.

9. Tarumi K, Koga H, Lida M et al. Colonic aphthoid erosions as the only manifestation of tuberculosis: case report. Gastrointest Endosc. 2002;55:743–5.
10. Hugot J-P, Alberti C, Berrebi D, Bingen E, Cézard J-P. Crohn's disease: the cold chain hypothesis. Lancet. 2003;362:2012–15.
11. Berkelhammer C, Ekambaram A, Silva RG. Low-volume oral colonoscopy bowel preparation sodium phosphate and magnesium citrate. Gastrointest Endosc. 2002;56:89–94.
12. Goldstein NS, Leon-Armin C, Mani A. Crohn's colitis-like changes in sigmoid diverticulitis specimens is usually an idiosyncratic inflammatory response to the diverticulosis rather than Crohn's colitis. Am J Surg Pathol. 2000;24:668–75.
13. Rutgeerts P, Colombel JF, Van Deventer S et al. Endoscopic healing induced by infliximab maintenance therapy correlates with long-term clinical response in patients with active Crohn's disease. Results of endoscopic substudy of ACCENT 1. Am J Gastroenterol. 2002; 97:S260.
14. Daperno M, D'Haens G, Van Assche G et al. Development and validation of a new, simplified endoscopic activity score for Crohn's disease: the SES-CD. Gastrointest Endosc. 2004;60(4):505–12.
15. Eliakim R, Adler SN. Capsule video Endoscopy in Crohn's disease – the European experience. Gastrointest Endosc. Clin N Am. 2004;14:129–37.
16. Reddy DN, Kaffes AJ, Sriram PVJ, Venkat Rao G. Capsule endoscopic features of Crohn's disease. Dig Endosc. 2004;16:138–42.
17. Mow WS, Lo SK, Targan SR et al. Initial experience with wireless capsule enteroscopy in the diagnosis and management of inflammatory bowel disease. Clin Gastroenterol Hepatol. 2004;2:31–40.
18. Swain P. Wireless capsule endoscopy and Crohn's disease. Gut. 2005;54:323–6.
19. Fireman Z, Mahajna E, Broide E et al. Diagnosing small bowel Crohn's disease with wireless capsule endoscopy. Gut. 2003;52:390–2.
20. Herrerias JM, Caunedo A, Rodriguez-Tellez M, Pellicer F, Herrerias JM Jr. Capsule endoscopy in patients with suspected Crohn's disease and negative endoscopy. Endoscopy. 2003;35:564–8.
21. Mary JY, Modigliani R. Development and validation of an endoscopic index of the severity for Crohn's disease: a prospective multicentre study. Groupe d'Etudes Therapeutiques des Affections Inflammatoires du Digestif (GETAID). Gut. 1989;30:983–9.
22. Hommes DW, Van Deventer SJ. Endoscopy in inflammatory bowel diseases. Gastroenterology. 2004;126:1561–73.

# 3
# Colitis diagnosis and therapeutic strategies – how, what and when to biopsy

**B. F. WARREN**

## INTRODUCTION

It is not straightforward to lay down rules about what should and should not be biopsed. It is more helpful to suggest methods of interpretation of biopsies taken at particular times in the disease history, and within the context of which they are taken. This chapter attempts to do that. Above all, the utility and value of gastrointestinal mucosal biopsies in inflammatory bowel disease (IBD) will depend upon the level of communication between the endoscopist and the pathologist. The context of the gastrointestinal biopsy in IBD is all-important. Biopsy of normal-looking mucosa may be extremely useful in some circumstances. A biopsy taken at a particular time in the evolution or resolution of the disease will have its own characteristic appearances. Some modern drug and/or surgical treatments may produce confusing histological appearances, causing one IBD to mimic the other, or to mimic other causes of chronic inflammation in the gut. It is not sufficient to say the biopsy has come from a colon affected by IBD; we need to know much more than this to be able put it into context.

Biopsies of ulcers, polyps and other lesions are very tempting things to take; indeed they are important things to take, but it must be remembered that, to help to put them into context histologically, biopsies of surrounding flat mucosa and more distant flat mucosa or other lesions in the colon are equally and crucially important. The endoscopic distribution of the colitis is extremely important and the significance of diverticular sigmoid colitis will be explored, as will unusual patterns of ulcerative colitis (UC) such as the skip lesion in the appendix or the caecal patch lesion.

Postsurgical biopsies generate their own problems. Biopsies from ileostomy ends will always have chronic inflammation and non-specific changes, and ileoscopy with biopsy from further along the ileum will usually be more rewarding. Biopsies from the proximal side in Crohn's disease (CD) show activity, but whether this is of clinical significance is difficult to assess. Biopsies from the stomach and duodenum may reveal focal active gastritis and duodenitis and granulomas in CD, but minor change may also be seen in patients with UC. Diversion of the faecal stream in inflammatory bowel disease produces different effects according to the starting diagnosis. Diversion of pre-existing normal large bowel produces diversion proctocolitis. Diversion of pre-existing UC produces diversion on top of UC with more severe inflammation than previously present. Diversion in CD is often about resolution of inflammatory changes. Biopsies from the pelvic ileal reservoir and pouch mucosa are useful when coupled with the clinical history and then endoscopic appearances to aid the diagnosis of pouchitis. It is probably more important to exclude other causes of inflammation within the pouch. When the patient has symptoms of pouchitis, but clearly does not have pouchitis, biopsies of the pre-pouch ileum and columnar cuff within the anal canal may yield the answer. Biopsies in dysplasia will be discussed, in particular localized versus widespread lesions of the dysplasia and management.

## BIOPSIES EARLY IN THE COURSE OF CHRONIC IBD

Biopsies within 6 weeks of onset of symptoms in IBD will rarely show much crypt architecture and distortion, and it may sometimes be difficult to distinguish early changes of IBD from infective colitis. Surrawicz and Belic[1] helped with their studies some years ago by identifying some of the changes, which may indicate the very early stages of chronic IBD. These include basal plasmacytosis and basal lymphoid aggregates or follicles. Superficial oedema in the lamina propria and neutrophils would be more in keeping with infective colitis[2], but this distinction is not always easy, and *Campylobacter* may produce a colitis which closely mimics IBD. It also has to be noted that in severe UC superficial oedema and clusters in the superficial part of the lamina propria are not uncommon.

## NORMAL HISTOLOGICAL VARIATIONS WHICH MAY CAUSE DIAGNOSTIC CONFUSION

There are several features in the normal mucosa which may be misinterpreted histologically as abnormal. One of these is the presence of normal racemosely branched crypts. These occur at approximately one to seven crypts. The other point of difficulty in the normal large bowel mucosa is the appearance of the normal density of cells in the right side of the colon. In the caecum the lamina propria is filled out to its full thickness by a mixture of chronic inflammatory cells. This is perfectly normal and would be unusual and abnormal at any other site within the colon. If histopathologists do not appreciate this there will be gross overdiagnosis of inflammation in the caecum. In a patient with no other findings at colonoscopy this clearly appends an unwelcome and incorrect label of IBD. In some patients with UC it may lead to an erroneous assessment of the extent of colonic involvement in the disease.

## DIARRHOEA WITH NORMAL COLONOSCOPY

Diarrhoea with a normal colonoscopy may have several explanations. Minimal change colitis[3] refers to an UC which has a normal or near-normal colonoscopy but the histological features may be those of classical UC and the treatment is the same as for UC. Other important causes are microscopic colitis, lymphocytic or collagenous colitis or some newer variants[4]. The diagnosis of microscopic colitis depends on presentation with persistent watery bloodless diarrhoea and no obvious endoscopic findings and typical histological findings of collagenous colitis or one of the newer variants. Focal active colitis is another important consideration[5]. Here the focal collections of neutrophils are causing destruction of part of a crypt wall and this may be seen commonly on the right side of the colon in association with bowel preparation, drugs or infection and the lesions are quite focal. Very few adults with this condition turn out to have CD whereas in the paediatric series by Greenson et al.[6] some of the children did turn out to have CD even though these were small in number.

Patients with CD causing diarrhoea may have a normal colonoscopy but the biopsy may reveal an isolated granuloma in the absence of active inflammation.

## BIOPSIES OF ULCERS

Ulcers may be part of IBD or they may be part of a superimposed or primary infection such as cytomegalovirus, amoebae or other unusual infection. Patients with IBD may occasionally have rectal mucosal prolapse, but this is unusual. Patients with solitary ulcer/prolapse syndrome may be misdiagnosed as IBD due to the presence of inflammation in the biopsies taken from the ulcerated region in the rectum, which shows the importance of taking biopsies from the ulcer, and the mucosa away from the ulcer; of course IBD may be complicated by carcinoma.

## BIOPSY OF POLYPS

In IBD one expects to find a benign inflammatory polyp quite commonly. Lipomas may be found in the ascending colon. Cytomegalovirus has been mentioned as a cause of ulcers; both it and amoebae are common causes of polyps. In long-standing chronic IBD amyloid may deposit as a polyp. When patients with IBD get older they may enter the adenoma age group and patients with inflammatory bowel disease may also have adenomas. These may sometimes be difficult to distinguish from DALMS[7], and both may give rise to adenocarcinoma.

## SIGMOID COLITIS

Sigmoid colitis causes considerable diagnostic difficulty. The commonest cause of isolated colitis within the sigmoid colon is the relationship to diverticular disease[8]. A very small proportion of patients with diverticular colitis may develop UC. If the sigmoid colitis alone is biopsied or resected and submitted for histological examination the histological appearances may be quite confusing. They may mimic CD, UC or mucosal prolapse. It is very important when taking a biopsy from the mucosa from sigmoid colitis to also biopsy the rectum, since diverticula do not occur in the rectum; this will instantly exclude UC if the rectum is normal.

## VARIATION IN APPEARANCES IN UC

The biopsy in UC may have varying degrees of severity according to the quantity of neutrophils and the amount of epithelial damage brought about by the neutrophils. The epithelial damage may result in crypt abscesses and crypt rupture or in surface erosions or ulcers. Several scoring systems have been devised to try to quantify the damage and activity in UC[9]. These are not in routine clinical use. They are quite useful in drug trials where one wishes to put numbers on to levels of improvement in relation to UC histology. The only time a scoring system is really useful in routine clinical practice is in evaluating acute inflammatory changes in the pouch mucosa, to decide whether they are severe enough to correlate with a clinical and endoscopic diagnosis of pouchitis[10]. The biopsy pathology in UC varies with time and treatment, as has been stated earlier there has been little crypt architectural distortion in the first 6 weeks, making diagnosis difficult. Later in the course of the disease, after treatment, UC may become quite patchy and may resemble CD. There are mainly microscopic areas of patchiness and occasionally skip lesions may be seen in UC. Skip lesions are the hallmark of CD. There are only two acceptable skip lesions in UC; one is in the appendix as described by Davidson and Dixon[11], and the other is the caecal patch as described by D'Haens[12]. Both these are acceptable in the spectrum of UC, and are not contraindications to pouch surgery.

## MUCOSAL BIOPSIES IN CD

In CD the large bowel mucosal biopsy may be normal or may have isolated mucosal granulomas. If there is inflammation with granulomas in relation to crypt damage this may cause confusion, and may lead to an erroneous diagnosis of CD. Granulomas may form in relation to crypt damage in all manner of forms of colitis. Intra-observer variation is great in the biopsy diagnosis of chronic IBD but the only feature usually agreed upon in intra-observer studies is the patchiness and acute and chronic inflammatory changes in CD. The classical features of CD[13] in the mucosa are focal erosion, focal inflammation and focal architectural change with relatively little mucin

17

depletion. Abscess ulcers are seen very early in the course of the disease. Resections are easier to interpret since one may see perineural chronic inflammation and transmural granulomas along with transmural chronic inflammation in the form of lymphoid aggregates. Transmural inflammation in lymphoid aggregates cannot be seen by biopsy. They can be seen in diverticular disease, but usually they appear somewhat different in that they may be associated with individual diverticula rather than being diffuse and distributed throughout the bowel. Resected CD particularly in the small bowel, has the advantage of also having fat wrapping[14], and is more difficult to judge in the large bowel due to anatomical considerations.

The terminal ileum in CD will have patchy deep inflammatory changes. The terminal ileum in backwash ileitis in UC usually has diffuse mucosal disease, although to my knowledge there is no systematic study being done of these differences.

## MIMICRY OF CD BY UC

Ulcerative colitis may closely mimic Crohn's colitis when there are granulomas in response to crypt damage and when there are cryptolytic granulomas (crypt damaging granulomas). When there is patchiness of disease after treatment it may also mimic CD when there is resolution of histological changes after treatment, or when there is severe or fulminant colitis[15]. Diversion proctitis in the three-stage pouch procedure in UC develops many of the changes of CD[16], and again this is not a contraindication to pouch surgery. The skip lesions mentioned above are also mimics of CD.

Mucosal granulomas are a problem. Those occurring in response to crypt damage contain neutrophils, mucin and epithelial remnants. The cryptolytic granuloma mentioned above, and described by Lee et al.[17], has small areas of crypt damage but is brought about by granulomas. This was reported originally to have a high specificity for the diagnosis of CD, but subsequent studies by Price have shown that it may occur in all manner of forms of colitis and is not at all specific of CD[18].

## UPPER GASTROINTESTINAL TRACT BIOPSIES

There has been much excitement about the specificity of focal inflammatory changes in the upper gastrointestinal tract when the endoscopy is normal, to differentiate CD from UC[19]. The value of this finding is not absolute in that some cases of focal inflammatory changes have also been reported in UC[20].

It may be particularly difficult to differentiate Crohn's from UC in the case of fulminant colitis, after treatment, or where rare variants of UC are not recognized. The follow-up of post-treatment biopsies in IBD – the duty of the pathologist when looking at these biopsies – is to establish whether IBD/UC or CD is still the diagnosis; has it got better; was it IBD originally? Is it now complicated by infection? It is often important to go back to the whole patient and to the original pretreatment series. The most important forms of superimposed infection are pseudomembranous colitis and cytomegalovirus[15.]

Quiescent UC may produce inflammatory polyps. It is important to biopsy the polyps and the flat mucosa. Biopsies from the ileostomy may show specific changes in CD and anastomotic biopsies in CD usually show recurrence proximal to the site of the anastomosis.

## MIMICRY OF UC BY CD

Diversion in UC will mimic CD. Diversion in CD may mimic UC or show complete resolution[21,22].

## POUCHITIS

Pouchitis is diagnosed and based on clinical symptoms of diarrhoea, discharge and systemic upset with endoscopic diffuse severe ulceration and histological features of ulceration and severe/acute inflammation[10]. These are required to correlate with a clinical diagnosis of colitis. Most pouch biopsies show merely adaptive changes in the pouch mucosa, which may include some acute inflammatory cells[23]. The histopathologist has a duty to exclude mimics of pouchitis when the pouch mucosa is inflamed. Secondary pouchitis may occur in response to localized inflammation outside the pouch, such as an abscess or tumour. Mucosal prolapse may occur within the pouch since the pouch is a neo-rectum and may develop changes seen in the normal rectum. Cytomegalovirus has been mentioned as a complication of IBD; it may be seen in irregular Crohn's-like ulcers in the pouch, and this is not CD. Pouch granulomas may be seen, and these are quite non-specific. CD may undoubtedly occur within the pouch, but it is a difficult place to make a confident diagnosis since many of the histological changes of CD may be seen in patients with pouchitis who have had UC.

Granulomas which one sees in pouch mucosa may be seen in relation to crypt rupture or within lymphoid follicles. They do not appear to be related to pouchitis and may be totally asymptomatic.

Ulcer-associated cell lineage may be seen in pouches following ulceration[23]. This may be important in that the patient who gets better after pouchitis whose biopsy shows ulcer-associated cell lineage can indicate ulceration previously, but one cannot be certain it was due to pouchitis since in the light of suitable symptoms it is likely to be a helpful association. In the patient with symptoms of pouchitis in whom one does not identify pouchitis one most consider the columnar cuff of the anal canal below the pouch, which may become inflamed and dysplastic, and also the ileum above the pouch. These should be inspected carefully and biopsied[24,25].

## DYSPLASIA IN UC

Dysplasia in UC is a difficult area. It is important to make an accurate diagnosis, not to overdiagnose the dysplasia and to put it into context. It has now become recognized that locally dysplastic lesions resembling adenomas may respond very well to local excision provided there is careful colonoscopy to exclude other lesions and careful colonoscopic follow-up[26]. Cyclosporin related changes may closely mimic dysplasia[27].

## SUMMARY

All biopsies in chronic IBD must be viewed in context, and must be from known biopsy sites. One should consider iatrogenic disease and normal or unusual variants of disease. It is also very important to consider what a biopsy from this site at this time will tell you with regard to the patient's prognosis and treatment. It is also important to think about which site you need to biopsy to answer your current question. It is crucial, when a lesion is visualized at colonoscopy, to biopsy the lesion and apparent normal mucosa to put it into context with its background. If your patient with IBD is failing to get better it is important to reconsider the diagnosis of IBD, and to see whether there is a superimposed infection. Often repeat biopsies are forgotten as an important way of excluding infections complicating UC in someone who is receiving more and more immunosuppressive therapy, but failing to get better. It is crucial for a pathologist to work closely with clinicians in managing IBD patients, and to have regular meetings to review biopsy and resection material for optimal management for these complex cases.

## References

1.  Surawicz CM, Belic L. Rectal biopsy helps to distinguish acute self-limited colitis from idiopathic inflammatory bowel disease. Gastroenterology. 1984;86:104–13.
2.  Day DW, Mandal BK, Morson BC. The rectal biopsy in *Salmonella* colitis. Histopathology. 1978;2:117–31.
3.  Elliott PR, Williams CB, Lennard-Jones JE et al. Colonoscopic diagnosis of minimal change colitis in patients with a normal sigmoidoscopy and normal air contrast barium enema. Lancet. 1982;20:650–1.
4.  Edwards CM, Warren BF, Travis SPL. Microscopic colitis: classification and terminology. Histopathology. 2002;40:374–6.
5.  Greenson JK, Stern RA, Carpenter SL, Barnett JL. The clinical significance of focal active colitis. Hum Pathol. 1997;28:729–33.
6.  Xin W, Brown PI, Greenson JK. The clinical significance of focal active colitis in pediatric patients. Am J Surg Pathol. 2003;27:1134–8.
7.  Geboes K. How is dysplasia recognised. In: Jewell DP, Warren BF, Mortensen NJ, editors. Challenges in Inflammatory Bowel Disease. Oxford: Blackwell, 2001:193–276.
8.  Shepherd NA. Diverticular disease and chronic idiopathic inflammatory bowel disease: associations and masquerades. Gut. 1996;38:801–2.
9.  Geboes K, Riddell RH, Ost A, Jensfelt B, Persson T, Lofberg R. A reproducible grading scale for histological assessment of inflammation in ulcerative colitis. Gut. 2000;47:404–9.
10. Shepherd NA, Jass JR, Duval I, Moskowitz RL, Nicholls RJ, Morson BC. Restorative proctocolectomy with ileal reservoir: pathological and histochemical study of mucosal biopsy specimens. J Clin Pathol. 1987;40:601–7.
11. Davison AM, Dixon MF. The appendix as a skip lesion in ulcerative colitis. Histopathology. 1990;16:93–5.
12. D'Haens G, Geboes K, Peeters M, Baert F, Ectors N, Rutgeerts P. Patchy caecal inflammation associated with distal ulcerative colitis: a prospective endoscopic study. Am J Gastroenterol. 1997;92:1275–9.

13. Warren BF. Classic pathology of ulcerative and Crohn's colitis. J Clin Gastroenterol. 2004;38(Suppl. 5):S33.
14. Sheehan AL, Warren BF, Gear MWL, Shepherd NA. Fat wrapping in Crohn's disease; pathological basis and relevance to surgical practice. Br J Surg. 1992;79:955–8.
15. Price AB. Overlap in the spectrum of non-specific chronic inflammatory bowel disease: colitis indeterminate. J Clin Pathol. 1978;31:567–77.
16. Warren BF, Shepherd NA, Bartolo DCC, Bradfield JWB. Pathology of the defunctioned rectum in ulcerative colitis. Gut. 1993;34:514–16.
17. Lee FD, Maguire C, Obeidat W, Russell RI. Importance of cryptolytic lesions and pericryptal granulomas in inflammatory bowel disease. J Clin Pathol. 1997;50:148–52.
18. Warren BF, Shepherd NA, Price AB, Williams GT. Importance of cryptolytic lesions and pericryptal granulomas in inflammatory bowel disease. J Clin Pathol. 1997;50:888.
19. Oberhuber G, Hirsch M, Stolte M. High incidence of upper gastrointestinal tract involvement in Crohn's disease. Virchows Arch. 1998;432:49–52.
20. Furusu H, Murase K, Nishida Y et al. Accumulation of mast cells and macrophages in focal active gastritis of patients with Crohn's disease. Hepatogastroenterology. 2002;49:639–43.
21. Harper PH, Lee EC, Kettlewell MGW, Bennett MK, Jewell DP. Role of faecal stream in the maintenance of Crohn's colitis. Gut. 1985;26:279–84.
22. Edwards CM, George BD, Jewell DP, Warren BF, Mortensen NJ, Kettlewell MGW. Role of a defunctioning stoma in the management of large bowel Crohn's disease. Br J Surg. 2000;87:1063–6.
23. Warren BF, Shepherd NA. Surgical pathology of the intestines: the pelvic ileal reservoir and diversion proctocolitis. In: Lowe DG, Underwood JCE, editors. Recent Advances in Histopathology, vol. 18. Edinburgh: Churchill Livingstone, 1999:63–88.
24. Thompson-Fawcett MW, Mortensen NJ, Warren BF. 'Cuffitis' and inflammatory changes in the columnar cuff, anal transitional zone, and ileal reservoir after stapled pouch-anal anastomosis. Dis Colon Rectum. 1999;42:348–55.
25. Thompson-Fawcett MW, Warren BF, Mortensen NJ. A new look at the anal transitional zone with reference to restorative proctocolectomy and the columnar cuff. Br J Surg. 1998;85:1517–21.
26. Odze RD, Farraye FA, Hecht JL, Hornick JL. Long-term follow-up after polypectomy treatment for adenoma-like dysplastic lesions in ulcerative colitis. Clin Gastroenterol Hepatol. 2004;2:534–41.
27. Hyde GM, Jewell DP, Warren BF. Histological changes associated with the use of intravenous cyclosporin in the treatment of severe ulcerative colitis may mimic dysplasia. Colorectal Dis. 2002;4:455–8.

# Section II
# Microscopic colitis

**Chair: T. TYSK and B.F. WARREN**

# 4
# Epidemiology of microscopic colitis

## F. FERNÁNDEZ-BAÑARES

## CASE DEFINITION

Collagenous colitis (CC) and lymphocytic colitis (LC) are diseases included into the spectrum of microscopic colitis syndrome[1]. Another disease which would be included is microscopic colitis with giant cells[2]. Patients with similar clinical characteristics but with colonic biopsies showing chronic inflammation in the lamina propria with or without an increase in intraepithelial lymphocytes (without achieving the limits required for LC) are referred to as microscopic colitis NOS (not otherwise specified) until we know more about classification and aetiology[1].

These diseases are characterized by chronic watery diarrhoea, normal radiological and endoscopic appearances, and microscopic abnormalities in the colon. The diagnosis of both CC and LC is based on a compatible clinical picture and well-established objective histological criteria[1]. Clinical criteria include chronic or recurrent watery diarrhoea of at least 1 month duration, and grossly normal or slightly abnormal (mild erythema and/or oedema) full colonoscopy. The histological criteria[1,3] are: (1) increased chronic inflammatory infiltrate (plasma cells, eosinophils and lymphocytes) in the lamina propria; (2) increased number of intraepithelial lymphocytes (IEL) (normal $<7$ per 100 epithelial cells); and (3) damage to surface epithelium, with flattening of epithelial cells and/or epithelial loss and detachment, and minimal crypt architecture distortion. Histological diagnosis of CC requires the additional presence of an abnormal surface subepithelial collagen layer with a thickness $\geqslant 10$ μm, which entraps superficial capillaries and with an irregular lacy appearance of the lower edge of the basement membrane. A number of IEL higher than 20 lymphocytes per 100 epithelial cells in the absence of a thickened subepithelial collagen layer ($<10$ μm) is necessary to diagnose LC.

Case definition will affect incidence values, and different clinical and histopathological criteria cause problems when comparing epidemiological studies. In some studies, different criteria have been used: only histopathological criteria and a thickness $\geqslant 15$ μm to define CC[4]; increase in IEL $> 10\%$ to define LC[5]. In Spanish and Swedish studies, case definitions were similar[6–8].

## DESCRIPTIVE EPIDEMIOLOGY

### Incidence and prevalence rates

The incidence of collagenous colitis has been estimated in several population-based studies performed mostly in Europe in the past two decades[4-9]. The diagnostic awareness of these conditions by physicians in the geographical area of interest impacts the likelihood of diagnosis and, therefore, incidence and prevalence. The symptoms of microscopic colitis have frequently been attributed to functional diarrhoea, and the diagnosis of the disease is performed only if the physician in charge refers the patient for colonoscopy, and if the endoscopist takes multiple colonic biopsies in all patients referred for colonoscopy due to recurrent or chronic diarrhoea, in which the macroscopic appearance of the colonic mucosa was normal or mildly abnormal (mild oedema or erythema). In this sense it is not clear if geographical differences in the incidence of microscopic colitis reflect a true difference in frequency or simply better case ascertainment.

The reported mean annual incidence of CC ranges from 0.6 to 6.1 per 100 000 inhabitants-year (Table 1). The lowest incidences were reported in a preliminary report from northern France published only in abstract form in 1994[9], and in the first 5-year population-based study from Sweden (1984-88)[6]. Later Swedish studies showed increased incidences which in 1996-98 reached the highest incidence reported. As mentioned, it is not clear if there is a true increase in incidence or better disease awareness.

Peak incidence is observed in older women (up to 26.9 per 100 000 in women aged 60-69 years in Swedish studies). Median age at diagnosis in the different population-based studies ranges from 58 to 68 years, and the female/male ratio ranges from 4.8:1 to 9.0:1.

The reported mean incidence of LC has ranged from 3.7 to 9.8 cases per 100 000 inhabitants-year (Table 1). The highest rate described comes from a study performed in the USA but published only as an abstract[5]. As mentioned above, the definition of LC was less strict than in earlier European studies. On the other hand, Swedish studies suggest an increase of incidence in recent years. As before, it is not clear if there is a true increase in incidence or better disease awareness.

**Table 1** Mean annual incidence of microscopic colitis per 100,000 inhabitants-year in population-based epidemiological studies

| Geographical area and years | CC | LC |
|---|---|---|
| Örebro, Sweden, 1984-93[6] | 1.8 | |
| Franche-Comté, France, 1987-92[9] | 0.6 | |
| Uppsala, Sweden, 1992-94* | 1.9 | |
| Terrassa, Spain, 1993-97[7] | 2.3 | 3.7 |
| Örebro, Sweden, 1993-98[8] | 4.9 | 4.4 |
| Olmsted County, Minnesota, 1994-2001[5] | 5.1 | 9.8 |
| Iceland, 1995-99[4] | 5.2 | 4.0 |

*Referenced in Olesen et al.[8]

Peak incidence is also observed in elderly or middle-aged women. Median age at diagnosis ranges from 59 to 70 years, and the female:male ratio seems to be less marked, at 2.1:1 to 5.0:1.

Combined rates of CC and LC are close to values reported for Crohn's disease, and are approaching the incidence of ulcerative colitis in areas in which inflammatory bowel disease is considered common. The clinical relevance is that microscopic colitis should be suspected in patients presenting with chronic non-bloody diarrhoea. In this sense microscopic colitis is diagnosed at a rate of 10 per 100 normal-looking colonoscopies performed in patients with chronic watery diarrhoea, and of almost 20% of those older than 70 years[8].

Data on the prevalence of microscopic colitis are scarce. The prevalence of CC in Örebro, Sweden in 1993 was approximately 16 cases per 100 000 persons[6], and in Olmsted County (MN, USA) in 2001 the figure was 36 per 100 000 persons[5]. With these rates the disease is included in the list of 'rare diseases' of the European Community, which are defined as life-threatening or chronically debilitating diseases which are of such low prevalence that special combined efforts are needed to address them. As a guide, a low prevalence is taken as prevalence of less than 5 per 10 000 persons.

The only prevalence figure available for LC is from the USA study, in which a less strict definition of LC was used; this showed 64 cases per 100 000 persons[5]. There are no data from European studies but the results should be similar to those described in CC.

## Mortality and morbidity

Microscopic colitis has not been associated with increased mortality, and does not appear to have a malignant colonic potential. However, an increase in relative risk of lung cancer in CC has been described[10], suggesting a possible role of smoking in this disorder.

Life-threatening diarrhoea is extremely rare, and the clinical course is, in general, benign with few serious complications[11–14]. However, colonic perforation has been reported in 16 patients requiring a laparotomy; it seems to be a rare complication with a frequency in the Swedish register of CC of less than 1%[15]. Only two of the 16 cases occurred spontaneously, and the others after a colonoscopy or barium enema. Mucosal tears – described as long, shallow, linear or serpiginous mucosal ulcers, resembling a 'fracture' – could be the cause of colonic perforation in such cases. It has been hypothesized that decreased distensibility of the colon caused by extensive subepithelial and submucosal collagen deposition renders it susceptible to mucosal 'fractures' during colonoscopy air insufflation[16].

## RISK FACTORS AND MICROSCOPIC COLITIS

Identification of risk factors is an important goal for epidemiologists because better understanding of pathological mechanisms may result in new concepts of causation and treatment.

## Environmental risk factors

### Cigarette smoking

Data on a possible relationship between smoking and microscopic colitis are scarce and controversial. It has been suggested that patients with CC are more likely to be active smokers, and patients with LC more likely to be ex-smokers[13,17], suggesting a relationship similar to that observed in inflammatory bowel disease (IBD): Crohn's disease is positively associated with cigarette smoking, while a negative association exists between smoking and ulcerative colitis. However, a recent study in LC did not find a higher proportion of ex-smokers than current smokers[14]. Case–control studies are required to further characterize this effect.

### Drug consumption

There seems to be an association between non-steroidal anti-inflammatory drugs (NSAID) and CC, reported in several case reports as well as in a case–control study. In that study the use of NSAID was significantly more common among CC patients (61%) than in a control group (irritable bowel syndrome or colonic diverticular disease) (13%)[18]. However, other authors did not find NSAID consumption more frequent in CC (Table 2). Patients with CC often have concomitant arthrosis[12], which is more frequent in elderly people; thus NSAID use may simply be a marker of joint pain. However, it is considered that there is a well-established association between NSAID and microscopic colitis since in some cases there is an association with the introduction, as well as with the withdrawal, of the drug; in addition, in at least one case with CC, rechallenge was followed by clinical relapse. On the other hand, it is well known that NSAID can cause colonic inflammation and exacerbate IBD. Therefore, NSAID use should be discouraged in patients with CC. Data concerning a possible relationship between NSAID and LC are scarce. In one study 61% of patients with LC were taking aspirin or other NSAID[17], whereas in other reports the frequency of use was 18–36%[12,13].

**Table 2**  Consumption of NSAID (and aspirin) in patients with microscopic colitis

| Reference | | CC | LC |
|---|---|---|---|
| Riddell et al., 1992[18] | CC: | 19/31 (61%) | |
| | Controls: | 4/31 (13%) | |
| Veress et al., 1995[19] | | 4/24 (16.7%) | |
| Bohr et al., 1996[11] | | 35/104 (33.6%) | |
| Mullhaupt et al., 1998[20] | | | 5/27 (18.5%) |
| Baert et al., 1999[13] | | 27/96 (28%) | 19/80 (36.2%) |
| Pardi et al., 2002[17] | | | 129/170 (61%) |
| Abdo et al., 2002[21] | | 15/62 (24%) | |
| Fernández-Bañares et al., 2003[12] | | 13/37 (35%) | 8/44 (18%) |

To date at least 16 drugs have been reported with the onset of LC (recently reviewed in Olesen et al.[14] and Cappell[22]). Ticlopidine is more often reported, with more than 30 cases, followed by Cyclo 3 fort (a venotonic drug), flutamide, and lansoprazole. In most cases the onset of LC has been associated with the introduction of a drug, followed by clinical remission after its withdrawal. However, no association has been proved. Diarrhoea is a well-known side-effect of most of these drugs. Thus, whether these drugs induce diarrhoea in patients with previously non-symptomatic LC, or if they are the cause of LC, is unknown.

## Infection

A variety of infectious triggers have been proposed (*Yersinia* sp, *Campylobacter jejuni, Clostridium difficile*), but remain unproved[23-25].

LC shares many features with 'Brainerd diarrhoea', or epidemic chronic diarrhoea. This condition is characterized by acute watery diarrhoea of prolonged duration and was described in central Minnesota associated with the ingestion of raw milk[26,27]. Histopathological analysis of colonic biopsies shows a resemblance to LC. Epidemiological data suggest an infectious cause of 'Brainerd diarrhoea', but no causative organism has been identified. These similarities raise the possibility of an infectious aetiology also for LC.

A sudden onset of symptoms in a subset of patients with both LC and CC, and a clinical course with a single attack in around 70% of patients[12,14], may support the theory of an infectious cause in some patients with microscopic colitis. However, the limited number of reported family clusters argues against a contagious organism.

## Genetic risk factors

There is very little information suggesting a role for genetic factors in the aetiology of microscopic colitis. There are only a few reports of familial occurrence of microscopic colitis[28,29]. Familial aggregation has been evaluated in a recent large series of patients with LC. A family history of CC was seen in 1% of LC patients; however, none had a family history of LC[14]. In contrast, there were no patients with a family history of LC or CC in another recent large series of patients with LC[17].

It is noteworthy that a family history of ulcerative colitis or Crohn's disease was seen in 7% of LC patients in the Swedish series[14], and in 2% in the US series[17]. Progression of microscopic colitis to Crohn's disease or ulcerative colitis has also been reported[12,30-32]. These are intriguing observations suggesting the existence of an underlying common abnormality predisposing to both microscopic colitis and IBD.

On the other hand, a predisposition to coeliac disease has also been described, but the magnitude of this association remains controversial. Variable percentages of coeliac disease ranging from 0% to 40% have been described. In some studies a bias in the selection of cases including patients with severe forms of microscopic colitis, either protracted diarrhoea or debilitating disease, may explain the observed high percentages of coeliac

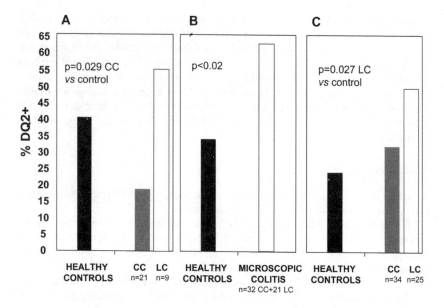

**Figure 1** Frequency of HLA-DQ2 in patients with microscopic colitis as compared to healthy controls. **A:** ref. 33; **B:** ref. 35; **C:** ref. 36

disease. In this sense the frequency of coeliac disease ranges from 0% to 17% in large series[8,11–14,17]. Nevertheless, the range remains wide, suggesting that a different prevalence of coeliac disease in the geographical areas where the studies were performed might account for the result.

One study of HLA haplotypes showed an increase in HLA-A1 and HLA-DRW53 in LC and a decrease in HLA-DQ2 in CC[33]. The same group later reported increased HLA-A1 and decreased HLA-A3 in LC, and no HLA associations in CC[34]. Another study showed an increase in HLA-DQ2 and HLA-DQ1,3 in both LC and CC[35], similar to the pattern observed in coeliac disease, thus suggesting a relationship between these entities. All these studies used serological assays to evaluate HLA status. A recent study assessed HLA-DQ2 and HLA-DQ8 using polymerase chain reaction, which is considered the most sensitive assay, showing an increase in HLA-DQ2 in LC, but not in CC (Figure 1)[36]. Since HLA class II molecules are implicated in the binding of peptide antigens, HLA-immunoregulated inflammatory reactions could have a role in the susceptibility of at least LC. On the other hand, the association with coeliac-predisposing genes might explain the observed relationship with coeliac disease.

# References

1.  Warren BF, Edwards CM, Travis SPL. 'Microscopic colitis': classification and terminology. Histopathology. 2002;40:374–6.
2.  Libbrecht L, Croes R, Ectors N, Staels F, Geboes K. Microscopic colitis with giant cells. Histopathology. 2002;40:335–8.
3.  Lazenby AJ, Yardley JH, Giardiello FM et al. Lymphocytic ('microscopic') colitis: a comparative histopathologic study with particular reference to collagenous colitis. Hum Pathol. 1989;20:18–28.
4.  Agnarsdottir M, Gunnlaugsson O, Orvar KB et al. Collagenous and lymphocytic colitis in Iceland. Dig Dis Sci. 2002;47:1122–8.
5.  Pardi DS, Smyrk TC, Kammer P et al. The epidemiology of microscopic colitis: a population-based study in Olmsted County, MN. Gastroenterology. 2004;126(Suppl. 2): A124 (Abstract).
6.  Bohr J, Tysk C, Eriksson S et al. Collagenous colitis in Örebro, Sweden, an epidemiological study 1984–1993. Gut. 1995;37:394–7.
7.  Fernández-Bañares F, Salas A, Forné M, Esteve M, Espinós J, Viver JM. Incidence of collagenous and lymphocytic colitis: a five-year population-based study. Am J Gastroenterol. 1999;94:418–23.
8.  Olesen M, Eriksson S, Bohr J, Järnerot G, Tysk C. Microscopic colitis: a common diarrheal disease. An epidemiological study in Örebro, Sweden, 1993–1998. Gut. 2004;53:346–50.
9.  Raclot G, Queneau PE, Ottignon Y et al. Incidence of collagenous colitis. A retrospective study in the east of France. Gastroenterology. 1994;106:A23 (Abstract).
10. Chan JL, Tersmette AC, Offerhaus GJ, Gruber SB, Bayless TM, Giardello FM. Cancer risk in collagenous colitis. Inflamm Bowel Dis. 1999;5:40–3.
11. Bohr J, Tysk C, Eriksson S et al. Collagenous colitis: a retrospective study of clinical presentation and treatment in 163 patients. Gut. 1996;39:846–51.
12. Fernández-Bañares F, Salas A, Esteve M et al. Collagenous and lymphocytic colitis: evaluation of clinical and histological features, response to treatment, and long-term follow up. Am J Gastroenterol. 2003;98:340–7.
13. Baert F, Wouters K, D'Haens G et al. Lymphocytic colitis: a distinct clinical entity? A clinicopathological confrontation of lymphocytic and collagenous colitis. Gut. 1999;45: 375–81.
14. Olesen M, Erikson S, Bohr J et al. Lymphocytic colitis: a retrospective clinical study of 199 Swedish patients. Gut. 2004;53:536–41.
15. Bohr J, Larsson JG, Eriksson S, Järnerot G, Tysk C. Colonic perforation in collagenous colitis: an unusual complication. Eur J Gastroenterol Hepatol. 2005;17:121–4.
16. Sherman A, Ackert JJ, Rajapaksa R, West AB, Oweity T. Fractured colon? An endoscopically distinctive lesion associated with colonic perforation following colonoscopy in patients with collagenous colitis. J Clin Gastroenterol. 2004;38:341–5.
17. Pardi DS, Ramnath VR, Loftus EV, Trmaine WJ, Sandborn WJ. Lymphocytic colitis: clinical features, treatment, and outcomes. Am J Gastroenterol. 2002;97:2829–33.
18. Riddell RH, Tanaka M, Mazzoleni G. Non-steroidal anti-inflammatory drugs as a possible cause of collagenous colitis: a case–control study. Gut. 1992;33:683–6.
19. Veress B, Lofberg R, Bergman L. Microscopic colitis syndrome. Gut. 1995;36:880–6.
20. Mullhaupt B, Güller U, Anabitarte M, Güller R, Freid M. Lymphocytic colitis: clinical presentation and long term course. Gut. 1998;43:629–33.
21. Abdo A, Raboud J, Freeman HJ et al. Clinical and histological predictors of response to medical therapy in collagenous colitis. Am J Gastroenterol. 2002;97:1164–8.
22. Cappell MS. Colonic toxicity of administered drugs and chemicals. Am J Gastroenterol. 2004;99:1175–90.
23. Bohr J, Nordfelth R, Järnerot G, Tysk C. *Yersinia* species in collagenous colitis: a serologic study. Scand J Gastroenterol. 2002;37:711–14.
24. Khan MA, Brunt E, Longo WE, Presti ME. Persistent *Clostridium difficile* colitis: a possible etiology for the development of collagenous colitis. Dig Dis Sci. 2000;45:998–1001.
25. Perk G, Ackerman Z, Cohen P et al. Lymphocytic colitis: a clue to an infectious trigger. Scand J Gastroenterol. 1999;34:110–12.
26. Bryant DA, Mintz ED, Puhr ND et al. Colonic epithelial lymphocytosis associated with an epidemic of chronic diarrhea. Am J Surg Pathol. 1996;20:1102–9.

27. Osterholm MT, McDonald KL, White KE et al. An outbreak of a newly recognized chronic diarrhea syndrome associated with raw milk consumption. J Am Med Assoc. 1986;256: 484–90.
28. van Tilburg AJP, Lam HGT, Seldenrijk CA et al. Familial occurrence of collagenous colitis. A report of two families. J Clin Gastroenterol. 1990;12:279–85.
29. Jarnerot G, Hertervig E, Grano C et al. Familial occurrence of microscopic colitis: a report on five families. Scand J Gastroenterol. 2001;36:959–62.
30. Aquel B, Bishop M, Krishna M, Cangemi J. Collagenous colitis evolving into ulcerative colitis: a case report and review of the literature. Dig Dis Sci. 2003;48:2323–7.
31. Chandratre S, Bramble MG, Cooke WM, Jones RA. Simultaneous occurrence of collagenous colitis and Crohn's disease. Digestion. 1987;36:55–60.
32. Giardiello FM, Jackson FW, Lazenby AJ. Metachronous occurrence of collagenous colitis and ulcerative colitis. Gut. 1991;32:447–9.
33. Giardiello FM, Lazenby AJ, Bayless TM, et al. Lymphocytic (microscopic) colitis. Clinicopathological study of 18 patients and comparison to collagenous colitis. Dig Dis Sci. 1989;34:1730–8.
34. Giardiello FM, Lazenby AJ, Yardley JH et al. Increased HLA1 and diminished HLA A3 in lymphocytic colitis compared to controls and patients with collagenous colitis. Dig Dis Sci. 1992;37:496–9.
35. Fine KD, Do K, Schulte K et al. High prevalence of celiac sprue-like HLA-DQ genes and enteropathy in patients with the microscopic colitis syndrome. Am J Gastroenterol. 2000; 95:1974–82.
36. Fernández-Bañares F, Esteve M, Farré C et al. Predisposing HLA-DQ2 and HLA-DQ8 haplotypes of celiac disease and associated enteropathy in microscopic colitis. Eur J Gastroenterol Hepatol. (In press).

# 5
# Microscopic colitis: histological classification

## K. GEBOES, G. DE HERTOGH, P. VAN EYKEN and K. P. GEBOES

## INTRODUCTION

Diarrhoea (three or more bowel movements per day) lasting more than 4 weeks is a common symptom in adults. The prevalence is approximately 1–5%, making it a major cause of disability[1]. Many patients do not seek medical attention unless the diarrhoea is associated with other symptoms such as weight loss. Nevertheless, the effect of chronic diarrhoea on quality of life and health-care expenses is considerable[2]. Patients with chronic diarrhoea, with or without the passage of blood, are likely to be fully investigated, including one or other form of endoscopy with biopsy. Whether this is cost-effective has not been established. The results of such studies tend to depend largely upon the social security systems of the different countries. However, several studies show that colonoscopy and biopsy is useful in the investigation of patients with chronic diarrhoea, yielding a histological diagnosis in 22–31% of patients who had a macroscopically normal colon at colonoscopy[3–6]. Histological diagnosis includes a variety of conditions such as spirochaetosis, pseudomelanosis coli, collagenous colitis and microscopic colitis. Various forms of colitis can thus be present in the absence of radiological and endoscopic lesions or features of colitis (Table 1). Because of the limitations on the patterns of tissue response to a varied range of insults, the evaluation of tissue samples and the histological diagnosis of colitis requires good knowledge of the different aetiological possibilities and of the microscopic features which allow a diagnosis of colitis. In 1993 a French and an American research group suggested the use of 'microscopic colitis' as an umbrella term to cover any form of colitis in which there was histological but no endoscopic or radiological abnormality[20,21]. The term 'microscopic colitis' had been introduced earlier in 1980, for a condition characterized by chronic diarrhoea and a mild increase in inflammatory cells in the colonic mucosa which was macroscopically normal[22]. In a comparative histopathological study it was later shown that the most distinctive feature of this condition was a marked increase in the number of intraepithelial lymphocytes (IEL)[23]. The condition was therefore renamed 'lymphocytic colitis'. It appeared to be different from 'collagenous colitis', a condition first

**Table 1**  Normal colonoscopy and abnormal histology

---

Infections
    Spirochaetosis[7]
    Post-infectious irritable bowel syndrome[8]
    Miscellaneous infections: *C. difficile, Campylobacter coli, E. coli* etc.[9]

Drug-related colitis
    Pseudomelanosis coli
    Drug-related lymphocytic and collagenous colitis
    Miscellaneous

Inflammatory bowel diseases (IBD) (Crohn's disease and ulcerative colitis)
    Minimal change colitis[10]
    IBD in remission

Microscopic colitis
    Lymphocytic colitis: idiopathic, coeliac disease-related, colonic epithelial lymphocytosis
    associated with an epidemic outbreak of diarrhoea[11] (drug-related)

    Collagenous colitis: idiopathic, (drug-related), (infection-related), (IBD-related)

    Variants: microscopic colitis with giant cells[12,13], microscopic colitis with granulomatous
    inflammation[14], pauci-IEL lymphocytic colitis[15], pseudomembranous variant of
    collagenous colitis[16], microscopic colitis not otherwise specified (NOS)[17], apoptotic
    colopathy[48], mastocytic (entero)colitis[49]

    Atypical cases: cryptal lymphocytic colitis[18]

Allergy-associated colitis[19]
    Eosinophilic cryptitis/colitis

---

reported in 1976. In this report histopathological examination of rectal biopsies from a woman presenting with chronic watery diarrhoea and an endoscopically normal rectal mucosa revealed a markedly thickened subepithelial collagen layer and an increase of inflammatory cells in the lamina propria[24]. Collagenous colitis and lymphocytic colitis were the two first types of microscopic colitis to be recognized. Since then, various other types have been reported[12–17], which might or might not be distinct nosological entities[25]. Collagenous colitis and lymphocytic colitis are similar but not identical; the clinical presentation is slightly different. Patients with lymphocytic colitis present somewhat earlier and symptoms are milder. The histology is clearly different although overlapping histological features may be present in collagenous colitis (increase in IEL in 28% of patients) and lymphocytic colitis (thickening of subepithelial collagen layer in 26% of patients)[26]. Cases of lymphocytic colitis with a thin, but structurally abnormal layer of subsurface collagen, evident by trichrome stain but not in sections stained with haematoxylin and eosin, have been referred to as 'minimal collagenous colitis'[27].

## DEFINITION

The diagnosis of microscopic colitis is a clinicopathologic one. A typical patient has a chronic intermittent disease course with watery diarrhoea, weight loss and abdominal pain as the main symptoms. Routine blood tests are non-diagnostic. Radiographic and endoscopic examinations are normal or show non-specific abnormalities. Mucosal granularity and irregularity of the rectosigmoid on double-contrast barium enema have occasionally been reported in collagenous colitis[28]. Endoscopically, erythema or oedema have been reported in up to one-third of cases. Mucosal tears, haemorrhagic lacerations and submucosal dissection on insufflation have been reported in a minority of the patients[29,30]. Mucosal biopsies show evidence of inflammation of the lamina propria and variable alterations of the epithelial compartment.

## HISTOPATHOLOGY

The histological diagnosis of microscopic colitis is based upon a combination of several features (Table 2)

**Table 2**   Histological features to be assessed for a diagnosis of 'microscopic colitis'

Inflammation
   Lamina propria cellularity
      Intensity: increased
      Composition: mononuclear (lymphocytes, plasma cells); + eosinophils
      (collagenous colitis); neutrophils (rare)

   Intraepithelial lymphocytes
      Increased in surface epithelium ( > 20 per 100 surface epithelial cells);
      mandatory in lymphocytic colitis (occasionally only in crypt epithelium)

   Miscellaneous
      Giant cells: rare
      Granulomas: rare

Subepithelial collagen layer
   Thickening ( > 10 μm): patchy; mandatory in collagenous colitis

Epithelial compartment
   Surface epithelium
      Flattening: common
      Detachment: common
      Presence of neutrophils: uncommon

   Crypt epithelium
      Presence of neutrophils (cryptitis; crypt abscess; cryptolytic granulomas): rare
      Crypt distortion: focal: rare
      Paneth cell metaplasia: uncommon

## Inflammation

The inflammation is recognized by an increase in cellularity in the lamina propria compared to the normal colon due to inflammatory cells, and through the presence of IEL. Counting lamina propria cells is not feasible in routine practice. The presence of plasma cells at the base of the mucosa, just above the muscularis mucosae in more than one well-oriented biopsy, represents a loss of the normal gradient and is considered abnormal[17]. The infiltrate is predominantly mononuclear, consisting mainly of plasma cells and lymphocytes. Most of the lymphocytes are CD4$^+$ T cells. A significant decrease in inflammatory cells can be noted after treatment[31]. A marked increase in mononuclear cells, particularly T cells, has been observed in samples from patients obtained following acute *Campylobacter* enteritis and in the post-dysenteric irritable bowel syndrome[8]. These cases may be erroneously over-diagnosed as microscopic colitis[17]. Usually, the epithelial compartment is normal in these cases; furthermore, CD68$^+$ foamy histiocytic cells may be more common[8]. The presence of these cells has been explained as an indication of a previous injury[32]. In collagenous colitis there is also an increase in the number of eosinophils, often in association with the subepithelial collagen layer[33]. Neutrophils are rarely seen. Colitis characterized by a marked eosinophilic infiltrate ($\geqslant 20$ per high-power field) is also observed in drug reactions and in food intolerance in children. It can be responsible for rectal bleeding but also for diarrhoea with normal colonoscopy. It can be distinguished from microscopic collagenous or lymphocytic colitis by the lack of increase of mononuclear cells[34].

A diffuse increase in the number of IEL is mandatory in lymphocytic colitis. The required number varies between 10 and 20 per 100 surface epithelial cells (normal number = 4). In a series of 59 patients with lymphocytic colitis and a subepithelial collagen layer $> 10$ μm, three to five biopsy samples were examined. The number of IEL varied between 10 and 65 (median 30). There was no tendency for a more prominent increase in a particular segment of the colon[26]. For epidemiological studies a number of $> 20$ is often used. Patients with a mean of $\geqslant 10$ IEL/100 enterocytes have been diagnosed as 'pauci-IEL lymphocytic colitis'. They can have clinicopathological associations similar to those in classic lymphocytic colitis patients[15]. The low number can be explained in some patients by a symptomatic treatment. Occasional cases with absence of increased IEL in the surface epithelium, and of epithelial injury with increased IEL in the cryptal epithelium, have been reported as cryptal lymphocytic colitis[18]. In these cases endoscopy can be abnormal and cryptal lymphocytic colitis probably represents 'atypical cases'. In collagenous colitis the number of IEL is often, but not always, increased. The number of IEL in ulcerative colitis, Crohn's colitis and infectious colitis is usually not increased, although a focal increase and a lymphocytic colitis-like pattern in Crohn's disease have been described. The lymphocytic colitis-like pattern may precede the eventual clinical pathological diagnosis of Crohn's disease[35].

The number of IEL is also increased in biopsy samples from patients obtained following acute *Campylobacter* enteritis and in post-dysenteric irritable bowel syndrome. In common with CD3$^+$ lymphocytes in the lamina propria, the number of IEL decreases over time[8]. Some of the patients with pauci-IEL lymphocytic colitis may rather have a post-dysenteric irritable bowel syndrome.

Accumulation of giant cells just beneath the surface epithelium has been reported in a small number of patients with a clinical and endoscopic presentation suggestive of microscopic colitis. It is not clear if this so-called 'microscopic colitis with giant cells' is really a distinct pathological entity (Figure 1) Response to therapy is comparable with that observed for collagenous and lymphocytic colitis[12,13]. A granulomatous inflammation, characterized by scattered non-necrotizing granulomas, often closely associated with crypt epithelium (cryptolytic granulomas) has also been reported in patients presenting with a history suggestive of microscopic colitis. The pattern must not be confused with Crohn's disease[14].

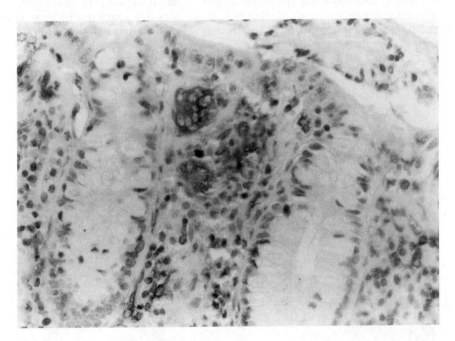

**Figure 1** Microphotograph showing a rectal biopsy from a patient presenting with chronic watery diarrhoea. Accumulation of giant cells underneath the surface epithelial cells is shown with an immunohistochemical staining using antibodies directed against CD68. The proposed diagnosis was 'microscopic colitis with giant cells'

Surface intraepithelial neutrophils are usually few in number but active crypt inflammation is relatively common. The occurrence of pseudomembranous colitis superimposed on otherwise typical collagenous colitis has been described in isolated case reports. This does not necessarily signify a separate disorder, however; but may instead represent an unusual histological variant[16].

## Subepithelial collagen layer

The most characteristic feature of collagenous colitis is thickening of the subepithelial collagen layer (SCL), consisting of collagen type I, III and VI in addition to the glycoprotein tenascin, separated from the epithelial cells by the apparently normal basal membrane composed of collagen type IV (Figures 2 and 3) The thickness of the SCL in the normal colorectal mucosa is <4 μm with small regional variations[36]. Normal values reported in the literature vary between 2–3 and 3–7 μm. The most common minimum thickness for a diagnosis of collagenous colitis is 10 μm, but the SCL often measures 15–30 μm or more (up to 70 μm). Diarrhoea is most commonly noted when the SCL is more than 15 micrometer. The thickening of the SCL is often patchy (the transverse colon usually having the thickest band), both within a biopsy specimen and between specimens from different regions of the colon. Thickening increases towards the right side of the colon and can be absent in the sigmoid colon and rectum. The rectum is spared is approximately 30% of cases[37]. The thickening may persist after treatment[31].

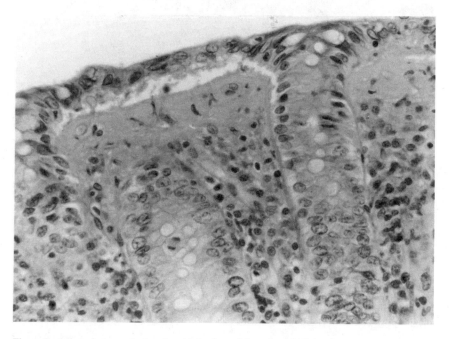

**Figure 2** Microphotograph showing thickening of the subepithelial collagen layer in a biopsy from a patient with collagenous colitis

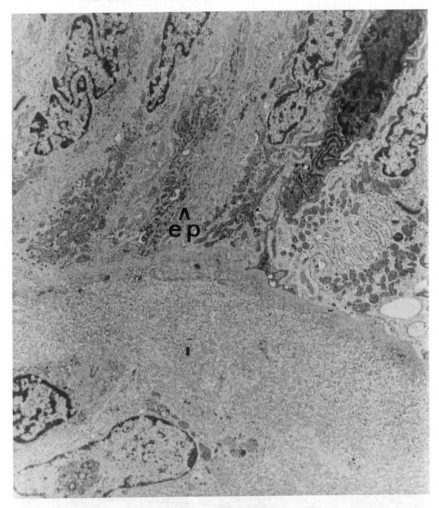

**Figure 3** Transmission electron microscopy confirms the accumulation of collagen underneath the basement membrane. ep = epithelium; ∧ indicates the position of the epithelium

Biopsies from patients with persistent watery bloodless diarrhoea, normal colonoscopy and chronic inflammation in the absence of a thickened collagen band or increased IEL are referred to as microscopic colitis not otherwise specified (NOS)[17]. These patients either have genuine microscopic colitis (but they received treatment with, for instance, topical steroids) or they may belong to the group of the post-dysenteric irritable bowel patients.

## Epithelial compartment

The surface epithelium is usually focally or more diffusely abnormal. Flattening of the epithelial cells, partial or complete detachment, mucin depletion and vacuolization of the cytoplasm are common features. Crypt distortion is uncommon and, when present, focal. More widespread crypt distortion is observed in 'minimal change colitis' which usually behaves as does ulcerative colitis[10,17]. Paneth cell metaplasia is more common in collagenous colitis (44%) than in lymphocytic colitis (14%). In collagenous colitis, Paneth cell metaplasia is noted more frequently in those patients whose symptoms are ongoing or recurrent, and it has been suggested that its presence may be used as a marker to predict more persistent or severe disease[38].

## THE SMALL INTESTINE

The small intestine can be involved in microscopic colitis. The number of IEL is often significantly increased in the terminal ileum in patients with lymphocytic and collagenous colitis compared to controls (Figure 4) There are a few reports of microscopic colitis patients with ileal villous atrophy, of which at least some were assessed as primary[39]. Duodenal abnormalities were reported in up to 70% of patients with microscopic colitis (of whom only 7% had positive anti-endomysial antibodies).

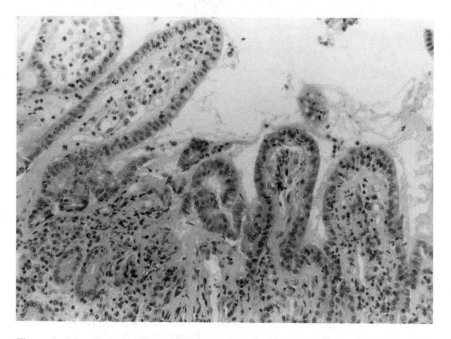

**Figure 4** Microphotograph showing a diffuse increase of intraepithelial cells in a biopsy obtained in the ileum. The patient had 'lymphocytic ileocolitis'

## INFLAMMATORY BOWEL DISEASE (IBD) AND MICROSCOPIC COLITIS

A focal lymphocytic colitis-like pattern was observed in four patients who were eventually diagnosed with Crohn's disease. In one patient with Crohn's disease the biopsies showed a collagenous colitis morphology. Colonoscopic abnormalities were, however, found in four of these patients, making a diagnosis of microscopic colitis less likely[35]. In a comment on this paper it was stressed that colonic epithelial lymphocytosis without a thickened SCL can be found in a clinically heterogeneous group of patients[40]. In a review of patients with colonic biopsies at the Mayo Clinic between 1978 and 1998, 15 patients (nine female, six male) were identified who had both a histological diagnosis of classic IBD and a histological diagnosis of microscopic colitis. The mean age of the patients at the time of the microscopic colitis was 61 years; 13 patients had collagenous colitis. NSAID use was documented in 11 patients. In 12 patients the IBD was ulcerative colitis. Either IBD or microscopic colitis may precede the onset of the other. In this series the association of microscopic colitis was found predominantly in patients with pancolonic involvement[41]. Progression of collagenous colitis to ulcerative colitis was observed in two further patients, testing positive for perinuclear antineutrophil cytoplasmic antibodies[42]. We have identified 11 additional cases using a questionnaire with data from 12 IBD centres (five in North America and seven in Europe). Four patients presented initially with collagenous colitis and later developed ulcerative pancolitis. Two patients were taking NSAID. Two patients with initial collagenous colitis developed Crohn's disease. In summary it seems reasonable to assume that there is a rare association between microscopic colitis and IBD, especially ulcerative colitis and collagenous colitis. Many of the patients with progression towards ulcerative colitis have been treated with NSAID.

## COELIAC DISEASE AND MICROSCOPIC COLITIS

Gluten has been associated with microscopic colitis, more particularly lymphocytic colitis. In a study by Wolber et al. 12 out of 39 (31%) patients with newly diagnosed coeliac disease had a simultaneous diagnosis of lymphocytic colitis[43]. Treatment with gluten-free diet in 10 of these patients resulted in a clinical improvement in nine of them. Rectal gluten challenge in patients with coeliac disease has shown a rapid increase of the number of IEL in the rectum[44]. It is thus possible that gluten is responsible for the histopathological changes corresponding to lymphocytic colitis in some cases of coeliac disease.

## AETIOLOGY AND CLASSIFICATION

The aetiology of lymphocytic and collagenous colitis is largely unknown and probably multifactorial. At least 16 drugs have been associated with lymphocytic colitis and/or collagenous colitis (including ticlodipine and related compounds, Cyclo 3 fort, lansoprazole, non-steroidal anti-inflammatory drugs, simvostatin and cimetidine). Several enteric infections such as *Clostridium difficile* (collagenous colitis), *Campylobacter jejuni* (lymphocytic colitis) and *Yersinia enterocolitica* (collagenous colitis) have also been associated with the onset of microscopic colitis[45]. With regard to the aetiology, microscopic colitis therefore seems to be a heterogeneous condition. Collagenous colitis can be subdivided into idiopathic cases, drug-related cases, infection-related cases and IBD-related cases. In lymphocytic colitis, idiopathic cases, drug-related disease, infection-related conditions, coeliac disease-associated cases and, less likely, IBD-related patients must be considered.

## CONCLUSION

Microscopic colitis is an umbrella term used to cover any form of colitis in which there is histological but no endoscopic or radiological abnormality. Abnormal histology and a normal endoscopy is seen in a large variety of conditions. Therefore, most commonly 'microscopic colitis' is used to designate collectively two major subtypes, namely lymphocytic and collagenous colitis. The histological diagnostic features of these conditions are summarized in Table 3. These two conditions are relatively common[46,47]. Several variants of both of these types of microscopic colitis, such as microscopic colitis with giant cells and with granulomatous inflammation, have been described, but it is not clear if these are specific entities. The different variants seem, however, to be rare disorders. Aetiologically, microscopic colitis is a heterogeneous condition. Drugs, infections and coeliac disease must be considered as possible causative agents. It might therefore be more appropriate to consider the conditions as 'microscopic colitis syndrome' because 'collagenous colitis' or 'lymphocytic colitis' is a histological diagnosis, for which different aetiologies and hence treatments can be considered.

**Table 3**   Diagnostic histopathological criteria

Collagenous colitis
   A diffusely (not all samples should be involved) distributed and thickened subepithelial collagen layer $\geq 10$ μm

   Epithelial flattening and detachment

   Inflammation in the lamina propria with mainly mononuclear cells

   Increased number of intraepithelial lymphocytes may be present

Lymphocytic colitis
   Increased number of intraepithelial lymphocytes (IEL) $\geq 20$ per 100 surface epithelial cells

   Epithelial flattening and detachment

   Inflammation in the lamina propria with mainly mononuclear cells

   Thickening ($< 10$ μm) of the subepithelial collagen layer may be present

# References

1    Schiller LR. Diarrhea. Med Clin N Am. 2000;84:1259–74.
2.   Schiller LR. Chronic diarrhea Gastroenterology. 2004;127:287–93.
3.   Prior A, Lessels AM, Whorwell PJ. Is biopsy necessary if colonoscopy is normal? Dig Dis Sci. 1987;32:673–6.
4.   Whithead R. Colitis: problems in definition and diagnosis. Virchows Arch Pathol Anat. 1990;417:187–90.
5.   Marshall JB, Singh R, Diaz-Arias AA. Chronic, unexplained diarrhea: are biopsies necessary if colonoscopy is normal? Am J Gastroenterol. 1995;90:372–6.
6.   Shah RJ, Fenoglio-Preiser C, Bleau BL, Giannella RA. Usefulness of colonoscopy with biopsy in the evaluation of patients with chronic diarrhea. Am J Gastroenterol. 2001;96: 1091–5.
7.   Alsaigh N, Fogt F. Intestinal spirochetosis: clinicopathological features with review of the literature. Colorect Dis. 2002;4:97–100.
8.   Spiller RC, Jenkins D, Thornley JP et al. Increased rectal mucosal enteroendocrine cells, T lymphocytes, and increased gut permeability following acute *Campylobacter* enteritis and in post-dysenteric irritable bowel syndrome. Gut. 2000;47:804–11.
9.   Dickinson RJ, Gilmour HM, McClelland DB. Rectal biopsy in patients presenting to an infectious disease unit with diarrhoeal disease. Gut. 1979;20:141–8.
10.  Elliott PR, Williams CB, Lennard-Jones JE et al. Colonoscopic diagnosis of minimal change colitis in patients with normal sigmoidoscopy and normal air-contrast barium enema. Lancet. 1982;I:650–1.
11.  Bryant DA, Mintz ED, Puhr ND, Griffin PM, Petras RE. Colonic epithelial lymphocytosis associated with an epidemic of chronic diarrhea. Am J Surg Pathol. 1996;20:1102–9.
12.  Libbrecht L, Croes R, Ectors N, Staels F, Geboes K. Microscopic colitis with giant cells. Histopathology. 2002;40:335–8.
13.  Sandmeier D, Bouzourene H. Microscopic colitis with giant cells: a rare new histopathologic subtype? Int J Surg Pathol. 2004;12:45–8.
14.  Saurine TJ, Brewer JM, Eckstein RP. Microscopic colitis with granulomatous inflammation. Histopathology. 2004;45:82–6.
15.  Bhanot P, Goldstein NS. Patients with pauci-IEL lymphocytic colitis are similar to classic lymphocytic colitis: broadening the morphologic definition of lymphocytic colitis. Mod Pathol. 2003;16:111A.
16.  Fiel MI, Robbins D, Harpaz N. Pseudomembranous variant of collagenous colitis. Mod Pathol. 2003;16:118 (Abstract).
17.  Warren BF, Edwards CM, Travis SPL. Microscopic colitis: classification and terminology. Histopathology. 2002;40:374–6.
18.  Rubio CA, Lindholm J. Cryptal lymphocytic coloproctitis: a new phenotype of lymphocytic colitis? J Clin Pathol. 2002;55:138–40.
19.  Muller S, Schwab D, Aigner T, Kirchner T. Allergy-associated colitis. Characterization of an entity and its differential diagnosis. Pathology. 2003;24:28–35.
20.  Flejou JF, Bogomoletz WV. Microscopic colitis: collagenous colitis and lymphocytic colitis. A single concept? Gastroenterol Clin Biol. 1993;17:28–32.
21.  Levison DA, Lazenby AJ, Yardley JH. Microscopic colitis cases revisited. Gastroenterology. 1993;105:1594–6.
22.  Read NW, Krejs GJ, Read MG, Santa Ana CA, Morawski SG, Fordtran JS. Chronic diarrhea of unknown origin. Gastroenterology. 1980;78:264–71.
23.  Lazenby AJ, Yardley JH, Giardiello FM, Jessurun J, Bayless TM. Lymphocytic ('microscopic') colitis: a comparative histophatologic study with particular reference to collagenous colitis. Hum Pathol. 1989;20:18–28.
24.  Lindström CG. Collagenous colitis with watery diarrhoea – a new entity? Pathol Eur 1976; 11:87–9.
25.  Rotimi O, Rodrigues MG, Lim C. Microscopic colitis with giant cells – is it really a distinct pathological entity? Histopathology. 2004;44:502–14.
26.  Baert F, Wouters K, D'Haens G et al. Lymphocytic colitis: a distinct clinical entity? A clinicopathological confrontation of lymphocytic and collagenous colitis. Gut. 1999;45: 375–81.

27. Xin W, Evans LT, Appelman HD, Anderson MA, McKenna BJ. Minimal collagenous colitis: microscopic colitis with minimal subsurface collagen is appropriately diagnosed as collagenous colitis. Mod Pathol. 2005;18:A561

28. Feczko PJ, Mezwa DG. Nonspecific radiographic abnormalities in collagenous colitis. Gastrointest Radiol. 1991;16:128–32.

29. Cruz-Correa M, Milligan F, Giardiello FM et al. Collagenous colitis with mucosal tears on endoscopic insufflation: a unique presentation. Gut. 2002;51:600–1.

30. Poupardin-Moulin C, Atlani M, Sabate JM, Coffin B. Ulcérations coliques au cours de la colite collagène. Gastroenterol Clin Biol. 2004;28:310–11.

31. Baert F, Schmit A, D'Haens G et al. Budesonide in collagenous colitis: a double-blind placebo-controlled trial with histologic follow-up. Gastroenterology. 2002;122:20–5.

32. Bejarano PA, Aranda-Michel J, Fenoglio-Preiser C. Histochemical and immunohistochemical characterization of foamy histiocytes (muciphages and xanthelasma) of the rectum. Am J Surg Pathol. 2000;24:1009–15.

33. Fasoli R, Talbot I, Reid M, Prince C, Jewell DP. Microscopic colitis: can it be qualitatively and quantitatively characterized? Ital J Gastroenterol. 1992;24:393–6.

34. Machida HM, Catto Smith AG, Gall DG, Trevenen C, Scott RB. Allergic colitis in infancy: clinical and pathologic aspects. J Pediatr Gastroenterol Nutr. 1994;19:22–6.

35. Goldstein NS, Gyorfi T. Focal lymphocytic colitis and collagenous colitis: patterns of Crohn's colitis? Am J Surg Pathol. 1999;23:1075–81.

36. Van den Oord JJ, Geboes K, Desmet VJ. Collagenous colitis: an abnormal collagen table? Two new cases and review of the literature. Am J Gastroenterol. 1982;77:377–81.

37. Offner FA, Jao RV, Lewin KJ, Havelec L, Weinstein WM. Collagenous colitis: a study of the distribution of morphological abnormalities and their histological detection. Hum Pathol. 1999;30:451–7.

38. Goff JS, Barnett JL, Peike T, Appelman HD. Collagenous colitis: histopathology and clinical course. Am J Gastroenterol. 1997;92:57–60.

39. Marteau P, Lavergne-Slove A, Lemann M et al. Primary ileal villous atrophy is often associated with microscopic colitis. Gut. 1997;41:561–4.

40. Goldblum J, Wang N. Lymphocytic and collagenous colitis as possible patterns of Crohn's colitis. Am J Surg Pathol. 2000;24:755–6.

41. Panaccione R, Tremaine WJ, Batts KW, Sandborn WJ. Diagnosis of lymphocytic or collagenous colitis in patients with ulcerative colitis or Crohn's disease. Gastroenterology. 1999;116:A833.

42. Pokorny CS, Kneale KL, Henderson CJA. Progression of collagenous colitis to ulcerative colitis. J Clin Gastroenterol. 2001;32:435–8.

43. Wolber R, Owen D, Freeman H. Colonic lymphocytosis in patients with celiac sprue. Hum Pathol. 1990;21:1092–6.

44. Loft DE, Marsh MN, Crowe PT. Rectal gluten challenge and diagnosis of coeliac disease. Lancet. 1990;335:1293–5.

45. Olesen M. Microscopic colitis: studies of epidemiology, clinical features and nitric oxide. Linköping Univ Med Dissert. 2004;830:2–3.

46. Nielsen OH, Vainer B, Schaffalitzky de Muckadell OB. Microscopic colitis: a missed diagnosis? Lancet. 2004;364:2055–7.

47. Bohr J, Tysk C, Eriksson S, Jarnerot G. Collagenous colitis in Orebro, Sweden; an epidemiological study 1984–1993. Gut. 1995;37:394–7.

48. McKenna BJ, Eldeiry P, Odze RD et al. Apoptotic colopathy: a new variant of microscopic diarrheal disease? Mod Pathol. 2001;14:91A.

49. Jakate S, John R, Keshavarzian A, Demeo M. Mastocytic enterocolitis: another possible cause for intractable diarrhea in adults. Mod Pathol. 2005;18:488A.

# 6
# Mechanisms of pathogenesis in microscopic colitis

J. BOHR

## AETIOLOGY

The cause of microscopic colitis (MC) is unknown. At present both collagenous colitis (CC) and lymphocytic colitis (LC), are considered to be abnormal immunological reactions to various mucosal insults in predisposed individuals.

### Genetics and HLA

Nine familial cases with CC and LC, and with mixed CC and LC, have been reported[1-5]. Twelve per cent of patients with LC reported a family history of other bowel disorders such as inflammatory bowel disease, coeliac disease or CC[6]. Whether these associations are due to genetics, environmental factors or chance cannot be assessed.

There are reports of an increased frequency of HLA-A1, HLA-DRW53 in LC, and decreased HLA-DQ2 in CC[7], and HLA-A3 was later reported decreased in LC[8]. In a third report HLA-DQ2 and HLA DQ1,3, which are also asociated with coeliac disease, were reported increased in CC and LC[9]. Conclusions must await more consistent data.

### Reaction to a luminal agent

Faecal stream diversion by an ileostomy normalizes or reduces the characteristic histopathological changes in CC. This observation is the basis of the theory that CC is caused by an agent in the faecal stream[10]. There is an increased number of T lymphocytes in the epithelium, and this supports the theory that CC is an abnormal immunological reaction to a luminal agent[11-13]. Moreover, abnormalities of colonic histology resembling LC have been reported in untreated coeliac disease[14], and in patients with coeliac disease who had been given a gluten enema[15].

## Infectious aetiology

The sudden onset of the disease in some patients, and the effect of various antibiotics, support a possible infectious cause[16]. An association with MC and infections with *Campylobacter jejuni*[17] and *Clostridium difficile*[18-20] have been reported. In another study, *Yersinia enterocolitica* was detected in three of six patients prior to CC diagnosis, and a serological study showed that antibodies to *Yersinia* species were more common in CC patients than in healthy controls[21,22]. LC has many similarities to 'Brainerd diarrhoea', a condition with chronic watery diarrhoea characterized by acute onset and prolonged duration, and colonic biopsies in these patients show lesions similar to LC. An infectious cause in Brainerd diarrhoea is suspected but not verified.

## Drugs

There are several reports on drug-induced microscopic colitis, especially in LC (Table 1). Most reports concern ticlopidine and Cyclo 3 fort. In a case–control study the use of NSAID was significantly more common among CC patients than in controls, and discontinuation of NSAID was followed by improvement of the diarrhoea in some patients[23]. Others have found that use of NSAID at presentation was associated with a greater need for 5-ASA and steroid therapy, possibly reflecting a more resistant form of disease, but withdrawal of NSAID did not improve clinical symptoms in that study[24]. It is, however, important to assess concomitant drug use in the patients, and consider withdrawal of drugs that might worsen the condition.

**Table 1**  Drugs reported associated with microscopic colitis

| *Lymphocytic colitis* | *Collagenous colitis* |
|---|---|
| Ticlopidine[46-48] | Lanzoprazole[49-51] |
| Cyclo 3 Fort[52-54] | NSAID[23] |
| Ranitidine[55] | Cimetidine[56] |
| Vinburnine[49] | |
| Tardyferon[57] | |
| Flutamide[48] | |
| Acarbose[58] | |
| Piroxicam[59] | |
| Levodopa-benserazide[60] | |
| Carbamazepine[6] | |
| Sertraline[6] | |
| Paroxetine[6] | |
| Oxetorone[61] | |
| Lanzoprazole[50, 62] | |

## Autoimmunity and hormonal status

Both CC and LC are associated with autoimmune diseases. An autoimmune pathogenesis has therefore been proposed, possibly initiated by a foreign luminal agent, which causes an immunological crossreaction with an endogenous antigen. A study of autoantibodies and immunoglobulins in CC showed that the mean level of IgM in CC patients was significantly increased[25], similar to primary biliary cirrhosis. A specific autoantibody in CC has not been reported. CC are more frequent in women, and has been reported to improve during pregnancy, which indicates that hormonal factors are of influence in CC[16].

## Bile acids

Data on bile acid malabsorption in MC are conflicting. In one study no association was found, whereas others found bile acid malabsorption in 27–44% of patients with CC and in 9–60% of patients with LC[26–29]. The coexistence of bile acid malabsorption seems to worsen the diarrhoea in patients with CC[27]. These observations are the basis for bile acid binding treatment. Even patients without bile acid malabsorption may respond to this treatment. This emphasizes the importance of the faecal stream, and the therapeutic effect may possibly be related to binding of luminal toxins[30].

## Smoking

An association with cigarette smoking has been reported in CC[31], and might be more frequent even in LC than in the background population[6]. These data need to be confirmed.

## PATHOPHYSIOLOGY

### The collagenous layer and inflammatory mediators

Studies on collagen metabolism in CC show a decreased degradation of collagen[32]. Transforming growth factor-β, basic fibroblast growth factor and vascular endothelial growth factor, which stimulate collagen synthesis, are up-regulated in CC[33–35]. This all leads to excess deposition of collagen, and possibly takes place simultaneously.

Except for nitric oxide (NO)[36–38] and prostaglandins[39,40], inflammatory mediators were previously not reported in CC. Lately, however, NF-κB was shown to be equally activated in CC and ulcerative colitis[41]. This finding is interesting as NF-κB has earlier been suspected of initiating the macroscopic mucosal lesions seen in IBD, which is not found in MC. NF-κB seems to have diverse, almost opposite, roles in inflammatory bowel disease[42], and need to be further studied in MC.

## Nitric oxide

NO production is greatly increased in active MC caused by an up-regulation of inducible NO synthase (iNOS) in the colonic epithelium[36–38]. The levels of NO correlate with clinical activity and histopathological status of the colonic mucosa; i.e. patients in histopathological remission had normal levels of colonic NO in contrast to increased levels in patients with histologically active disease[38]. NO is involved in the diarrhoeal pathophysiology as infusion in the colon of $N^G$-monomethyl-L-arginine, an inhibitor of NOS, reduced colonic net secretion by 70% and the addition of L-arginine increased colonic net secretion by 50%[43]. NO is possibly an inflammatory mediator, but whether its role is proinflammatory or protective remains unclear.

## Secretory or osmotic diarrhoea

Diarrhoeal pathophysiology in CC has been regarded as secretory, caused by the epithelial lesions, the inflammatory infiltrate in the lamina propria and the collagenous band that might be a barrier for reabsorption of electrolytes and water[44]. Furthermore, an impaired epithelial barrier function due to down-regulation of tight junction molecules was found to contribute to diarrhoeal pathophysiology[44]. Studies on the influence of fasting on diarrhoea in CC indicated, however, that osmotic diarrhoea was predominant[45]. Many patients report that fasting reduces their diarrhoea in accordance with this observation.

## Disease mechanism

The disease mechanism of CC is not firmly established. It could be speculated that the subepithelial collagenous layer in the colon normally acts as a defence barrier in a dynamic process, in which the layer is thickened as a result of various mucosal injuries or agents, in order to avoid noxious effects on the colon and the rest of the body. According to this theory, patients with CC respond with an uncontrolled immunological reaction to certain agents, which results in excess deposition of collagen in or adjacent to the basement membrane. In line with this hypothesis, LC could be an early stage of CC. Conversion from LC to CC, however, is not frequent; thus LC is possibly rather a related disease, with a different pathological immunological reaction to an agent in the faecal stream.

## References

1.  van Tilburg AJ, Lam HG, Seldenrijk CA et al. Familial occurrence of collagenous colitis. A report of two families. J Clin Gastroenterol. 1990;12:279–85.
2.  Järnerot G, Hertervig E, Gränö C et al. Familial occurrence of microscopic colitis: a report on five families. Scand J Gastroenterol. 2001;36:959–62.
3.  Abdo AA, Zetler PJ, Halparin LS. Familial microscopic colitis. Can J Gastroenterol. 2001; 15:341–3.
4.  Freeman HJ. Familial occurrence of lymphocytic colitis. Can J Gastroenterol. 2001;15: 757–60.

5. Thomson A, Kaye G. Further report of familial occurrence of collagenous colitis. Scand J Gastroenterol. 2002;37:1116.
6. Olesen M, Eriksson S, Bohr J, Jarnerot G, Tysk C. Lymphocytic colitis: a retrospective clinical study of 199 Swedish patients. Gut. 2004;53:536–41.
7. Giardiello FM, Lazenby AJ, Bayless TM et al. Lymphocytic (microscopic) colitis. Clinicopathologic study of 18 patients and comparison to collagenous colitis. Dig Dis Sci. 1989;34:1730–8.
8. Giardiello FM, Lazenby AJ, Yardley JH et al. Increased HLA A1 and diminished HLA A3 in lymphocytic colitis compared to controls and patients with collagenous colitis. Dig Dis Sci. 1992;37:496–9.
9. Fine KD, Do K, Schulte K et al. High prevalence of celiac sprue-like HLA-DQ genes and enteropathy in patients with the microscopic colitis syndrome. Am J Gastroenterol. 2000; 95:1974–82.
10. Järnerot G, Tysk C, Bohr J, Eriksson S. Collagenous colitis and fecal stream diversion. Gastroenterology. 1995;109:449–55.
11. Giardiello FM, Lazenby AJ. The atypical colitides. Gastroenterol Clin N Am. 1999;28:479–90.
12. Stampfl DA, Friedman LS. Collagenous colitis: pathophysiologic considerations. Dig Dis Sci. 1991;36:705–11.
13. Armes J, Gee DC, Macrae FA, Schroeder W, Bhathal PS. Collagenous colitis: jejunal and colorectal pathology. J Clin Pathol. 1992;45:784–7.
14. Fine KD, Lee EL, Meyer RL. Colonic histopathology in untreated celiac sprue or refractory sprue: is it lymphocytic colitis or colonic lymphocytosis? Hum Pathol. 1998;29: 1433–40.
15. Dobbins WO, Rubin CE. Studies of the rectal mucosa in celiac sprue. Gastroenterology. 1964;47:471–9.
16. Bohr J, Tysk C, Eriksson S, Abrahamsson H, Järnerot G. Collagenous colitis: a retrospective study of clinical presentation and treatment in 163 patients. Gut. 1996;39: 846–51.
17. Perk G, Ackerman Z, Cohen P, Eliakim R. Lymphocytic colitis: a clue to an infectious trigger. Scand J Gastroenterol. 1999;34:110–12.
18. Vesoulis Z, Lozanski G, Loiudice T. Synchronous occurrence of collagenous colitis and pseudomembranous colitis. Can J Gastroenterol. 2000;14:353–8.
19. Khan MA, Brunt EM, Longo WE, Presti ME. Persistent Clostridium difficile colitis: a possible etiology for the development of collagenous colitis. Dig Dis Sci. 2000;45:998–1001.
20. Byrne MF, McVey G, Royston D, Patchett SE. Association of Clostridium difficile infection with collagenous colitis. J Clin Gastroenterol. 2003;36:285.
21. Makinen M, Niemela S, Lehtola J, Karttunen TJ. Collagenous colitis and Yersinia enterocolitica infection. Dig Dis Sci. 1998;43:1341–6.
22. Bohr J, Nordfelth R, Järnerot G, Tysk C. Yersinia species in collagenous colitis: a serologic study. Scand J Gastroenterol. 2002;37:711–4.
23. Riddell RH, Tanaka M, Mazzoleni G. Non-steroidal anti-inflammatory drugs as a possible cause of collagenous colitis: a case–control study. Gut. 1992;33:683–6.
24. Abdo A, Raboud J, Freeman HJ et al. Clinical and histological predictors of response to medical therapy in collagenous colitis. Am J Gastroenterol. 2002;97:1164–8.
25. Bohr J, Tysk C, Yang P, Danielsson D, Järnerot G. Autoantibodies and immunoglobulins in collagenous colitis. Gut. 1996;39:73–6.
26. Eusufzai S, Löfberg R, Veress B, Einarsson K, Angelin B. Studies on bile acid metabolism in collagenous colitis: no evidence of bile acid malabsorption as determined by the SeHCAT test. Eur J Gastroenterol Hepatol. 1992;4:317–21.
27. Ung KA, Gillberg R, Kilander A, Abrahamsson H. Role of bile acids and bile acid binding agents in patients with collagenous colitis. Gut. 2000;46:170–5.
28. Ung KA, Kilander A, Willen R, Abrahamsson H. Role of bile acids in lymphocytic colitis. Hepatogastroenterology. 2002;49:432–7.
29. Fernandez-Banares F, Esteve M, Salas A et al. Bile acid malabsorption in microscopic colitis and in previously unexplained functional chronic diarrhea. Dig Dis Sci. 2001;46: 2231–8.
30. Andersen T, Andersen JR, Tvede M, Franzmann MB. Collagenous colitis: are bacterial cytotoxins responsible? Am J Gastroenterol. 1993;88:375–7.

31. Pardi DS. Microscopic colitis: an update. Inflamm Bowel Dis. 2004;10:860–70.
32. Aigner T, Neureiter D, Muller S, Kuspert G, Belke J, Kirchner T. Extracellular matrix composition and gene expression in collagenous colitis. Gastroenterology. 1997;113:136–43.
33. Stahle-Backdahl M, Maim J, Veress B, Benoni C, Bruce K, Egesten A. Increased presence of eosinophilic granulocytes expressing transforming growth factor-beta1 in collagenous colitis. Scand J Gastroenterol. 2000;35:742–6.
34. Taha Y, Raab Y, Larsson A et al. Mucosal secretion and expression of basic fibroblast growth factor in patients with collagenous colitis. Am J Gastroenterol. 2003;98:2011–17.
35. Taha Y, Raab Y, Larsson A et al. Vascular endothelial growth factor (VEGF) – a possible mediator of inflammation and mucosal permeability in patients with collagenous colitis. Dig Dis Sci. 2004;49:109–15.
36. Lundberg JON, Herulf M, Olesen M et al. Increased nitric oxide production in collagenous and lymphocytic colitis. Eur J Clin Invest. 1997;27:869–71.
37. Perner A, Nordgaard I, Matzen P, Rask-Madsen J. Colonic production of nitric oxide gas in ulcerative colitis, collagenous colitis and uninflamed bowel. Scand J Gastroenterol. 2002; 37:183–8.
38. Olesen M, Middelveld R, Bohr J et al. Luminal nitric oxide and epithelial expression of inducible and endothelial nitric oxide synthase in collagenous and lymphocytic colitis. Scand J Gastroenterol. 2003;38:66–72.
39. Rask-Madsen J, Grove O, Hansen MG, Bukhave K, Scient C, Henrik-Nielsen R. Colonic transport of water and electrolytes in a patient with secretory diarrhea due to collagenous colitis. Dig Dis Sci. 1983;28:1141–6.
40. Raclot G, Queneau PE, Ottignon Y et al. Incidence of collagenous colitis. A retrospective study in the east of France. Gastroenterology. 1994;106:A23.
41. Andresen L, Jorgensen VL, Perner A, Hansen A, Eugen-Olsen J, Rask-Madsen J. Activation of nuclear factor kappaB in colonic mucosa from patients with collagenous and ulcerative colitis. Gut. 2005;54:503–9.
42. Schreiber S. The complicated path to true causes of disease: role of nuclear factor kappaB in inflammatory bowel disease. Gut. 2005;54:444–5.
43. Perner A, Andresen L, Normark M et al. Expression of nitric oxide synthases and effects of L-arginine and L-NMMA on nitric oxide production and fluid transport in collagenous colitis. Gut. 2001;49:387–94.
44. Burgel N, Bojarski C, Mankertz J, Zeitz M, Fromm M, Schulzke JD. Mechanisms of diarrhea in collagenous colitis. Gastroenterology. 2002;123:433–43.
45. Bohr J, Järnerot G, Tysk C, Jones I, Eriksson S. Effect of fasting on diarrhoea in collagenous colitis. Digestion. 2002;65:30–4.
46. Brigot C, Courillon-Mallet A, Roucayrol AM, Cattan D. Lymphocytic colitis and ticlopidine. Gastroenterol Clin Biol. 1998;22:361–2.
47. Berrebi D, Sautet A, Flejou JF, Dauge MC, Peuchmaur M, Potet F. Ticlopidine induced colitis: a histopathological study including apoptosis. J Clin Pathol. 1998;51:280–3.
48. Baert F, Wouters K, D'Haens G et al. Lymphocytic colitis: a distinct clinical entity? A clinicopathological confrontation of lymphocytic and collagenous colitis. Gut. 1999;45:375–81.
49. Chauveau E, Prignet JM, Carloz E, Duval JL, Gilles B. Lymphocytic colitis likely attributable to use of vinburnine (Cervoxan). Gastroenterol Clin Biol. 1998;22:362.
50. Thomson RD, Lestina LS, Bensen SP, Toor A, Maheshwari Y, Ratcliffe NR. Lansoprazole-associated microscopic colitis: a case series. Am J Gastroenterol. 2002;97:2908–13.
51. Wilcox GM, Mattia A. Collagenous colitis associated with lansoprazole. J Clin Gastroenterol. 2002;34:164–6.
52. Pierrugues R, Saingra B. Lymphocytic colitis and Cyclo 3 fort: 4 new cases. Gastroenterol Clin Biol. 1996;20:916–7.
53. Beaugerie L, Luboinski J, Brousse N et al. Drug induced lymphocytic colitis. Gut. 1994;35:426–8.
54. Bouaniche M, Chassagne P, Landrin I, Kadri N, Doucet J, Bercoff E. Lymphocytic colitis caused by Cyclo 3 Fort. Rev Med Interne. 1996;17:776–8.
55. Beaugerie L, Patey N, Brousse N. Ranitidine, diarrhoea, and lymphocytic colitis. Gut. 1995;37:708–11.

56. Duncan HD, Talbot IC, Silk DB. Collagenous colitis and cimetidine. Eur J Gastroenterol Hepatol. 1997;9:819–20.
57. Bouchet-Laneuw F, Deplaix P, Dumollard JM et al. Chronic diarrhea following ingestion of Tardyferon associated with lymphocytic colitis. Gastroenterol Clin Biol. 1997;21:83–4.
58. Piche T, Raimondi V, Schneider S, Hebuterne X, Rampal P. Acarbose and lymphocytic colitis. Lancet. 2000;356:1246.
59. Mennecier D, Gros P, Bronstein JA, Thiolet C, Farret O. Chronic diarrhea due to lymphocytic colitis treated with piroxicam beta cyclodextrin. Presse Med. 1999;28:735–7.
60. Rassiat E, Michiels C, Sgro C, Yaziji N, Piard F, Faivre J. Lymphocytic colitis due to Modopar. Gastroenterol Clin Biol. 2000;24:852–3.
61. Macaigne G, Boivin JF, Chayette C, Cheaib S, Deplus R. Oxetorone-associated lymphocytic colitis. Gastroenterol Clin Biol. 2002;26:537.
62. Ghilain JM, Schapira M, Maisin JM et al. Lymphocytic colitis associated with lansoprazole treatment. Gastroenterol Clin Biol. 2000;24:960–2.

# 7
# Microscopic colitis: treatment

## A. TROMM

## INTRODUCTION

The umbrella term microscopic colitis is used for both collagenous and lymphocytic colitis[1]. Reviewing the literature in this field it is important to highlight three remarks:

1. The majority of recommendations and trials has been made for collagenous colitis.

2. The cardinal clinical symptom of microscopic colitis is watery diarrhoea; thus, the main therapeutic goal is to improve stool frequency and consistency.

3. The aetiology and pathogenesis of the diseases are unknown. In this regard treatment will be almost symptomatic.

A variety of therapeutic agents have been used in collagenous colitis[2-4]. However, most regimens are supported only by case reports or small, non-controlled series[5]. Thus, past recommendations for therapy remain empirical.

Treatment regimes vary and have included antidiarrhoeal agents, aminosalicylates, antibiotics, systemic corticosteroids, bismuth subsalicylate or subnitrate, cholestyramine, ketotifen, verapamil, pentoxifylline, spasmolytics, azathioprine, methotrexate, cyclosporine and octreotide[5]. The role of a disturbed absorption of bile acids remains controversial and needs to be evaluated in controlled studies. In some cases therapy with proton pump inhibitors might precede the clinical manifestation of collagenous colitis. The cessation of treatment leads to a rapid clinical improvement in the majority of patients. However, the mechanism has not yet been investigated.

Recently we conducted an open-label design to monitor the clinical effects of *Escherichia coli* Nissle 1917 (EcN) on stool frequency and stool consistency in 14 patients[6]. Due to the open-label protocol EcN was administered at different doses (one to six capsules per day containing $2.5-25 \times 10^9$ viable bacteria). Except for two patients who discontinued treatment, therapy duration was at least 4 weeks. The results indicate a marked clinical response due to the oral administration of EcN with a reduction of the stool frequency $\geqslant 50$ % in $9/14$ (64%) patients. Stool frequency clearly ($p = 0.034$) decreased from $7.6 \pm 4.8/$ day to $3.7 \pm 5.8/$day at the end of therapy (between 4 and 18 weeks). Moreover stool consistency changed in $7/14$ patients from watery or slimy to soft (six patients) and normal (one patient), respectively.

Surgery is described as an ultimate, but very rarely applied, alternative in severe, unresponsive collagenous colitis. It has been shown that ileostomy leads to a reduction of the collagen band and lymphocytic infiltrate in collagenous colitis. These data indicate the possible influence of a luminal agent in collagenous colitis.

## BISMUTH SUBSALICYLATE

Fine and Lee[7] published a pilot trial indicating that $11/12$ patients achieved clinical remission within 8 weeks of treatment with bismuth subsalicylate (BSS). In addition, BSS has been tested in a placebo-controlled study in 14 patients with collagenous ($n = 9$) *and* lymphocytic ($n = 5$) colitis, which is published in abstract form[8]. BSS was given as a daily dose of nine tablets with 262 mg BSS each for 8 weeks. Non-responders were treated in a cross-over regimen subsequently. The primary response rate was $7/7$ in the bismuth group, and $5/6$ in the non-responder group.

## PREDNISOLONE

Systemic corticosteroids are effective in reducing stool frequency; however, therapy is limited by the large number of undesired effects related to high bioavailability. Prednisolone (50 mg) daily was not superior to placebo in a controlled clinical trial[9]. Limitations of this study are the small number of patients ($n = 12$) and the short duration of therapy (2 weeks).

## BUDESONIDE

Budesonide is a lipophilic steroid with a high receptor binding affinity and a high first-pass effect in the liver. Thus, the bioavailability of budesonide is rather low ($\approx 11\%$). With respect to the location of the subepithelial collagen layer and the lymphocytic infiltrate in collagenous colitis the pharmacological profile of budesonide seems to be suitable for a rational luminal therapy of collagenous colitis. The local efficacy of budesonide in the ileum is realized by a pH-dependent delivery of budesonide due to a eudragit layer.

Case reports and non-controlled pilot trials have revealed evidence that budesonide is effective in collagenous colitis, and have led to recent controlled randomized clinical trials aimed at evaluating the efficacy and safety of budesonide on clinical data generated under controlled conditions.

## Non-controlled clinical trials and case reports

Janetschek and Böckmann[10] and Tromm et al.[11] reported the effective use of budesonide (3 mg t.i.d.) in the treatment of collagenous colitis in a total of three and seven patients, of whom three and two patients, respectively, were ineffectively treated previously with metronidazole, mesalazine, or prednisolone. The results indicate a rapid and sustained clinical response in all patients, with clinical improvement achieved within the first 10 days and diarrhoea ceasing after 7 weeks at latest[11].

In the pilot trial, including seven cases, daily stool frequency significantly decreased from $10.43 \pm 5.56$ to $3.3 \pm 1.2$ after 10 days and to $1.86 \pm 0.69$ after 10 weeks. Stool consistency was markedly improved[11]. Three patients in total were biopsied. In all patients a highly significant reduction of the collagen layer, as well as of the lymphoplasmatic infiltrate, was observed (for overview see Table 1).

No relapse was reported in all three patients for a period with a maximum of 11 months[11]. In 3/7 patients who participated in the pilot trial, no diarrhoea recurred within 7, 12, or 15 months after budesonide was terminated.

Retrospective case reports revealed clinical remission in 2/2 patients on budesonide[2].

Comparable results have been obtained in three patients refractory to prednisone treatment. After administration of budesonide (3 mg t.i.d.), clinical symptoms resolved immediately. The mean follow-up after starting with budesonide was 11 months (7–18 months). One case has been kept symptom-free on a lower budesonide dose (3 mg b.i.d.), and one patient has been in remission for more than 1 year after a 3-month budesonide treatment course[12].

In an open pilot trial, five patients received budesonide (9 mg/day) for 3–24 months. Complete response as defined by less than three normal stools/day was achieved in 3/5 patients, and partial response in 2/5 patients, which was defined as $\geqslant 50\%$ reduction in stool frequency and minimal abdominal pain not interfering with daily activities. Duration to response ranged between 3 and 6 weeks[13].

## Controlled clinical trials and meta-analysis

The primary outcome measure in nearly all trials was clinical remission or improvement as characterized by decreased faecal frequency, stool weight or stool consistency. Moreover, a decrease of further accompanying complaints has been also considered.

Histological response was implemented as a secondary outcome measure and has been classified as a decrease in inflammation activity or thickness of collagen band in the lamina propria.

The Belgian IBD Research Group conducted a placebo-controlled, multi-centre double-blind study in which a total of 28 patients were randomly allocated to budesonide 9 mg o.d. ($n = 14$) or placebo ($n = 14$) over a period of 8 weeks. Subsequently, non-responders received open-label budesonide treatment for another 8 weeks; all patients were followed up for the entire 16-week study period[14].

**Table 1** Pilot study and case reports on budesonide in collagenous colitis

| Reference | Design | Duration | Treatment regime | Patients (n) | Objectives |
|---|---|---|---|---|---|
| Janetschek & Böckmann[10] | Pros, op; case report | 7–9 weeks | Budesonide* 9 mg/day | 3 | Clinical response Histological response |
| Delarive et al.[13] | Pros, op; case report | 3–24 months | Budesonide# 9 mg o.d. | 5 | Clinical response |
| Tromm et al.[6] | Pros, op; pilot trial | 10 weeks | Budesonide* 3 mg t.i.d. | 7 | Clinical response Histological response |
| Lanyi et al.[12] | Pros, op; case report | 3–7 months | Budesonide# 3 mg t.i.d. | 3 | Clinical response |
| Bohr et al.[2] | Retros, op; case report | n.r. | Budesonide (dose n.r.) | 2 | Clinical response |

Pros: prospective; retros: retrospective; op: open-label; co: crossover; ext: extension; o.d.: once daily; t.i.d.: thrice daily; n.r.: not reported.
*Budenofalk® 3-mg capsules (Falk Pharma); #Entocort® 3-mg capsules (Astra Zeneca).

All patients included showed at least three semi-loose to loose stools per day and a subepithelial collagen band exceeding 10 μm. Clinical response was defined by a 50% drop in the disease activity score (number of bowel movements during the past 7 days) at week 8 compared to week 0. According to this stringent definition, eight of 14 budesonide patients and only three of 14 placebo patients responded to therapy (intention-to-treat (ITT) analysis; $p = 0.05$). Maximal clinical efficacy was already reached within the first 2 weeks and was maintained throughout the 8-week study period. Clinical response was accompanied by improved stool consistency. Of the remaining six patients on budesonide not matching the definition of clinical response, two showed a favourable outcome considered as clinical response by themselves and their physicians. The low baseline disease activity scores in some patients can explain the disagreement. With exclusion of these patients not meeting the entry criterion of 21 stools/week at week 0 (three on budesonide, two on placebo), eight of 11 budesonide patients and only three of 12 placebo patients ($p = 0.02$) responded to therapy.

Histological evaluation of biopsies available at week 8 revealed no significant differences with regard to thickness of the subepithelial collagen band between the two groups, although a remarkable reduction was found in a subgroup. However, there was a highly significant reduction of the infiltrate of the lamina propria in the budesonide group (Table 2).

**Table 2**  Clinical improvement – budesonide vs placebo[17]

| Study | Budesonide (n = 47) | Placebo (n = 47) | Weight (%) | Peto odds ratio* (95% CI) |
|---|---|---|---|---|
| Baert et al.[14] | 8/11 | 3/12 | 25.0 | 6.23 (1.26–30.92) |
| Bonderup et al.[16] | 10/10 | 2/10 | 21.1 | 23.73 (4.15–135.72) |
| Miehlke et al.[15] | 20/26 | 3/25 | 53.8 | 13.08 (4.39–38.99) |
| Total | 38/47 | 8/47 | 100.00 | 12.32 (5.53–27.46) |

* <1 favours placebo, >1 favours budesonide; CI: confidence interval.

In a double-blind study, a total of 51 patients with histologically proven collagenous colitis were randomly assigned to budesonide (9 mg o.d., $n = 23$) or placebo ($n = 22$) for 6 weeks[15]. Complete colonoscopy and histopathological assessment was performed before and after treatment. Clinical symptoms were assessed by standardized questionnaires.

The rate of clinical remission, as defined by three or less soft or solid stools/day, was significantly higher on budesonide than on placebo (per-protocol (PP): 86.9% vs 13.6%; (ITT): 76.9% vs 12.0%; $p < 0.001$). The median time period until clinical remission occurred among all patients on budesonide was 13 days (2–30 days).

Histological improvement was observed in 14 patients on budesonide (60.9%) and in one patient on placebo (4.5%; $p < 0.001$). On budesonide,

**Table 3**  Histologic improvement – budesonide vs placebo[17]

| Study | Budesonide (n = 47) | Placebo (n = 47) | Odds ratio (fixed)* (95% CI) |
|---|---|---|---|
| Baert et al.[14] | 10/11 | 4/12 | 20.00 (1.85–216.19) |
| Bonderup et al.[16] | 10/10 | 3/10 | 45.00 (2.01–1006.80) |
| Miehlke et al.[15] | 14/26 | 1/25 | 28.00 (3.28–238.91) |

*Less than 1 favours placebo, more than 1 favours budesonide; CI: confidence interval.

inflammation of the lamina propria was markedly reduced virtually throughout the entire colon, and degenerated surface epithelium was restored (Table 3).

Reduction of the thickness of the collagen band was observed in a similar proportion in both treatment groups. Clinical remission correlated positively with histological improvement in 12 patients on budesonide.

The clinical and histological effects of budesonide in collagenous colitis have also been the subject of a placebo-controlled double-blind trial[16]. For a treatment period of 8 weeks a total of 20 patients were randomized to receive placebo (n = 10) or budesonide (n = 10; 9 mg o.d. to 3 mg o.d.). Stool frequency and weight were registered before and after treatment. Sigmoidoscopy was performed before and after treatment, and biopsies at fixed locations were obtained for morphometric analysis. All 10 patients on budesonide had a reduction in stool frequency or stool weight of $\geqslant 50\%$, whereas only two patients on placebo showed a similar response ($p < 0.001$). On budesonide, stool weight was reduced from 574 g/day to 200 g/day and stool frequency was reduced from 6.2/day to 1.9/day ($p < 0.01$).

The histological inflammation grade in the sigmoid mucosa and the thickness of collagen layer were significantly reduced. A correlation between the grade of inflammation as well as collagen layer thickness and stool weight was found. Eight of 10 patients had relapse of symptoms within 8 weeks after stopping treatment.

As shown in a total of three appropriately conducted controlled clinical trials in collagenous colitis[14–16], in a combined analysis[17] budesonide proved to be very effective in inducing clinical and histological remission in collagenous colitis. Budesonide is the only intervention for which strong clinical evidence of benefit exists for clinical as well as histological improvement in collagenous colitis.

The study by Madisch et al.[18] revealed evidence that budesonide improves the gastrointestinal quality of life index (GIQLI) in patients with collagenous colitis.

Bajor et al.[19] presented a poster at the DDW 2003 indicating that the 75SeHCAT values increased in all but one patient after 8 weeks of budesonide treatment. Thus, the clinical effect of budesonide may be mediated by an up-regulation of the active bile acid uptake in the terminal ileum leading to a reduced bile acid load to the colon. Furthermore, levels of vascular endothelial growth factor (VEGF) significantly decreased after treatment with budesonide[20].

In conclusion, as has been shown in a recently published meta-analysis[17] of the randomized controlled clinical trials available, budesonide (9 mg o.d. for 6–8 weeks) is effective in the treatment of collagenous colitis with very high clinical (81% vs 17%) and histological (61–100% vs 4–33%) response rates as compared to placebo. The number needed to treat (NNT) has been calculated to be 1.58 (95 % CI ± 1.86) in a second meta-analysis[21].

Budesonide has recently been licensed in the United Kingdom for the treatment of collagenous colitis.

The long-term-treatment of collagenous colitis is still under discussion. The recurrence rates after termination of the acute-phase therapy with budesonide are high. In this regard the important questions to be answered in the near future are: Is there an indication for a maintenance treatment of collagenous colitis? Which drug should be used? At what dose?

## References

1. Lazenby AJ, Yardley JH, Giardiello FM, Jessurun J, Bayless TM. Lymphocytic (microscopic) colitis: a comparative histopathological study with particular reference to collagenous colitis. Hum Pathol. 1989;20:18–28.
2. Bohr J. A review of collagenous colitis. Scand J Gastroenterol. 1998;33:2–9.
3. Tromm A, Bayerdörffer E, Delarive J, Blum AL, Stolte M. Diagnostik und Therapie der kollagenen Kolitis. Leber Magen Darm. 1999;29:169–76.
4. Zins BJ, Sandborn WJ, Tremaine WJ. Collagenous and lymphocytic colitis: subject review and therapeutic alternatives. Am J Gastroenterol. 1995;90:1394–400.
5. Stroehlein JR. Microscopic colitis. Curr Opin Gastroenterol. 2004;20:27–31.
6. Tromm A, Niewerth U, Khoury M et al. The probiotic E. coli strain Nissle 1917 for the treatment of collagenous colitis: first results of an open label trial. Z Gastroenterol. 2004;42:365–9.
7. Fine KD, Lee EL. Efficacy of open-label bismuth-subsalicylate for the treatment of microscopic colitis. Gastroenterology. 1998;114:29–36.
8. Fine KD, Ogunji F, Lee EL, Lafon G, Tanzi M. Randomized, double-blind, placebo-controlled trial of bismuth subsalicylate for microscopic colitis. Gastroenterology. 1999;116:A40 (Abstract).
9. Munck LK, Kjeldsen J, Phlipsen E, Fischer Hansen B. Incomplete remission with short-term prednisolone treatment in collagenous colitis. Scand J Gastroenterol. 2003;38:606–10.
10. Janetschek P, Böckmann U. Budesonide – a new highly effective therapeutic approach to collagenous colitis. Digestion. 1998;59(S3):159.
11. Tromm A, Griga Th, Möllmann HW, May B, Müller K-M, Fisseler-Eckhoff A. Budesonide for the treatment of collagenous colitis: first results of a pilot trial. Am J Gastroenterol. 1999;94:1871–5.
12. Lanyi B, Dries V, Dienes H-P, Kruis W. Therapy of prednisone-refractory collagenous colitis with budesonide. Int J Colorect Dis. 1999;14:58–61.
13. Delarive J, Saraga E, Dorta G, Blum A. Budesonide in the treatment of collagenous colitis. Digestion. 1998;59:364–6.
14. Baert F, Schmit A, D'Haens G et al. and Belgian IBD Research Group and Codali Brussels, Belgium. Budesonide in collagenous colitis – a double-blind placebo-controlled trial with histologic follow-up. Gastroenterology. 2002;122:20–5.
15. Miehlke S, Heymer P, Bethke B et al. Budesonide treatment for collagenous colitis – a randomized, double-blind, placebo-controlled, multicenter trial. Gastroenterology. 2002;123:978–84.
16. Bonderup OK, Hansen JB, Birket-Smith L, Vestergaard V, Teglbjaerg PS, Fallingborg J. Budesonide treatment of collagenous colitis – a randomised, double blind, placebo controlled trial with morphometric analysis. Gut. 2003;52:248–51.
17. Chande N, McDonald JWD, MacDonald JK. Interventions for treating collagenous colitis. Cochrane Database Syst Rew. 2004;1:CD003575.

18. Madisch A, Heymer P, Voss C et al. Oral budesonide therapy improves quality of life in patients with collagenous colitis. Int J Colorectal Dis. 2004;11 (Epub).
19. Bajor A, Kilander A, Gälman C, Rudling M, Ung K-A. The effects of budesonide in collagenous colitis may be promoted by low concentrations of bile acids in the colon due to stimulated active absorption in the ileum. Gastroenterology. 2003;124(S1):A146 (Abstract).
20. Griga T, Tromm A, Schmiegel W, Pfisterer O, Müller K-M, Brasch F. Collagenous colitis: implications for the role of vascular endothelial growth factor in repair mechanism. Eur J Gastroenterol Hepatol. 2004;16:397–402.
21. Feyen B, Wall GC, Finnerty EP, Dewitt JE, Reyes RS. Meta-analysis: budesonide for collagenous colitis. Aliment Pharmacol Ther. 2004;20:745–9.

# Section III
# Predicting outcomes

**Chair: M.A. KAMM and M. KEIGHLEY**

# 8
# Predicting the natural history of inflammatory bowel disease

S. VERMEIRE

## INTRODUCTION

Not only are the initial presentations of inflammatory bowel disease (IBD) patients very different, the disease itself in a given patient is dynamic and phenotypically evolves with time. Predicting the disease course may be very difficult and unpredictable. Nevertheless, at the time of diagnosis, or during the further follow-up, patients will want answers to important questions as to how the disease will progress and what the likelihood of a surgical intervention will be, what the risks of complications and cancer are, etc.

This chapter gives an overview of the natural history of IBD, and will address important questions with which physicians are confronted by their patients.

## WHAT IS THE LIKELIHOOD OF A FLARE IN ANY GIVEN YEAR?

Both Crohn's disease (CD) and ulcerative colitis (UC) are characterized by flare-ups alternating with periods of remission (Figure 1). This means that most patients will have to take medication (mostly for maintenance of remission and intermittently additional induction therapy for treating a flare) for a large part of their lives. Population-based data from Denmark ($n = 373$) showed that, after the first year of diagnosis, the majority of CD patients in any population is in remission (55%) or has only a mild disease activity (15%)[1]. Nevertheless, up to a third of patients will have highly active disease. Very similar data from Silverstein et al. showed that 64.4% of the follow-up time of CD patients is characterized by medical or surgical remission[2]. A full year of remission is followed by a 80% chance of remission in the following year, whereas a patient experiencing a recent flare has only a 30% chance of remission in the following year[3].

For UC, approximately 50% of patients will be in clinical remission every year at any point in time[4]. After 25 years of follow-up, however, the cumulative probability of a relapsing disease course amounts to 90%. Langholz et al. also showed that active disease in the first 2 years after diagnosis indicates with 70–80% probability an increased probability of 5 consecutive years of active disease[4].

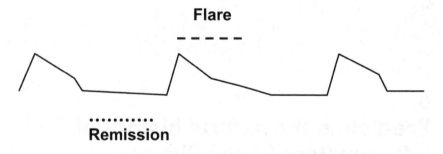

**Figure 1** The natural course of IBD is characterized by flares alternating with periods of remission

## WHAT IS THE RISK OF A PATIENT NEEDING STEROIDS?

With the introduction of novel biological therapies such as infliximab, the hope is that corticosteroids could be avoided as much as possible in the future. Figures from Copenhagen County illustrated that 56% of patients require corticosteroids, and data from Olmsted County are similar, with 43% requirement of corticosteroids for CD patients and a somewhat lower (34%) rate for UC patients[5,6]. The short-term outcome (30 days) of a first course of steroids is such that approximately 60% of patients will have a complete response, 30% a partial response, and 10–15% will be non-responders. At 1 year only 32% of CD patients and 49% of UC patients will have a prolonged response[6]. Moreover, 28% (CD) and 22% (UC) will become steroid-dependent.

## WILL THE LOCATION AND BEHAVIOUR OF THE DISEASE REMAIN STABLE OVER TIME?

The majority of patients will present with extended ileocolonic disease at the time of diagnosis. The study by Farmer et al. showed 30% isolated small bowel disease, 28% pure colonic disease and 42% ileocolitis[7]. The location of the disease changes only minimally over time. At 10 years only 15% of patients will show a change in location[8].

In contrast to this, the disease behaviour is susceptible to changes with increasing disease duration. Whereas the majority of patients (90%) present with inflammatory, non-stricturing and non-penetrating disease at diagnosis, after 10 years approximately one-third of patients are classified within each of the three recognized disease behaviours (inflammatory, stricturing or penetrating)[8]. French data showed that, over a 20-year period, patients have a 88% risk of developing stricturing disease (18%) or penetrating disease (70%)[9].

The location of the disease determines behaviour: ileal disease is associated with stricturing disease and colonic disease with inflammatory or penetrating disease[7–9].

Molecular markers may prove useful in the future to predict the natural history. Whereas patients carrying two mutations in the CARD15 gene had a 7-fold increased risk for stricturing disease, as shown by Brant et al., this risk further increased to 17 in the presence of ileal disease[10].

## WHAT IS THE LIKELIHOOD OF A SURGICAL INTERVENTION?

At 1 year following the start of corticosteroid therapy, 40% of CD patients and 30% of UC patients will need surgery[6]. It is well known that surgery will not cure CD, and that the disease recurs in almost all patients[11]. Greenstein et al. studied 770 CD patients undergoing intestinal resection for perforating or non-perforating indications, and demonstrated that 77% of perforating patients and 71% of non-perforating patients who underwent a second surgery had that surgery for the same indication as for their first operation[12]. Patients with perforating disease had a more rapid recurrence, whereas stricturing disease patients showed a slower recurrence. Looking in the long term, Bernell et al. studied 1936 CD patients and showed that the cumulative risk of surgery at 15 years was over 80%[13].

Smoking is a well-known risk factor for CD, for various reasons: it is not only associated with an increased risk for the disease itself, but smokers also have a more aggressive disease course and an increased risk for surgery and postoperative recurrence. Smoking, on the other hand, is protective against UC.

Another established risk factor is appendectomy. A recent meta-analysis on a total of 2770 UC patients showed that appendectomy decreases the risk of UC by 70% (adjusted OR 0.292; 95% CI 0.224–0.379)[14]. More recent data suggested that appendectomy may delay the onset of UC. In this study, patients with previous appendectomy ($n$ =20) had a mean age at onset which was approximately 10 years older (42.5 years) compared to the patients ($n$ =239) without previous appendectomy (mean age at onset 32.1 years)[15]. There was no influence of appendectomy on disease extent, need for immunosuppressive therapy or colectomy rates. The latter is in contrast to the French study by Cosnes et al. showing that UC patients with appendectomy had a lower risk of colectomy compared to non-appendectomized patients[16]. In the same study, previous appendectomy (OR 0.40) and current smoking (OR 0.60) were independent factors protecting against colectomy. The authors also assessed the incidence of flares prospectively between 1997 and 2000, and showed that appendectomy was associated with a less severe disease course.

## ARE CURRENT THERAPIES ABLE TO ALTER THE NATURAL HISTORY?

With the therapeutic options available for the treatment of IBD, physicians are able to bring patients into remission and keep them off steroids, to maintain remission and to induce mucosal healing. Although the use of immunosuppressive therapies in particular has dramatically risen over the past 25 years, this was not paralleled by a reduced risk for surgery, as recently shown[17]. The preliminary data from the Benelux step-up/top-down trial in CD suggest that infliximab might change the natural history of the disease. Induction therapy with infliximab and azathioprine maintenance resulted in a remission rate without steroids of 75% at 6 months compared to 41% for the step-up treatment arm ($p = 0.006$)[18]. The full results of this trial are expected soon.

## WHAT IS THE RISK OF COLORECTAL CANCER?

When looking at the available studies on colorectal cancer in IBD, there is a great variability in cancer incidence between hospital studies and population-based studies. At 30 years, hospital studies showed cumulative cancer rates up to 40%, whereas in population studies the figure was much lower (13.5%)[19]. The current hypothesis for the increased risk in patients with IBD is that long-standing inflammation in the colon is responsible for dysplastic changes in the mucosa. It is therefore logical that the risk increases with longer disease duration and with greater extent of disease. The latter was nicely shown by Ekbom and colleagues in a population-based study from Sweden[20]. A total of 3117 UC patients were followed for 1–60 years after diagnosis. The RR for cancer increased from 1.7 (proctitis) to 2.8 (left-sided) to 14.8 (pancolitis) (Figure 2). Other risk groups that were identified included young age at onset, UC patients with a familial risk and concomitant primary sclerosing cholangitis (PSC)[20].

The risk of colorectal cancer in patients with UC, but also in patients with Crohn's colitis, begins to increase at 8 years from diagnosis. There are two approaches to prevent this either total colectomy or endoscopic surveillance. The current cancer surveillance guidelines suggest the following strategy, based on the location and extent of the disease and disease duration. For UC proctitis there are no data to support special recommendations beyond those for the general population; for pancolitis or left-sided colitis <8 years, the same surveillance guidelines as those applied in the general population hold; finally, for pancolitis or left-sided colitis >8 years, a colonoscopy every 1–2 years with two to four biopsies every 10 cm or prophylactic colectomy are proposed. In the absence of prospective studies and cost-effectiveness analyses, the choice must be made on an individual basis[21].

## IS THE LIFE EXPECTANCY OF IBD PATIENTS ALTERED?

Population-based data from Copenhagen County in Denmark showed no increased mortality for UC patients overall, nor for men or women separately, as compared to the background population[22,23]. However, patients >50 years at diagnosis, and those with extensive colitis at diagnosis, tended to have a lower life expectancy.

In contrast, a number of studies have shown that the life expectancy of CD patients is slightly lower, with standardized mortality rates varying between

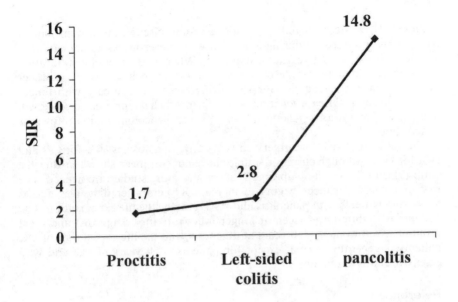

**Figure 2** Cancer risk in patients with UC according to disease extent. The Y-axis shows the standardized incidence ratio (SIR), which is defined as the ratio of observed to expected cases (from ref. 20)

**Table 1** Studies on mortality rates in patients with Crohn's disease

| Reference | Region | Mortality | Standardized mortality rate |
|---|---|---|---|
| Persson et al.[24] | Sweden | ↑ | 1.40 |
| Loftus et al.[25] | Olmsted County | ↑ | |
| Palli et al.[26] | Florence | ↑ | 1.50 |
| Ekbom et al.[27] | Uppsale Region | ↑ | 1.60 |
| Probert et al.[28] | Leicestershire | = | 0.70 |
| Munkholm et al.[29] | Copenhagen County | = | |
| Jess et al.[30] | Copenhagen County | ↑ | 1.30 |

0.70 and 1.60 (Table 1)[24–30]. However, this slightly decreased survival rate is observed only at longer follow-up after diagnosis, and is most pronounced in women <50 years at diagnosis.

## SUMMARY

Although IBD is considered a chronic relapsing disease, more than half of patients are in remission during any given year. Nevertheless, many will need steroids during the first year after diagnosis. Whereas the anatomical location of the disease remains stable over time, the disease behaviour changes over time, with an increasing risk for stricturing/penetrating disease with longer disease duration. Disease location will influence behaviour: ileal disease will tend to evolve towards stricturing disease and ileocolonic/colonic towards penetrating.

The cumulative risk for surgery 15 years after diagnosis is 80% for CD and 30% for UC. Although current therapies have not (yet) been shown to alter the natural history, the follow-up time is short and more studies are needed. The risk of colorectal cancer begins to increase 8 years after diagnosis and is greatest in patients with pancolitis and PSC. Finally, the life expectancy of CD patients is slightly lower (seen at longer follow-up after diagnosis) and most pronounced in women < 50 years at diagnosis, and the life expectancy of UC patients is generally normal except for patients > 50 years of age and with extensive colitis at diagnosis

## References

1. Munkholm P, Langholz E, Davidsen M, Binder V. Disease activity courses in a regional cohort of Crohn's disease patients. Scand J Gastroenterol. 1995;30:699–706.
2. Silverstein MD, Loftus EV, Sandborn WJ et al. Clinical course and costs of care for Crohn's disease: Markov model analysis of a population-based cohort. Gastroenterology. 1999;117: 49–57.
3. Veloso FT, Ferreira JT, Barros L, Almeida S. Clinical outcome of Crohn's disease: analysis according to the Vienna classification and clinical activity. Inflamm Bowel Dis. 2001;7:306–13.
4. Langholz E, Munkholm P, Davidsen M, Binder V. Course of ulcerative colitis: analysis of changes in disease activity over years. Gastroenterology. 1994;107:3–11.
5. Munkholm P, Langholz E, Davidsen M, Binder V. Frequency of glucocorticoid resistance and dependency in Crohn's disease. Gut. 1994;35:360–2.
6. Faubion WA Jr, Loftus EV Jr, Harmsen WS, Zinsmeister AR, Sandborn WJ. The natural history of corticosteroid therapy for inflammatory bowel disease: a population-based study. Gastroenterology. 2001;121:255–60.
7. Farmer RG, Whelan G, Fazio VW. Long-term follow-up of patients with Crohn's disease. Relationship between the clinical pattern and prognosis. Gastroenterology. 1985;88:1818–25.
8. Louis E, Collard A, Oger AF, Degroote E, Aboul Nasr El Yafi FA, Belaiche J. Behaviour of Crohn's disease according to the Vienna classification: changing pattern over the course of the disease. Gut. 2001;49:777–82.
9. Cosnes J, Cattan S, Blain A et al. Long-term evolution of disease behavior of Crohn's disease. Inflamm Bowel Dis. 2002;8:244–50.
10. Brant SR, Picco MF, Achkar JP et al. Defining complex contributions of NOD2/CARD15 gene mutations, age at onset, and tobacco use on Crohn's disease phenotypes. Inflamm Bowel Dis. 2003;9:281–9.
11. Rutgeerts P, Geboes K, Vantrappen G, Beyls J, Kerremans R, Hiele M. Predictability of the postoperative course of Crohn's disease. Gastroenterology. 1990;99:956–63.
12. Greenstein AJ, Lachman P, Sachar DB et al. Perforating and non-perforating indications for repeated operations in Crohn's disease: evidence for two clinical forms. Gut. 1988;29: 588–92.

13. Bernell O, Lapidus A, Hellers G. Risk factors for surgery and postoperative recurrence in Crohn's disease. Ann Surg. 2000;231:38–45.
14. Koutroubakis IE, Vlachonikolis IG. Appendectomy and the development of ulcerative colitis: results of a metaanalysis of published case-control studies. Am J Gastroenterol. 2000;95:171–6.
15. Selby WS, Griffin S, Abraham N, Solomon MJ. Appendectomy protects against the development of ulcerative colitis but does not affect its course. Am J Gastroenterol. 2002; 97:2834–8.
16. Cosnes J, Carbonnel F, Beaugerie L, Blain A, Reijasse D, Gendre JP. Effects of appendicectomy on the course of ulcerative colitis. Gut. 2002;51:803–7.
17. Cosnes J, Nion-Larmurier I, Beaugerie L, Afchain P, Tiret E, Gendre JP. Impact of the increasing use of immunosuppressants in Crohn's disease on the need for intestinal surgery. Gut. 2005;54:237–41.
18. Hommes D, Baert F, Van Assche G et al. A randomized controlled trial evaluating the ideal medical management for Crohn's disease (CD): top-down versus step-up strategies. Gastroenterology. 2005;128:A-577.
19. Hordijk ML, Shivananda S. Risk of cancer in inflammatory bowel disease: why are the results in the reviewed literature so varied? Scand J Gastroenterol (Supplement). 1989; 170:70–4; discussion 81–2.
20. Ekbom A, Helmick C, Zack M, Adami HO. Ulcerative colitis and colorectal cancer. A population-based study. N Engl J Med. 1990;323:1228–33.
21. Ekbom A, Helmick C, Zack M, Adami HO. Increased risk of large-bowel cancer in Crohn's disease with colonic involvement. Lancet. 1990;336:357–9.
22. Langholz E, Munkholm P, Davidsen M, Binder V. Colorectal cancer risk and mortality in patients with ulcerative colitis. Gastroenterology. 1992;103:1444–51.
23. Winther KV, Jess T, Langholz E, Munkholm P, Binder V. Survival and cause-specific mortality in ulcerative colitis: follow-up of a population-based cohort in Copenhagen County. Gastroenterology. 2003;125:1576–82.
24. Persson PG, Bernell O, Leijonmarck CE, Farahmand BY, Hellers G, Ahlbom A. Survival and cause-specific mortality in inflammatory bowel disease: a population-based cohort study. Gastroenterology. 1996;110:1339–45.
25. Loftus EV Jr, Silverstein MD, Sandborn WJ, Tremaine WJ, Harmsen WS, Zinsmeister AR. Crohn's disease in Olmsted County, Minnesota, 1940–1993: incidence, prevalence, and survival. Gastroenterology. 1998;114:1161–8.
26. Palli D, Trallori G, Saieva C et al. General and cancer specific mortality of a population based cohort of patients with inflammatory bowel disease: the Florence Study. Gut. 1998;42:175–9.
27. Ekbom A, Helmick CG, Zack M, Holmberg L, Adami HO. Survival and causes of death in patients with inflammatory bowel disease: a population-based study. Gastroenterology. 1992;103:954–60.
28. Probert CS, Jayanthi V, Wicks AC, Mayberry JF. Mortality from Crohn's disease in Leicestershire, 1972–1989: an epidemiological community based study. Gut. 1992;33: 1226–8.
29. Munkholm P, Langholz E, Davidsen M, Binder V. Intestinal cancer risk and mortality in patients with Crohn's disease. Gastroenterology. 1993;105:1716–23
30. Jess T, Winther KV, Munkholm P, Langholz E, Binder V. Mortality and causes of death in Crohn's disease: follow-up of a population-based cohort in Copenhagen County, Denmark. Gastroenterology. 2002;122:1808–14.

# 9
# Can we predict who develops extraintestinal manifestations?

## T. R. ORCHARD

## INTRODUCTION

Up to 30% of patients with inflammatory bowel disease (IBD) will develop extraintestinal manifestations (EIM). The commonest of these are musculoskeletal, dermatological and hepatic (primary sclerosing cholangitis). Much recent research has been devoted to trying to define specific clinical phenotypes within IBD, and to identify factors which may contribute to their pathogenesis or predict their prognosis. The EIM provide easily identifiable groups which can be studied in this way.

Many studies on EIM in the past have produced conflicting or inconclusive results, and this is largely due to study size and design. In order to identify successfully possible prognostic factors there are two important prerequisites. First the groups being studied must be clearly defined, and secondly the study must be of sufficient size to allow careful analysis of these groups. The major groups of EIM that have been studied are ankylosing spondylitis (AS), peripheral arthritis, erythema nodosum and uveitis, which form a group of musculoskeletal EIM, and primary sclerosing cholangitis (PSC), which is the major hepatic association of IBD. AS and PSC are clearly defined clinical syndromes, with recognized diagnostic criteria. The other groups, particularly peripheral arthritis, have previously been poorly defined, and studies have often included patients with both arthritis and arthalgia, and this has led to rather confused results.

The methods used to predict the development of EIM can be divided into clinical factors, serological markers and genetic associations, and studies of these factors have been made to a greater or lesser extent in all the major EIM.

## PRIMARY SCLEROSING CHOLANGITIS (PSC)

PSC is a progressive fibrotic liver disease which is characterized by fibrosis of the bile ducts, and ultimately leads to a secondary biliary cirrhosis. Its clinical course is extremely variable, and may be complicated by the development of cholangiocarcinoma. In terms of clinical predictors the condition occurs most frequently in males with extensive colitis. Indeed some authors have suggested that this colitis is itself phenotypically distinct form of classical ulcerative colitis (UC), as it tends to run a rather quiescent course, and may not even be diagnosed until after the PSC. The presence of PSC has been studied in relation to HLA status on a number of occasions, and has been associated with HLA-B8 and DR3[1] as part of the HLA-A1 B8 DR3 haplotype[2]; an association with HLA-DR2 has also been reported[3]. It has been suggested that the DR3 association seen in this group of patients may simply represent the association already discovered in UC between HLA-DR3 DQ2[4]. Indeed this association is strongest in males with extensive disease – the group at greatest risk of developing PSC. However, as many feel that the colitis seen in PSC patients may be different from classical UC, the association with HLA-DR3 may be a primary one. The wide variability of clinical course, and the relative infrequency of PSC in UC, make the determination of phenotype-determining genes within this group very difficult, due to small numbers. Mehal et al. have reported that patients who carry HLA-DR4 are at an increased risk of an aggressive clinical course, and the development of cholangiocarcinoma[5], and a more recent study has suggested HLA-DR3, DQ2 may be associated with rapid progression of disease[6]. None of these associations is secure enough to be clinically useful, and further work, ideally in large populations, will be required to settle the question of genetic influences. PSC does have a very strong association with the presence of pANCA, which is present in up to 75% of patients[7,8]. Its utility as a clinical predictor is hampered by the fact that pANCA is also common in UC, occurring in up to 70% of patients.

## ANKYLOSING SPONDYLITIS (AS)

There have been few studies of the clinical associations of AS in IBD. It appears to occur with about equal frequency in UC and Crohn's disease, with a prevalence of 1–5% depending on the study. Unlike idiopathic AS the male: female ratio is about equal, but no specific clinical subgroups appear to be particularly strongly associated with AS. Similarly there are no obvious serological correlates; however there is a strong genetic association with AS – that of HLA-B27.

In idiopathic AS 94% of Caucasian patients possess HLA-B27[9]. In IBD the prevalence is less, approximating 50–80% in most studies[10]. The reason for this is not clear, but it has been suggested that gut inflammation may lead to the genetic predisposition being overridden. Thus the intestinal inflammation allows sufficient quantity of pathogenic antigen to trigger an inflammatory reaction despite the fact that the HLA status is not favourable. Thus the negative predictive value of not possessing HLA-B27 is low, and patients who are HLA-B27 negative may still develop AS.

In addition to full-blown AS patients with IBD also have a substantial risk of developing isolated sacroiliitis – inflammation of the sacroiliac joints without the spinal ankylosis seen in AS. In the original radiographic surveys the prevalence was 18% in UC[11], but recent studies using more sensitive techniques such as CT and MRI scanning have suggested prevalences between 30% and 50%[12,13]. So far it has not been possible to identify those patients who will develop classical AS, as this appears to be a small minority. A recent small study from Oxford showed a prevalence of 35% for sacroiliitis in an unselected population of Crohn's disease patients. Interestingly the prevalence of HLA-B27 was not increased in the isolated sacroiliitis group[14]. However, all seven patients who possessed HLA-B27 in this study had MRI evidence of axial disease. This compares with estimates of between 1% and 10% for HLA-B27-positive subjects in the general population. This suggests that the positive predictive value of HLA-B27 in IBD may be high, and certainly higher than in the general population, meaning that a large proportion of IBD patients with HLA-B27 will have evidence of axial inflammation.

Studies of other predictors of axial disease have also been conducted in AS associated with IBD. HLA-DR1 is another association, but is probably related to the HLA-B27 association. CARD15 polymorphisms have also been associated with disease in some studies, but the results are not conclusive overall, and the effect is certainly substantially less important than that of HLA-B27.

## PERIPHERAL ARTHRITIS

The study of peripheral arthritis in IBD has been hampered by the fact that most studies have been very small. This is because in many cases the arthritis is short-lived, and nearly all the studies have been retrospective.

Peripheral arthritis has been reported in association with IBD for many years, but it was only in 1958 when the arthritis was proven to be inflammatory, and quite distinct from classical rheumatoid, being seronegative for rheumatoid factor[15].

The prevalence of peripheral arthropathy in IBD has been reported as between 10% and 20%, but the definitions of arthritis vary between studies, and often arthralgia in the absence of objective evidence of inflammation has been included. This is certainly common, and may relate to steroid reduction, or commencement of azathioprine. Recently the inflammatory peripheral arthritis in IBD has been classified, by studying only patients with objective evidence of joint swelling. This demonstrates two distinct types of arthropathy with different natural histories and articular distributions[16].

*Type 1 (pauciarticular)* affects less than five joints including a weightbearing joint. The swelling is acute and self-limiting and associated with relapse of the IBD in the majority of cases.

*Type 2 (polyarticular)* affects five or more joints, and affects a wide range of joints but particularly the metacarpophalangeal (MCP) joints. It may cause persistent problems with a median duration of 3 years.

The onset of arthritis may occur at any time during the course of the IBD or before it becomes clinically manifest. It is not related to disease extent in UC but in Crohn's disease it is reportedly more common in colonic disease. In both types of arthropathy there is little or no joint destruction and patients are seronegative.

In this series of 1459 patients the prevalence of type 1 was 3.6% in UC and 6.0% in Crohn's disease and for type 2 was 2.5% in UC and 4.0% in Crohn's disease. A further 5.3% of UC patients and 14.3% of Crohn's disease patients complained of arthralgia. These figures may underestimate the true prevalence, but it seems clear that the prevalence of all forms of peripheral arthritis in UC is between 5% and 10%, and significantly more in Crohn's disease – 10–20%.

Clinical predictors of peripheral arthritis are largely the presence of other mucocutaneous extraintestinal manifestations, particularly erythema nodosum (EN) and uveitis. There is an association between Crohn's disease affecting the colon and arthritis, but arthritis is also seen in pure ileal disease. It is rarely seen in purely proximal small bowel Crohn's disease. In UC there is no significant link with disease extent, and there are no other major clinical predictors. In Crohn's disease new-onset arthritis is extremely uncommon in patients who have undergone ileocaecal resection[17].

Genetic predictors of arthritis have been studied recently in the light of the two forms of peripheral arthritis, and distinct associations have been described. HLA-DR103 had previously been reported as being associated with arthritis in UC. In fact the association with HLA-DR103 is solely with type 1 arthritis, which is also associated with HLA-B27, whereas type 2 is associated with HLA-B44 (see Table 1)[18]. In patients with recurrent type 1 arthritis the prevalence of DR103 rises from 35% to 65%; however even at this level the positive predictive value is not really high enough to enable this to be a useful clinical tool.

Serological markers have not really been studied in this group of patients, with the exception of rheumatoid factor, which is not associated with peripheral arthritis in IBD. Studies of ASCA and ANCA in this group would be interesting.

**Table 1** HLA associations reported with extra-intestinal manifestations of inflammatory bowel disease

| Manifestation | HLA antigen | Affected patients (% with HLA) | IBD controls (% with HLA) |
|---|---|---|---|
| Type 1 arthritis | HLA-B27 | 26 | 7 |
| | HLA-B35 | 33 | 15 |
| | HLA-DR103 | 35 | 3 |
| Type 2 arthritis | HLA-B44 | 62 | 31 |
| Ankylosing spondylitis | HLA-B27 | 60 | 7 |
| Uveitis | HLA-B27 | 33 | 7 |
| | HLA-B58 | 13 | 3 |
| | HLA-DR103 | 20 | 3 |
| Erythema nodosum | HLA-B62 | 28 | 11 |

## ERYTHEMA NODOSUM (EN)

EN is the commonest skin manifestation. Its prevalence varies widely between studies, depending upon the nature of the study population and the type of study. It is reported in 1–9% of UC patients[19-21] and 6–15% of Crohn's disease patients[22-25], although the most comprehensive study, from Oxford, suggests a prevalence at the lower end of this range. However, all studies show a marked female preponderance with a F:M ratio of about 5:1.

EN is a characteristic condition of the skin which presents with painful raised erythematous lesions normally on the extensor surfaces of the limbs. The major clinical predictors of EN are the presence of type 1 arthritis or uveitis. Patients with type 1 arthritis and Crohn's disease have a 25% chance of developing EN, and in UC an 8% chance compared to 2% in Crohn's and 0.5% in UC without joint problems. In addition EN occurs with predominantly colonic disease. The genetic predictors of EN reflect the clinical situation in relation to type 1 arthritis. There is a small generalized rearrangement of HLA-B alleles in EN and a weak association with HLA-B62, but there is a much stronger association with a polymorphism in the promoter of the TNF-α gene. The −1031 polymorphism is associated with EN in 69% of EN patients compared to 34% of IBD controls[24]. This is of particular interest because EN associated with other disorders such as sarcoidosis has been linked with different polymorphisms in the same gene[26]. Thus this may represent a very important aetiological factor, but the strength of the association is still not sufficient to make it a worthwhile test in clinical practice. Serological studies in EN have not been undertaken.

## OCULAR INFLAMMATION

Ocular inflammation in IBD was first documented by Crohn in 1925. If left untreated it is a potential cause of blindness, but prompt treatment with topical steroids can minimize this risk.

The prevalence of ocular inflammation varies widely between studies – from 2% to 13% depending on the population and methodology. The manifestations range from conjunctivitis to more significant inflammation. This usually affects the anterior chamber, but may include iritis, episcleritis, scleritis and anterior uveitis. In a large retrospective study of 1459 patients (976 UC and 483 Crohn's disease patients) 3% of UC and 5% of Crohn's disease patients had these more serious eye complications[27]. The commonest were iritis (60%), episcleritis (30%) and uveitis (10%). The conditions affect females more than males with a ratio of approximately 3:1, and in about 30% of cases the patients suffered from recurrent episodes. Posterior segment eye disease has been described, including serous choroidoretinopathy and retinal detachment, but these are very rare, and it is not clear whether there is an increased incidence in IBD above that seen in the general population.

As with EN the major clinical predictor of ocular inflammation is the presence of other EIM – either form of arthritis or EN. Seventeen per cent of type 1 arthritis patients in both UC and Crohn's disease will develop ocular inflammation, and 17% and 26% of type 2 arthritis in UC and Crohn's disease respectively. This compares with 1.2% and 2.9% in patients without any form of arthritis.

Genetic studies of ocular inflammation in IBD have been justified by the association of idiopathic acute anterior uveitis with HLA-B*27 in a number of small studies[28]. Recently a large retrospective study in IBD demonstrated associations between ocular inflammation and several HLA alleles including HLAB*27 HLA-B*58 and HLA-DR*103[24] (see Table 1). Thus it appears that HLA genes may have an important role in the ocular complications of IBD. However, as with the other genetic associations described, these associations are not strong enough to be helpful clinical predictors. Studies of serological markers have investigated the role of antibodies to the antigenic form of tropomyosin expressed in both gut and eye[29], but the proposed antigen is expressed in the ciliary body (which is rarely affected) and not in the iris (which is often affected); this has yet to be widely replicated.

## SUMMARY

The extraintestinal manifestations of IBD are relatively common, and a number of studies have been performed which have demonstrated links with particular patterns of disease, certain genotypes, particularly in the HLA region, and some serological markers. However, none of these is sufficiently sensitive or specific to allow the accurate prediction of which patients will develop these complications, and if a patient has had one form of EIM the risk of developing others is certainly substantially greater than for other IBD patients. A high index of suspicion should be maintained.

## References

1. Leidenius M, Koskimies S, Kellokumpu I, K Hockerstedt K. HLA antigens in ulcerative colitis and primary sclerosing cholangitis. APMIS 1995;103:519–24.
2. Donaldson P, Farrant J, Wilkinson M, Hayllar K, Portmann B, Williams R. Dual association of HLA-DR2 and DR3 with primary sclerosing cholangitis. Hepatology. 1991;13:129–33.
3. Wilschanski M, Chait P, Wade J et al. Primary sclerosing cholangitis in 32 children: clinical, laboratory and radiographic features with survival analysis. Hepatology. 1995;22:1415–22.
4. Satsangi J, Welsh KI, Bunce M et al. Contribution of genes of the major histocompatibility complex to susceptibility and disease phenotype in inflammatory bowel disease. Lancet. 1996;347:1212–17.
5. Mehal WZ, Lo YD, Wordsworth BP et al. HLA DR4 is a marker for rapid disease progression in primary sclerosing cholangitis. Gastroenterology. 1994;106:160–7.
6. Boberg KM, Spurkland A, Rocca G et al. The HLA-DR3,DQ2 heterozygous genotype is associated with an accelerated progression of primary sclerosing cholangitis. Scand J Gastroenterol. 2001;36:886–90.
7. Gur H, Shen GQ, Sutjita M et al. Autoantibody profile of primary sclerosing cholangitis. Pathobiology. 1995;63:76–82.
8. Boberg KM, Lundin KEA, Schrumpf E. Etiology and pathogenesis in primary sclerosing cholangitis. Scand J Gastroenterol. 1994;29:47–58.
9. Brown MA, Pile KD, Kennedy LG et al. HLA class I associations of ankylosing spondylitis in the white population in the United Kingdom. Ann Rheum Dis. 1996;55:268–70.

10. Dekker-Saeys B, Meuwissen S, Berg-Loonen EVD et al. Clinical characteristics and results of histocompatibility typing (HLA B27) in 50 patients with both ankylosing spondylitis and inflammatory bowel disease. Ann Rheum Dis. 1978;37:36–41.
11. Wright V, Watkinson G. Sacroiliitis and ulcerative colitis. Br Med J. 1965;2:675–80.
12. Agnew JE, Pocock DG, Jewell DP. Sacroiliac joint uptake ratios in inflammatory bowel disease: relationship to back pain and to activity of bowel disease. Br J Radiol. 1982;55:821.
13. McEnif, N, Eustace S, McCarthy C, O'Malley M, Morain C, Hamilton S. Asymptomatic sacroiliitis in inflammatory bowel disease. Assessment by computed tomography. Clin Imag. 1995;19:258–62.
14. Orchard T, Holt H, Bradley L et al. Prevalence of sacroiliitis in Crohn's disease, and its correlation with clinical, radiologic and genotypic parameters. Gastroenterology. 2002;122: W1298.
15. Bywaters E, Ansell B. Arthritis associated with ulcerative colitis: a clinical and pathological study. Ann Rheum Dis. 1958;17:169–83.
16. Orchard T, Wordsworth B, Jewell D. The peripheral arthropathies of inflammatory bowel disease: their articular distribution and natural history. Gut. 1998;42:387–91.
17. Orchard TR, Jewell DP. The importance of ileocaecal integrity in the arthritic complications of Crohn's disease. Inflamm Bowel Dis. 1999;5:92–7.
18. Orchard TR, Thiyagaraja S, Welsh KI, Wordsworth BP, Hill Gaston JS, Jewell DP. Clinical phenotype is related to HLA genotype in the peripheral arthropathies of inflammatory bowel disease. Gastroenterology. 2000;118:274–8.
19. Schorr-Lesnick B, Brandt LJ. Selected rheumatologic and dermatologic manifestations of inflammatory bowel disease. Am J Gastroenterol. 1988;83:216–23.
20. Johnson ML, Wilson HTH. Skin lesions in ulcerative colitis. Gut. 1969;10:255–63.
21. Hossein Mir-Madjlessi S, Taylor JS, Farmer RG. Clinical course and evolution of erythema nodosum and pyoderma gangrenosum in chronic ulcerative colitis: a study of 42 patients. Am J Gastroenterol. 198;80:615–20.
22. Bernstein CN, Blanchard JF, Rawsthorne P, Yu N. The prevalence of extraintestinal diseases in inflammatory bowel disease: a population based study. Am J Gastroenterol. 2001;96:1116–22.
23. Greenstein A, Janowitz H, Sachar D. Extra-intestinal complications of Crohn's disease and ulcerative colitis. Medicine. 1976;55:401–12.
24. Orchard TR, Chua CN, Ahmad T, Cheng H, Welsh KI, Jewell DP. Uveitis and erythema nodosum in inflammatory bowel disease: clinical features and the role of HLA genes. Gastroenterology. 2002;123:714–18.
25. Veloso FT, Carvalho J, Magro F. Immune-related systemic manifestations of inflammatory bowel disease. A prospective study of 792 patients. J Clin Gastroenterol. 1996;23:29–34.
26. Labunski S, Posern G, Ludwig S, Kundt G, Brocker EB, Kunz M. Tumour necrosis factor-alpha promoter polymorphism in erythema nodosum. Acta Derm Venereol. 2001;81:18–21.
27. Orchard TR, Chua C, Cheng H, Jewell DP. Clinical features of erythema nodosum (EN) and uveitis assocaited with inflammatory bowel disease. Gastroenterology. 2000;118:755.
28. Lyons JL, Rosenbaum JT. Uveitis associated with inflammatory bowel disease compared with uveitis associated with spondyloarthropathy. Arch Ophthalmol. 1997;115:61–4.
29. Bhagat S, Das K. A shared and unique peptide in the human colon, eye and joint detected by a monoclonal antibody. Gastroenterology. 1994;107:103–8.

# 10
# Colitis: predicting outcomes – who gets cancer?

## A. FORBES

## INTRODUCTION

It is well established that the risk of colorectal carcinoma is increased in ulcerative colitis (UC). It is highly probable, although admittedly less well verified, that a similar increase in risk applies to patients with colonic Crohn's disease (CD). In both forms of inflammatory bowel disease (IBD) there remains doubt about the magnitude of the risk, and this naturally leads to controversy over the role of surveillance strategies, in terms of their intensity but also in respect as to whether they are justified at all. In the absence of controlled trials of surveillance these questions cannot be resolved entirely satisfactorily.

The emphasis in the IBD literature has understandably been on colorectal carcinoma, but there are important associations with other malignancies that should also be addressed.

## ANAL CARCINOMA IN IBD

There is a consensus that anal cancer is over-represented in CD but the magnitude of this excess is more controversial, ranging between no added risk and more than 20-fold excess. A recent review has tried to clarify this area[1]. Much of the paper was taken up with rectal cancer (which is definitely over-represented) but aspects specific to anal cancer with wide culling from the literature indicate that about 1% of all anal cancers occur in CD. Given the prevalence of CD this itself indicates an increased risk of about 10-fold. Those at most risk seem to be those with chronic perianal disease. Curiously the human papilloma virus HPV-16 does not seem especially prevalent in CD despite the damaged mucosa which one might have expected to permit easier infection.

A high index of suspicion should be maintained, with early recourse to biopsy of any unusual lesions if the present poor outcomes are to be improved upon.

# THERAPY-RELATED LYMPHOMA IN IBD

## Azathioprine

There is a large body of evidence indicating an increased risk of lymphoma in patients undergoing solid organ transplantation. A significant proportion of this risk can be attributed to immunosuppressive therapy, and azathioprine has been particularly implicated. Concern has therefore transferred to use of this drug in the IBD sphere. This has been addressed specifically by the Oxford group as well as less formally by a number of other major centres. Taking other publications into account, and incorporating their own data, they were able to conclude reasonably confidently that there was no increased risk of malignancy from azathioprine[2]. This conclusion applied equally to lymphoma and to other tumours. Neoplasia attributable to the underlying IBD was, however, confirmed. The overall rate of malignancy of 2.2% in azathioprine-treated patients compared favourably with the 2.8% in unexposed IBD patients, although of course this was not statistically significant.

## Infliximab

There was some anxiety about treatment-related lymphoma early in the clinical experience with infliximab, but this was considered more likely to reflect underlying disease (and especially rheumatoid arthritis in which lymphoma is markedly over-represented). Close scrutiny of post-marketing records has been maintained, and a reasonable belief has emerged that added risk is very low or absent in CD. However, recent Swedish data reveal a lymphoma incidence of 1.5% per year in infliximab-treated patients, which may well be higher than that to be expected in the initial cohorts of patients with severe CD in whom infliximab treatment would have been considered in its early days[3]. This was, after all, 3 patients from only 191 treated.

# CHOLANGIOCARCINOMA IN PRIMARY SCLEROSING CHOLANGITIS

A majority of patients with primary sclerosing cholangitis (PSC) has underlying IBD and the coupled association of PSC with IBD and colorectal carcinoma will be addressed later. However, PSC is also (and probably independently) associated with cholangiocarcinoma. The lifetime risk of biliary neoplasia has been estimated at anything from no increased risk to 42%, but a realistic composite risk taken from the various publications sets the risk at about 15%. An incidence rate of around 1.5% per annum in IBD patients with PSC seems a reasonable estimation[4]. Diagnosis is difficult and there are no obvious clinical risk factors or pointers other than that arising from the initial difficulty of diagnosing the PSC itself. As up to 40% of cholangiocarcinoma diagnoses are made within 12 months of establishment of PSC it is highly probable that large numbers of cancers are simply not recognized originally. Surveillance has been considered in liver centres caring for patients with PSC given that the results of any form of therapy for cholangiocarcinoma are poor, other than resection (or transplantation) when the tumour is very localized and almost pre-macroscopic. The scoring system from King's London depends on a rising CA19-9 and CEA (CA19-9 + (40 × CEA)). A score of 400 or more is said to have a positive predictive value for cholangiocarcinoma of 100%[5]; nonetheless, other units have disputed this and there is parallel interest in polymerase chain reaction (PCR) study of bile, looking for mutations of the k-ras oncogene, and preliminary studies of biliary positron emission (PET) scanning. It might now be considered reasonable to combine the King's score with routine laboratory investigation every 6 months, and add annual biliary imaging with MRCP (although some will advocate expert ultrasonographic scanning as sufficient).

## COLORECTAL CARCINOMA IN IBD

It will be assumed here that many (greater than 70%) examples of colorectal carcinoma (CRC) in IBD are preceded by dysplastic lesions. The precise numerical links between dysplasia and carcinoma remain controversial, however – especially when low-grade dysplasia is considered – and this area will be considered in another chapter of this volume. Fortunately most authors agree that the risk of neoplasia is time- and extent-related. In the case of UC we can conclude that a duration of greater than 10 years (from first symptoms rather than from the time of diagnosis) and a macroscopic extent to above the splenic flexure reliably pick out those at most risk. The data in Crohn's colitis are less robust but (mostly) referral centre studies suggest that the risks are similar in extensive colitis of long duration; in Crohn's the extent may conveniently be identified from those exhibiting disease of 50% or more of the entire colonic length.

Using published data to define population risk is surprisingly difficult given the wide differences in cancer incidence and mortality between centres. There is probably a risk of about 20% at 20 years in centres with relatively standard criteria for surgery for poor medical control. This equates to roughly six times the risk of CRC in the general population. Especially low frequencies are, however, seen in Denmark where there is a lower threshold for colectomy than in most IBD centres, and a lifetime risk of only three-fold is attributed in Sweden[6,7].

There does not appear to be an increased risk of CRC in IBD patients where the only colorectal involvement is of the rectosigmoid. Patients with UC limited to the left side appear to be at an intermediate risk between those with extensive colitis and normal controls. The tendency of distal colitis to progress proximally should be remembered in strategy planning. Approximately 20% of patients will develop colitis of at least one more proximal segment every 5 years.

## COLORECTAL ADENOMAS

There is of course a very well established association between colorectal adenomas and CRC. It is not certain that this risk is amplified further in IBD, but it seems probable. For the patient who has an adenoma in an unaffected part of the colon, and in whom this is removed endoscopically, there is probably very little additional cancer risk, and it may be sufficient to survey that patient subsequently at frequencies based only on the adenoma-attributable risk. Things are more complex when an adenoma is found in a colitis-affected area. This discussion is not for this volume. My practice is to arrange for the more rigorous surveillance than would be suggested for the patient according to colitis or adenoma risk alone, but not normally to be more aggressive than that except when completion of endoscopic excision is uncertain and when early repeat colonoscopy is clearly warranted.

## FAMILY HISTORY

There is no evidence that a family history of IBD has any impact on the likelihood of an index patient developing CRC.

A family history of CRC increases the risk of malignancy in IBD patients. The magnitude of this risk is different in different centres (highest in Leicestershire) but averages about 2.5-fold[8,9]. It is not clear that this is fully additive to the risks attributed to extensive colitis. Common sense would dictate otherwise, as a positive family history is frequent (around 10%) in the normal general population. Multiplying a 6-fold risk for extensive colitis with a 2.5-fold risk for positive family history would yield an implausible lifetime risk of over 50% for these patients.

## PSC AND CRC

PSC is the most important additional risk factor yet identified over and above the risks attributable to extent and duration of colitis. In meta-analyses there is an odds ratio of 4.8 for dysplasia or cancer (CI 3.6–6.4), and of 4.1 for confirmed cancer (CI 2.9–5.8)[10]. The risk persists into the postoperative situation for those undergoing liver transplantation for PSC. In a series of 57 IBD patients in whom the colon remained, and in whom liver grafting was performed, there were nine patients with dysplasia and three with colorectal carcinoma by 5 years' follow-up[11]. The odds ratio for this is 4.0 but the number of colitics needing transplantation is fortunately too small for significance to be reached. Survival (somewhat surprisingly) does not appear to be affected.

## OTHER IBD PATIENT GROUPS AT HIGHER RISK OF CRC

There are suggestions, but few data, to suggest increased risk of CRC in IBD patients with a range of anatomical features.

It has been felt that those with blind-ending or bypassed loops are at greater risk. This is probably only partly true, but these patients form a group deserving special attention because, of course, these loops are almost inevitably less accessible to standard imaging approaches and may in some cases have less opportunity to declare their new (neoplastic) features clinically.

Colonic strictures have also been thought alarming from their neoplastic potential. While it is true that strictures are indeed associated with malignant transformation the attributable risk is not that high. About 5% of UC patients will at some point develop a colonic stricture, but fewer than 25% of these have been shown to progress to CRC[12]. Standard surveillance strategies, coupled with intra-stricture cytology brushing and a radiological technique to examine more proximally, are suggested in the patient in whom the stricture cannot be negotiated endoscopically. Strictures most likely to transform (or to have transformed already) include those which are proximal, of late onset, and associated with intestinal obstruction. Strictures are, or become, malignant in about 60% of those first identified after 20 or more years of colitis compared to virtually none of those presenting in the first 10 years of illness. Strictures proximal to the splenic flexure are, or become, malignant in over 80% of cases, compared to 47% for sigmoid strictures and only 10% in the rectum. Almost all malignant strictures demonstrate obstructive features (clinically or radiologically) compared to only about 15% of those with benign lesions.

Colonic strictures are clearly much more common in CD affecting around 15% of all patients (and many more if ileocolic anastomotic strictures are also included). However, the risk of neoplastic transformation is lower than in UC as only about 7% of these strictures progress to cancer[13]. Malignancy is more likely in patients who present with stenosis only at older ages.

## IBD PATIENTS AT PREDICTABLY LOWER RISK OF CRC THROUGH MEDICATION

It is appropriate also for us to identify those at lower risk, both for their peace of mind and also to help in best targeting our surveillance efforts.

Almost all units and almost all studies agree that regular consumption of the 5-aminosalicylates helps to reduce the risk of CRC in patients with UC. The magnitude of the effect is difficult to establish with certainty given the very long time-frames under consideration and the necessary reliance on reportage with its strong potential for recall bias. It is probable that a standard (low) maintenance regime equivalent to mesalazine 1.6 g taken daily for 5 years or more is able to reduce relative cancer risk by some 30%. Patients should be advised accordingly.

A single centre has data worthy of dissemination in respect of ursodiol, but it looks as though this agent too may be effective in cancer prophylaxis, and sufficiently safe and well tolerated for this to be a reasonable strategy.

## FOLIC ACID

As in sporadic CRC it has been suggested that folic acid may have a protective effect against the condition in patients with UC. A meta-analysis of three rather poor studies concluded that lower rates of malignancy were to be observed[14]. Even in meta-analysis there is inadequate power to produce a significant result, but the authors make the point that four new negative studies would be necessary to reverse their conclusion. The best single study currently available is that of the Cleveland Clinic, which yielded an odds ratio of 0.5 for those on regular folate supplements[15]. This was achieved with an average daily intake of 1 mg with a probable dose effect and, perhaps importantly, a greater effect on cancer incidence than on surrogates such as dysplasia.

## THE QUESTION OF CHRONIC INFLAMMATION

It has not been clear whether the presence of chronic inflammation in IBD is itself an important component of the pathogenesis of associated CRC. The apparent negative correlation with aminosalicylate therapy would support such a link, but the absence of an increased cancer risk in chronic proctitis goes against it. We therefore undertook a case–control study including 68 patients with UC-related CRC[16]. Each case was paired with two colitics matched for age, sex, disease duration and era of diagnosis. Although the study was performed retrospectively it employed contemporaneously collected data, of which only histology was subsequently re-verified. Univariate analysis revealed highly significant correlations between future cancer and inflammation as judged by the endoscopist at the time of colonoscopies (odds ratio 2.5; $p = 0.001$), and for its presence histologically (odds ratio 5.1; $p < 0.001$). Univariate analysis also identified specific colonoscopic features as prognostically important. These included the presence of postinflammatory polyps (OR 2.1), strictures (OR 4.2), shortened colon (OR 10), tubular colon (OR 2.0), and severe segmental inflammation (OR 3.4). Conversely an endoscopic comment that the colon was actually or very nearly normal indicated a good prognosis for avoidance of neoplasia with an odds ratio of 0.40. The numbers involved were not sufficient to reach significance in this study, but we also showed numerical support for the adverse effects of PSC, and of a family history of CRC, and protection from aminosalicylates, azathioprine and folate supplements. On multivariate analysis the only secure conclusion was that the degree of histological inflammation was inversely related to the future risk of CRC. An increase of only one point in the standard histological grading increased the risk of neoplasia 4.7-fold (CI 2.1–10.5; $p < 0.001$). Confirmation of this result by another centre would permit its inclusion in surveillance strategy and allow a reduction in suggested colonoscopy frequency for such patients.

# CONCLUSION

Those with IBD at risk of CRC are those with extensive ($>50\%$) colitis (UC or CD) of a long ($>10$ years') duration. Some protection is afforded by prolonged regular ($>5$ years') administration of aminosalicylates and probably by folic acid (1 mg per day). Lower-risk patients may be identified histologically since those with lesser degrees of inflammation are protected. The cancer risk is modestly increased by a personal history of colonic adenomas, and by a family history of CRC, but not by one of IBD. The greatest additional risk is, however, from concurrent PSC, which quadruples the risk of neoplasia.

## References

1. Sjödahl RI, Myrelid P, Söderholm JD. Anal and rectal cancer in Crohn's disease. Colorectal Dis. 2003;5:490–3.
2. Fraser AG, Orchard TR, Robinson EM, Jewell DP. Long-term risk of malignancy after treatment of inflammatory bowel disease with azathioprine. Aliment Pharmacol Ther. 2002;16:1225–32.
3. Ljung T, Karlen P, Schmidt D et al. Infliximab in inflammatory bowel disease: clinical outcome in a population based cohort from Stockholm County. Gut. 2004;53:849–53.
4. Bergquist A, Ekbom A, Olsson R et al. Hepatic and extrahepatic malignancies in primary sclerosing cholangitis. J Hepatol. 2002;36:321–7.
5. Ramage JK, Donaghy A, Farrant JM, Iorns R, Williams R. Serum tumor markers for the diagnosis of cholangiocarcinoma in primary sclerosing cholangitis. Gastroenterology. 1995;108:865–9.
6. Ekbom A, Helmick CG, Zack M, Holmberg L, Adami HO. Survival and causes of death in patients with inflammatory bowel disease: a population-based study. Gastroenterology. 1992;103:954–60.
7. Langholz E, Munkholm P, Davidsen M, Binder V. Colorectal cancer risk and mortality in patients with ulcerative colitis. Gastroenterology. 1992;103:1444–51.
8. Nuako KW, Ahlquist DA, Mahoney DW, Schaid DJ, Siems DM, Lindor NM. Familial predisposition for colorectal cancer in chronic ulcerative colitis: a case–control study. Gastroenterology. 1998;115:1079–83.
9. Eaden J, Abrams K, Ekbom A, Jackson E, Mayberry J. Colorectal cancer prevention in ulcerative colitis: a case–control study. Aliment Pharmacol Ther. 2000;14:145–53.
10. Soetikno RM, Lin OS, Heidenreich PA, Young HS, Blackstone MO. Increased risk of colorectal neoplasia in patients with primary sclerosing cholangitis and ulcerative colitis: a meta-analysis. Gastrointest Endosc. 2002;56:48–54.
11. Loftus EV Jr, Aguilar HI, Sandborn WJ et al. Risk of colorectal neoplasia in patients with primary sclerosing cholangitis and ulcerative colitis following orthotopic liver transplantation. Hepatology. 1998;27:685–90.
12. Gumaste V, Sachar DB, Greenstein AJ. Benign and malignant colorectal strictures in ulcerative colitis. Gut. 1992;33:938–41.
13. Yamazaki Y, Ribeiro MB, Sachar DB, Aufses AH Jr, Greenstein AJ. Malignant colorectal strictures in Crohn's disease. Am J Gastroenterol. 1991;86:882–5.
14. Diculescu M, Ciocirlan M, Ciocirlan M et al. Folic acid and sulfasalazine for colorectal carcinoma chemoprevention in patients with ulcerative colitis: the old and new evidence. Rom J Gastroenterol. 2003;12:283–6.
15. Lashner BA, Provencher KS, Seidner DL, Knesebeck A, Brzezinski A. The effect of folic acid supplementation on the risk for cancer or dysplasia in ulcerative colitis. Gastroenterology. 1997;112:29–32.
16. Rutter M, Saunders B, Wilkinson K et al. Severity of inflammation is a risk factor for colorectal neoplasia in ulcerative colitis. Gastroenterology. 2004;126:451–9.

# Section IV
# Corticosteroid therapy

**Chair: J.F. COLOMBEL and A. FORBES**

# 11
# Mechanisms of steroid action and resistance in inflammatory bowel disease

## D. KELLEHER and R. McMANUS

## INTRODUCTION

Glucocorticoid drugs are the mainstay therapies of many inflammatory diseases. Their use is clearly indicated in the treatment of acute exacerbations of chronic inflammatory bowel disease, both Crohn's disease (CD) and ulcerative colitis (UC). However, a significant proportion of patients with both UC and CD may fail to respond to acute therapy with corticosteroids. Mechanisms for failure of the efficacy of corticosteroids may relate either to the activity of the disease due to pharmacogenomic effects, or alternatively, to potential mechanisms for steroid resistance related to the actions of corticosteroids (see Figure 1).

## MECHANISMS OF ACTIONS OF GLUCOCORTICOIDS IN INFLAMMATION

It is only in recent years that we are starting to develop an understanding of the complex pathways by which steroids mediate their effects. The glucocorticoid receptor is a cytosolic receptor which dimerizes on binding to its ligand before translocating to the nucleus to function as a transcription factor by binding to a glucocorticoid response (GR) element[1]. However, it has become clear that steroids can influence the regulation of gene function other than through the effects of GR. Hence, broadly, the actions of steroids have been divided into *transactivation* and *transrepression*[2] (Figure 2) . Transactivation through the GR results in the modulation of function of a range of genes including, for example, genes regulating the effects of steroids on bone, on glucose tolerance and on blood pressure[3]. Indeed, it is felt that many of the adverse effects of glucocorticoids relate to the role of GR in transactivation. It is furthermore apparent that many pro-inflammatory genes are down-regulated by glucocorticoids independently of the presence of a GR element (GRE) within

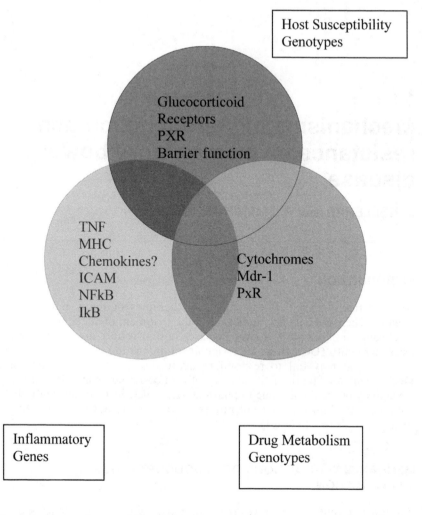

**Figure 1** Classes of genes which could impact on the outcome of steroid treatment of IBD illustrating the complexity of pharmacogenomics in this sector

those genes largely by transrepression[4]. Such genes include cytokines, such as IL-2 and IL-6, TNF-α, IL-1β, IFN-γ, chemokines including IL-8 and RANTES, enzymes such as cyclo-oxygenase and collagenase and adhesion molecules, including ICAM-1 and VCAM-1 (reviewed in ref. 5). The concept of transrepression means that the glucocorticoid receptor, as a monomer bound to a steroid, is capable of binding to transcription factors such as NF-κB and AP1, and hence functions to divert such transcription factors from mediating their pro-inflammatory actions[6–10].

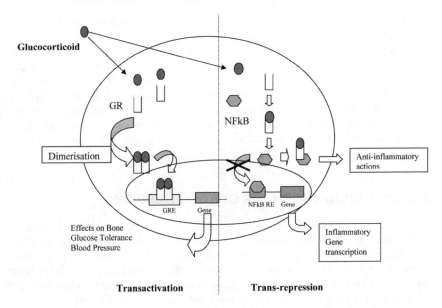

**Figure 2** Comparison between transactivation events and transrepression events mediated through glucocorticoid receptor. In transactivation the glucocorticoid interacts with a glucocorticoid receptor (GR) which then dimerizes. The complex is transcriptionally active on genes containing a glucocorticoid response element (GRE). Many such genes are involved in adverse effects of glucocorticoids. In transrepression monomeric GR interacts with the steroid. This complex may then interact with transcription factors such as NF-κB or AP-1, diverting them from their natural targets. Many anti-inflammatory effects of steroids are mediated through this route

In addition to the above mechanisms of action, recent studies have demonstrated effects of corticosteroids on messenger RNA stability[11], on histone deacetylation[12] and direct effects on the induction of I-κB[13], the inhibitor of NF-κB, a transcription factor critical for the induction of many inflammatory genes. It has also been reported that steroids may regulate mRNA stability through effects on MAP kinase (MAPK) regulation[14]. p38MAP kinase, an enzyme critically involved in the stabilization of cytokine messenger RNA, is inactivated by glucocorticoids. Specifically, glucocorticoids regulate the function of a phosphatase, known as MKP1, which dephosphorylates and inactivates p38MAPK. Hence, steroids have the capacity to destabilize the mRNA for a range of cytokines including, for example, tumour necrosis factor, IL-2 and many others. The rapid time course of many steroid effects *in vitro* is more compatible with effects on mRNA stability than with effects on transcriptional regulation[11].

A further mechanism of action of corticosteroids relates to the role of steroids in the regulation of histone deacetylation[15]. Histone deacetylase (HDAC), regulates inflammatory gene transcription through the control of histone structure[16]. Specifically, histone deacetylation results in gene repression by maintaining DNA in a coiled, inaccessible structure. Acetylation permits inflammatory gene transcription. Glucocorticoid receptors modulate both histone deacetylase and a steroid-binding protein, called CBP, with resultant reduced transcriptional capacity of inflammatory genes[17]. This mechanism of action of steroids is felt to be critically important in the response to steroids in chronic obstructive lung disease and asthma[18]. However, it is unclear whether this mechanism is functional in gastrointestinal tissue as the distribution of HDAC isoforms differs significantly between lung and the gastrointestinal tract.

## RATIONAL DRUG DESIGN FOR CORTICOSTEROIDS

Overall, therefore, the mechanisms of actions of corticosteroids are protean and complex, and this complexity has hindered the capacity to develop corticosteroids which are more specifically targeted with selectivity for anti-inflammatory properties. While steroids with dissociated functions have been synthesized and separation of anti-inflammatory effects (transrepression) from adverse effects (largely based on transactivation) has been observed *in vitro*[19], complex patterns of species specificity of steroid function have meant that it has been extremely difficult to assess such compounds in animal models of inflammation with consistent results[20]. Hence, while steroids which have potent anti-inflammatory properties, but no induction of glucose intolerance, have been reported, these have not yet reached clinical trials[19].

## PREVALENCE OF STEROID RESISTANCE IN INFLAMMATORY BOWEL DISEASE (IBD)

There is currently no clear universal definition for steroid resistance in IBD. Many patients treated with steroids fail to respond, and some may require radical surgery, such as total colectomy in the case of fulminant UC. In the course of their disease between 20% and 50% of patients will require surgery due to the failure of medical therapy. In the presence of a diarrhoeal disease, bioavailability of an orally administered agent may be a factor in initial steroid failure. However, there is also a significant failure rate with intravenous steroids. Several studies have attempted to define the prevalence of glucocorticoid resistance in IBD. In a retrospective study performed by Munkholm et al. 36% of patients were found to be steroid-dependent and 20% were steroid-resistant based on the long-term outcome at 1 year in CD patients with CD treated with their first course of oral prednisolone[20]. A high frequency of surgical intervention was reported in steroid-dependent patients (26%) and steroid-resistant patients (59%) within 1 month after glucocorticoid treatment. Steroid-resistance rates of 16% of CD and UC patients and steroid dependency in 28% and 22% of CD and UC patients respectively were reported by Faubion et al.[21]. Reinisch et al. have reported steroid dependency and resistance rates of 63% and 13% respectively using higher dosage schedules[22].

## MECHANISMS OF STEROID RESISTANCE IN IBD

There have been few studies on the potential mechanisms of steroid resistance. A study by Hearing et al. demonstrated that patients who have steroid-resistant disease also have steroid-resistant lymphocytes, with a failure to suppress lymphocyte proliferation despite high concentrations of dextramethasone seen in treatment failures. This study suggests that steroid resistance may relate to the failure of steroids to suppress activation and proliferation of their potential target cell, the T lymphocyte[23]. Nonetheless, it is not possible to utilize any single determinant of steroid responsiveness at this point in time to definitively predict steroid resistance.

There are many multiple potential mechanisms for resistance (see Table 1). Resistance may reflect innate mechanisms, such as genetic defects in receptor function, genetic defects in signalling function and pharmacogenetic defects in some of the pathways modulating steroid metabolism. In addition, it is possible that acquired mechanisms may also play a significant role, including mechanisms relating to high disease activity, altered signalling function or acquired alterations in drug kinetics. Multiple genes may contribute to the outcome of immunosuppressive therapy for any inflammatory disease, and such genes include not only genes involved in pharmacogenetics but also genes which are related innately to the severity of the inflammatory response, such as TNF-α genes[24], chemokine receptor genes[25], cytokine genes and MHC genes[26]. Indeed, in the case of IBD it has been previously demonstrated that genes in the MHC[27] and in the TNF region[28] may have a significant impact on the severity and distribution of disease. Hence, conceptually, a genetic profile contributing to an enhanced immune response may lead to an inflammatory reponse which is substantially more difficult to suppress using conventional immuno-suppressive agents.

**Table 1**  Mechanisms of steroid resistance

| |
| --- |
| Innate mechanisms |
|    Genetic defects in receptor function |
|    Genetic defect in signalling function |
|    Pharmacogenetic effects |
| |
| Acquired mechanisms |
|    Inflammation/high disease activity |
|    Altered signalling functions |
|    Alteration in drug kinetics |

## NF-κB AND STEROID RESISTANCE

One potential marker of inflammatory activity is the transcription factor, NF-κB. NF-κB controls many of the cytokines involved in the inflammatory response, including such cytokines as TNF and IL-1, and also the expression of adhesion molecules such as ICAM-1 and ELAM-1[29]. Epithelial NF-κB was found to be significantly elevated in patients with resistance to inflammatory

91

disease. This expression was specific to the epithelial cells of the gastrointestinal tract and correlated with failure of response to corticosteroids[30]. The effects on NF-κB levels in tissue may be genetic or acquired, and may relate to levels of inflammatory cytokines, such as TNF and IL-1, which regulate this gene. Genetic polymorphisms of an I-κB molecule with potential inhibitory effects on NF-κB, NF-κBIL1 (or I-κBL)[31] have been reported to be associated with myocardial ischaemic disease. Nonetheless, the finding that epithelial NF-κB was elevated, suggests that genes relating to the specific control of NF-κB in epithelial tissue might be implicated in the pathogenesis of resistant disease.

## GR FUNCTION AND STEROID RESISTANCE

GR dysfunction has been extensively studied in relationship to steroid-resistant asthma where altered receptor affinity and reduced receptor density have been postulated as resistance mechanisms[32]. Increased GR expression in peripheral lymphocytes has been reported in 83% of patients with steroid-resistant UC as compared to 9% of the steroid-responsive patients, and 10% of healthy volunteers in a Japanese study[33]. Similarly, in a Scandinavian study, GR mRNA in peripheral leucocytes has been reported to be higher in UC patients whose disease is in remission compared with controls, but levels did not differ between responders and non-responders who had required colectomy[34]. Thus, while receptor density may be associated with active disease, differences in GR density or GR mRNA levels do not appear to be important in determining glucocorticoid resistance in patients with UC.

Further prospective and longitudinal studies are required to assess the pathophysiological role of increase in the inhibitory GR-beta expression in UC. However, it is unlikely that this plays a significant role in the pathogenesis of steroid resistance. First, GR-beta is a relatively minor transcript, accounting for only 0.165% of total GR expression[35]. Secondly, transfection experiments have demonstrated that the GR-beta isoform has to be expressed in an at least 5–10-fold excess relative to GR-alpha to significantly inhibit glucocorticoid-mediated gene expression[36], and even this modest effect has not been ubiquitously reported. Thus, it is unlikely that the very low amounts of GR-beta found in UC patients[37] can exert a transdominant-negative effect.

## THE MULTI-DRUG RESISTANCE GENE MDR1

The activities of steroids and of other anti-inflammatory agents, such as cyclosporin, are potentially regulated through the effects of the P-glycoprotein 170 (PGP170) drug pump, which is the product of the MDR1 (or ABCB1) gene[38,38a]. The PGP170 pump is an ATP-dependent drug efflux pump, which is expressed on a wide variety of epithelial cells and cells of the immune system. The pump has promiscuous efflux activity, including activities relating to cytotoxic drugs, such as daunirubicin, and effects on cardiovascular drugs such as digoxin, effects on anti-inflammatory drugs such as steroids and cyclosporin and effects on the efflux of cytokines from inflammatory cells[39]. The MDR1 gene resembles many bacterial membrane transport genes and shares homology with the cystic fibrosis transmembrane regulator (CFTR) gene[40].

The role of PGP170 in inflammation has previously been studied in inflammatory diseases. Rheumatoid arthritis patients with high steroid requirements were found to have high expression of PGP170[41]. Similarly, in a prior study in renal allograft rejection, published in 1995, cyclosporin-treated patients with graft rejection were similarly found to have high PGP170 expression[42], hence contributing to drug efflux and failure of therapy. These studies were further supported by the finding that, in the MDR1 knockout mouse model, there is an eight-fold increase in tissue cyclosporin, steroid and digoxin levels[43]. We previously demonstrated that patients with IBD who fail medical therapy including such subgroups as patients who have total colectomy, refractory UC or patients with multiple surgical resections for CD, have increased levels of peripheral blood lymphocyte PGP170 expression, and that this expression appears to be relatively stable throughout the course of therapy for these conditions[44]. While these findings would suggest a significant role for MDR1/PGP170 in treatment responses to corticosteroids in IBD, this is compounded by the fact that mice deficient in MDR1 also acquire a form of IBD, which is dependent on the intestinal microflora. Hence, functional deficiency of MDR1 may impact on the progress of IBD, in addition to potential impacts on therapeutics.

To date at least 25 genetic variants of the MDR1 gene have been documented in Caucasian populations, although many of these occur at low frequency (i.e. less than the normal 2% cutoff to be considered a polymorphic allele). Several polymorphisms private to distinct populations have also been described. A polymorphism in exon 26 (C3435T) of the MDR1 gene has been the most extensively studied MDR1 polymorphism, and results are inconclusive regarding any impact it may have on gene expression. A number of initial studies showed it to be significantly correlated with levels of expression and function of PGP170 with healthy individuals homozygous for the C/C or 'resistant' genotype having significantly higher duodenal and natural killer T-cell MDR1 expression, 38% lower digoxin plasma levels and 17% more efflux of rhodamine dye from CD56[+] natural killer cells than volunteers with the T/T or 'responsive' genotype. The many subsequent studies have evinced a more complex picture of the relationship of C3435T with MDR1 expression and activity, with some confirming increased expression linked to the 3435C allele while others show no difference or even the reverse trend (reviewed in ref. 45). The relationship between MDR1 polymorphisms and function is similarly fraught with apparently contradictory outcomes[46]. Thus the relationship between this SNP and expression/activity of MDR1 appears complex and may relate to a number of issues such as tissue type and ethnicity. Substantial differences in the frequency of C3435T polymorphism have been reported between racial groups with a significantly higher frequency of the C/C genotype in West Africans (83%) and African Americans (61%) compared with 21% and 34% in German and Japanese populations respectively[47,48]. As noted earlier, the prevalence of glucocorticoid-unresponsiveness in several population-based cohorts of Caucasian IBD patients is approximately 20–40% which, while speculative, suggested that MDR1 pharmacogenetics might be implicated in steroid treatment failure.

Evidence of association of variants of the MDR1 gene with IBD has been sought in many sample populations from diverse geographical regions, and again the results are largely conflicting. Brandt et al.[49] showed that G2677 (Ala893) was associated with CD and to a lesser extent UC, while C3435T was not. Ho et al.[50] found the opposite, with the 3435T allele associated with UC only, and G2677T having no effect in either disease. Some studies have shown 3435T to be at least partially associated with UC[51,52] but not CD, while neither UC nor CD was associated in others[53,54]. However, it is interesting that MDR1 polymorphisms have been reported as being associated with disease severity in UC and CD (both the 2677T and 3435T sites[55]) and UC alone (3435T only[50]). Again, however, even though the Brandt and Potocnik studies agree on the association of the 2677 site, the direction of association is different. The complexity and apparently contradictory nature of these results points to the desirability of using comprehensive haplotype analyses rather than single SNP association, since this provides much more information as to the collective contribution of SNP in a gene. This will furthermore reduce the uncertainty caused by the selection of different markers in each study which currently makes comparisons difficult.

While the G2677T/A polymorphisms leads to non-synonymous substitutions (Ala893Ser/Thr) the association of 3435 is not in itself conclusive, as it affects a third base codon (wobble) residue, which does not change the coding sequence. Therefore the 3435T polymorphism may act as a surrogate for other MDR1 polymorphisms which have an impact on drug efflux and outcome of therapy, although it is interesting that Tang et al.[56] have shown evidence that both 2677 and 3435 polymorphisms may have experienced recent evolutionary selective pressure. Haplotypes composed of these markers differ markedly between reports and this may have implications for genetic studies in different populations[50,56]. In addition, while polymorphisms in MDR1 may be implicated in altering expression, it is also conceivable that polymorphisms in genes which regulate MDR1 may have a greater impact on expression of PGP170 (and indeed may regulate other proteins involved in steroid responsiveness), for example, the PXR gene, which is a potent regulator of MDR1 expression and is itself regulated by a variety of genetic and environmental factors[57]. In addition, the MDR1 gene has complex regulation with involvement of transcription factors, such as NP1, SP-1 and FY TCF and NF-R1[58]. Thus, it may be difficult to predict outcomes based on any single gene: more likely a complex of genetic polymorphisms may be involved in the regulation of expression. Reduced expression of PGP170 has been identified on a microarray study of IBD. It is clear, however, that PGP170 may be potently regulated by environmental factors, including for example many of the anti-retroviral drugs and hypericin/hyperforin, the active ingredient of the herbal remedy St John's Wort. We have demonstrated that St John's Wort strongly induces the expression of MDR1 with up to seven-fold increase in expression on sustained therapy[59]. Hence, it is clear that such induction has potential pharmacokinetic effects, which are far more potent than those associated with SNP in the MDR1 gene.

In conclusion, therefore, a wide range of genetic and environmental factors may contribute to steroid resistance in patients with IBD. While conceptually it has been suggested that array-based approaches with multiple algorithms may be utilized in the future to predict therapeutic outcomes in patients treated with this common drug, it is clear that the multiple factors affecting outcome are extremely complex. Hence, although gene chip approaches allowing analysis of drug metabolism, inflammatory and host receptor genotypes such as those of the glucocorticoid receptor and PXR may potentially be utilized to identify individuals likely to fail to respond to steroids, more detailed algorithms will be required in order for such an approach to have predictive value. In the interim it is critical that further research be performed in order to develop more specific steroids, and to develop new mechanisms of controlling the pharmacological and pharmacokinetic effects of existing steroid agents.

## References

1. Belvisi MG, Wicks SL, Battram CH et al. Therapeutic benefit of a dissociated glucocorticoid and the relevance of *in vitro* separation of transrepression from transactivation activity. J Immunol. 2001;166:1975–82.
2. Adcock IM, Lane SJ, Brown CR, Lee TH, Barnes PJ. Abnormal glucocorticoid receptor-activator protein 1 interaction in steroid-resistant asthma. J Exp Med. 1995;182:1951–8.
3. Dostert A, Heinzel T. Negative glucocorticoid receptor response elements and their role in glucocorticoid action. Curr Pharm Des. 2004;10:2807–16.
4. Gottlicher M, Heck S, Herrlich P. Transcriptional cross-talk, the second mode of steroid hormone receptor action. J Mol Med. 1998;76:480–9.
5. Heck S, Kullmann M, Gast A et al. A distinct modulating domain in glucocorticoid receptor monomers in the repression of activity of the transcription factor AP-1. EMBO J. 1994;13:4087–95.
6. Heck S, Bender K, Kullmann M, Gottlicher M, Herrlich P, Cato AC. I kappaB alpha-independent downregulation of NFkappaB activity by glucocorticoid receptor. EMBO J. 1997;16:4698–707.
7. De Bosscher K, Vanden Berghe W, Haegeman G. Mechanisms of anti-inflammatory action and of immunosuppression by glucocorticoids: negative interference of activated glucocorticoid receptor with transcription factors. J Neuroimmunol. 2000;109:16–22.
8. Diamond MI, Miner JN, Yoshinaga SK, Yamamoto KR. Transcription factor interactions: selectors of positive or negative regulation from a single DNA element. Science. 1990;249:1266–72.
9. Clark A. Post-transcriptional regulation of pro-inflammatory gene expression. Arthritis Res. 2000;2:172–4.
10. Delany AM, Brinckerho CE. Post-transcriptional regulation of collagenase and stromelysin gene expression by epidermal growth factor and dexamethasone in cultured human fibroblasts. J Cell Biochem. 1992;50:400–10.
11. Lasa M, Brook M, Saklatvala J, Clark AR. Dexamethasone destabilizes cyclooxygenase 2 mRNA by inhibiting mitogen-activated protein kinase p38. Mol Cell Biol. 2001;21:771–80.
12. Ito K, Barnes PJ, Adcock IM. Glucocorticoid receptor recruitment of histone deacetylase 2 inhibits interleukin-1 beta-induced histone H4 acetylation on lysines 8 and 12. Mol Cell Biol. 2000;20:6891–903.
13. Schmitz ML, Bacher S, Kracht M. I kappa B-independent control of NF-kappa B activity by modulatory phosphorylations. Trends Biochem Sci. 2001;26:186–90.
14. Kassel O, Sancono A, Kratzschmar J, Kreft B, Stassen M, Cato AC. Glucocorticoids inhibit MAP kinase via increased expression and decreased degradation of MKP-1. EMBO J. 2001;20:7108–116.
15. Ito K, Jazrawi E, Cosio B, Barnes PJ, Adcock IM. p65-activated histone acetyltransferase activity is repressed by glucocorticoids: mifepristone fails to recruit HDAC2 to the p65-HAT complex. J Biol Chem. 2001;276:30208–15.
16. Roth SY, Denu JM, Allis CD. Histone acetyltransferases. Annu Rev Biochem. 2001;70:81–120.

17. Ito K, Ito M, Elliott WM et al. Decreased histone deacetylase activity in chronic obstructive pulmonary disease. N Engl J Med. 2005;12:352(19):1967–76.
18. Barnes PJ. Anti-inflammatory actions of glucocorticoids: molecular mechanisms. Clin Sci (Lond). 1998;94:557–72.
19. Vayssiere BM, Dupont S, Choquart A et al. Synthetic glucocorticoids that dissociate transactivation and AP-1transrepression exhibit antiinflammatory activity *in vivo*. Mol Endocrinol. 1997;11:1245–55.
20. Munkholm P, Langholz E, Davidsen M, Binder V. Frequency of glucocorticoid resistance and dependency in Crohn's disease. Gut. 1994;35:360–2.
21. Faubion WA Jr, Loftus EV, Harmsen WS, Zinsmeister AR, Sandborn WJ. The natural history of corticosteroid therapy for inflammatory bowel disease: a population-based study. Gastroenterology. 2001;121:255–60.
22. Reinisch W, Gasche C, Wyatt J et al. Steroid dependency in Crohn's disease. Lancet. 1995;345:859.
23. Hearing SD, Norman M, Probert CS, Haslam N, Dayan CM. Predicting therapeutic outcome in severe ulcerative colitis by measuring *in vitro* steroid sensitivity of proliferating peripheral blood lymphocytes. Gut. 1999;45:382–8.
24. van Heel DA, Udalova IA, De Silva AP et al. Inflammatory bowel disease is associated with a TNF polymorphism that affects an interaction between the OCT1 and NF(-kappa)B transcription factors. Hum Mol Genet. 2002;11:1281–9.
25. Duerr RH. The genetics of inflammatory bowel disease. Gastroenterol Clin N Am. 2002;31:63–76.
26. Rector A, Vermeire S, Thoelen I et al. Analysis of the CC chemokine receptor 5 (CCR5) delta-32 polymorphism in inflammatory bowel disease. Hum Genet. 2001;108:190–3.
27 Orchard TR, Chua CN, Ahmad T, Cheng H, Welsh KI, Jewell DP. Uveitis and erythema nodosum in inflammatory bowel disease: clinical features and the role of HLA genes. Gastroenterology. 2002;123:714–18.
28. Sashio H, Tamura K, Ito R et al. Polymorphisms of the TNF gene and the TNF receptor superfamily member 1B gene are associated with susceptibility to ulcerative colitis and Crohn's disease, respectively. Imunogenetics. 2002;53:1020–7.
29. Tobler A, Meier R, Seitz M, Dewald B, Baggiolini M, Fey MF. Glucocorticoids downregulate gene expression of GM-CSF, NAP-1/IL-8, and IL-6, but not of M-CSF in human fibroblasts. Blood 199;79:45–51.
30. Bantel H, Schmitz ML, Raible A, Gregor M, Schulze-Ostho K. Critical role of NF-kappaB and stress-activated protein kinases in steroid unresponsiveness. FASEB J. 2002;16:1832–4.
31. Ozaki K, Ohnishi Y, Iida A et al. Functional SNPs in the lymphotoxin-alpha gene that are associated with susceptibility to myocardial infarction. Nat Genet. 2002;32:650–4.
32. Loke TK, Sousa AR, Corrigan CJ, Lee TH. Glucorticoidresistant asthma. Curr Allergy Asthma Rep. 2002;2:144–50.
33. Honda M, Orii F, Ayabe T et al. Expression of glucocorticoid receptor in lymphocytes of patients with glucocorticoid-resistant ulcerative colitis. Gastroenterology. 2000;118:859–66.
34. Flood L, Lofberg R, Stierna P, Wikstrom AC. Glucocorticoid receptor mRNA in patients with ulcerative colitis: a study of responders and nonresponders to glucocorticosteroid therapy. Inflamm Bowel Dis. 2001;7:202–9.
35. Leung DY, Hamid Q, Vottero A et al. Association of glucocorticoid insensitivity with increased expression of glucocorticoid receptor beta. J Exp Med. 1997;186:1567–74.
36. Bamberger CM, Bamberger AM, de Castro M, Chrousos GP. Glucocorticoid receptor beta, a potential endogenous inhibitor of glucocorticoid action in humans. J Clin Invest. 1995;95:2435–41.
37. Oakley RH, Jewell CM, Yudt MR, Bofetiado DM, Cidlowski JA. The dominant negative activity of the human glucocorticoid receptor β isoform. Specificity and mechanisms of action. J Biol Chem. 1999;274:27857–66.
38. Farrell RJ, Kelleher D. Glucocorticoid resistance in inflammatory bowel disease. J Endocrinol. 2003;178:339–46.
38a. Lum BL, Gosland MP. MDR expression in normal tissues. Pharmacologic implications for the clinical use of P-glycoprotein inhibitors. Hematol Oncol Clin N Am. 1995;9:319–36.

39. Tsuruoka S, Sugimoto KI, Ueda K, Suzuki M, Imai M, Fujimura A. Removal of digoxin and doxorubicin by multidrug resistance protein-overexpressed cell culture in hollow fiber. Kidney Int. 1999;56:54–63.

40. Lomri N, Fitz JG, Scharschmidt BF. Hepatocellular transport: role of ATP-binding cassette proteins. Semin Liver Dis. 1996;16:201–10.

41. Maillefert JF, Maynadie M, Tebib JG et al. Expression of the multidrug resistance glycoprotein 170 in the peripheral blood lymphocytes of rheumatoid arthritis patients. The percentage of lymphocytes expressing glycoprotein 170 is increased in patients treated with prednisolone. Br J Rheumatol. 1996;35:430–5.

42. Zanker B, Barth C, Menges AV, Lammerding P, Stachowski J, Baldamus CA. Expression of the MDR-1 in peripheral bloodmononuclear cells from cyclosporin-treated renal transplant recipients rejecting their graft. Transplant Proc. 1995;27:925–6.

43. Schinkel AH, Mayer U, Wagenaar E et al. Normal viability and altered pharmacokinetics in mice lacking mdr1-type (drug-transporting) P-glycoproteins. PNAS. 1997;94:4028–33.

44. Farrell RJ, Menconi MJ, Keates AC, Kelly CP. P-glycoprotein170 inhibition significantly reduces cortisol and cyclosporin efflux from human intestinal epithelial cells and T-lymphocytes. Ailment Pharmacol Ther. 2002;16:1021–31.

45. Kelleher D, Farrell R, McManus R. Pharmacogenetics of inflammatory bowel disease. Novartis Found Symp. 2004;263:41–53.

46. Woodahl EL, Ho RJ. The role of MDR1 genetic polymorphisms in interindividual variability in P-glycoprotein expression and function. Curr Drug Metab. 2004;5:11–19.

47. Cascorbi I, Gerlo T, Johne A et al. Frequency of single nucleotide polymorphisms in the P-glycoprotein drug transporter MDR1 gene in white subjects. Clin Pharmacol Ther. 2001;69:169–74.

48. Schaefeler E, Eichelbaum M, Brinkmann U et al. Frequency of C3435T polymorphism of MDR1 gene in African people. Lancet. 2001;358:383–4.

49. Brant SR, Panhuysen CI, Nicolae D et al. MDR1 Ala893 polymorphism is associated with inflammatory bowel disease. Am J Hum Genet. 2003;73:1282–92.

50. Ho GT, Nimmo ER, Tenesa A et al. Allelic variations of the multidrug resistance gene determine susceptibility and disease behavior in ulcerative colitis. Gastroenterology. 2005;128:288–96.

51. Schwab M, Schaeffeler E, Marx C et al. Association between the 3435T MDR1 gene polymorphism and susceptibility for ulcerative colitis. Gastroenterology. 2003;124:26–33.

52. Glas J, Torok HP, Schiemann U, Folwaczny C. MDR1 gene polymorphism in ulcerative colitis. Gastroenterology. 2004;126:367.

53. Croucher PJ, Mascheretti S, Foelsch UR, Hampe J, Schreiber S. Lack of association between the C3435T MDR1 gene polymorphism and inflammatory bowel disease in two independent Northern European populations. Gastroenterology. 2003;125:1919–20.

54. Gazouli M, Zacharatos P, Gorgoulis V, Mantzaris G, Papalambros E, Ikonomopoulos J. The C3435T MDR1 gene polymorphism is not associated with susceptibility for ulcerative colitis in Greek population. Gastroenterology. 2004;126:367–9.

55. Potocnik U, Ferkolj I, Glavac D, Dean M. Polymorphisms in multidrug resistance 1 (MDR1) gene are associated with refractory Crohn disease and ulcerative colitis. Genes Immun. 2004;5:530–9.

56. Tang K, Wong LP, Lee EJ, Chong SS, Lee CG. Genomic evidence for recent positive selection at the human MDR1 gene locus. Hum Mol Genet 2004;13:783–97.

57. Masuyama H, Suwaki N, Tateishi Y, Nakatsukasa H, Segawa T, Hiramatsu Y. The pregnane X receptor regulates gene expression in a ligand- and promoter-selective fashion. Mol Endocrinol. 2005;19:1170–80.

58. Xu D, Kang H, Fisher M, Juliano RL. Strategies for inhibition of MDR1 gene expression. Mol Pharmacol. 2004;66:268–75.

59. Hennessy M, Kelleher D, Spiers JP et al. St Johns wort increases expression of P-glycoprotein: implications for drug interactions. Br J Clin Pharmacol. 2002;53:75–82.

# 12
# Budesonide for ulcerative colitis

A. S. PEÑA and I. MARÍN-JIMÉNEZ

## INTRODUCTION

The frequent adverse effects associated with the use of glucocorticosteroids (GCS) prompted the development of a new group of drugs with equivalent efficacy and a more benign adverse event profile. The pharmacological development of novel GCS has been more difficult in ulcerative colitis (UC) because of variations in colonic pH, transit time, and bacterial metabolism. Prednisolone metasulphobenzoate, fluticasone propionate, tixocortol pivalate, beclomethasone dipropionate and budesonide have been evaluated[1]. The GCS budesonide, with high topical activity and a high rate of metabolism, has been administered in an oral controlled-release formulation. Because of the use of new drug delivery systems that target the bowel wall as the pharmacokinetic compartment of interest, budesonide has been called 'a model of targeted therapy'[2]. There are two commercially available enteric-coated pH-dependent release oral formulations (Entocord® EC and Budenofalk®). Budesonide in these galenic forms gives an overall treatment result in active UC approaching that of prednisolone but without suppression of plasma cortisol levels[3]. There have been many studies published on the effects of oral budesonide in Crohn's disease (CD)[4], but there is much less evidence on the efficacy of oral budesonide therapy in UC. In CD oral budesonide has been shown to be superior to mesalazine and placebo, and equivalent to prednisolone for the control of mild to moderately active ileocolonic CD, obtaining this beneficial therapeutic effect with less adrenal suppression and an improvement in the clinical adverse effect profile, compared to prednisolone. Similar studies in UC with the oral formulations are few. However, the efficacy and fewer side-effects of enema/foam preparations for the treatment of distal thesis are encouraging. We review the studies published so far with the available enteric-coated pH-dependent release oral formulations as well as the topical preparations for distal disease in UC.

## PHARMACOKINETIC PROPERTIES

Budesonide is a non-halogenated synthetic corticosteroid with the highest affinity for the glucocorticoid receptor if compared to other steroids (hydrocortisone, prednisolone, dexamethasone)[5]. Budesonide is a 1:1 mixture of the two epimers (22R and 22S), which are both rapidly eliminated with a terminal half-life of $2.7 \pm 0.6$ h[6]. Budesonide is extensively metabolized by hydroxylation, and the cytochrome P450 isoenzyme CYP3A4, expressed in high amounts in hepatocytes and in epithelial cells of the intestine wall, is mainly responsible for its rapid elimination[7].

Budesonide circulates in plasma mainly bound to proteins (88%), and over the dosage range of 3–15 mg/day it shows linear pharmacokinetic behaviour[8,9]. Due to the high clearance of budesonide, which approaches liver blood flow, a low oral bioavailability has to be expected. The vast majority of the drug is eliminated in the intestinal wall and during the first passage through the liver. After oral administration and absorption, budesonide undergoes a 90% first-pass hepatic metabolism[10] to form 6-beta-hydroxybudesonide and 16 alpha-hydroxyprednisolone; both of these have less than 1% of the parent compound's corticosteroid activity relative to the parent compound; that is why oral bioavailability is only 10%, which weakens the systemic action of budesonide. When the rectal administration is used in enemas, budesonide reaches the splenic flexure[11], and its bioavailability averages 15% in patients with UC. Some experiments[12] have revealed that budesonide has a longer residence time in colonic mucosa than systemic corticosteroids; 20 min and 4 h after perfusion of the rat colon higher concentrations of budesonide were detected as compared to prednisolone.

There are three different forms of oral controlled-released preparations of budesonide[13]: controlled-ileal release capsules, a pH-modified release formulation and a budesonide prodrug (budesonide-beta-D-glucuronide), this last is not commercially available[13]. The controlled-ileal release formulation (Entocort® EC) is composed of hard gelatin capsules, acid-resistant pellets Eudragit L 100-55, and has a delayed release at pH >5.5. The pH-modified release formulation (Budenofalk®) is also composed of gelatin capsules and acid-resistant pellets, but it has a composition of Eudragit L, S, LS, and RS, and has a delayed release at pH >6.4. Budesonide-beta-D-glucuronide is an oral prodrug targeted to deliver budesonide just to the colon, because the prodrug is not absorbed in the small intestine. This prodrug is hydrolysed by colonic bacterial and mucosal beta-glucuronidase to release free budesonide into the colon[14]. Hydrolysis rates of budesonide-beta-D-glucuronide in human faecal samples from patients with UC and normal volunteers are similar[15], but it is not clear if a reduction in pH in the colon in patients with inflammatory bowel disease (IBD) may inhibit bacterial deconjugation of the prodrug. Budesonide can also be administrated rectally by enemas or foams. This novel steroid has been evaluated for use in patients with IBD when administered either orally (3–9 mg/day) as a controlled-release formulation, or rectally as an enema or foam. It has a very positive profile of adverse glucocorticoid-related effects, and so is regarded as a useful agent for the treatment of IBD patients.

# STUDIES OF BUDESONIDE FOR ULCERATIVE COLITIS

## Topical budesonide: pharmacokinetic studies

Table 1 summarizes three studies that have evaluated different pharmacokinetic aspects of budesonide in UC patients[11,16,17]. The first[16] shows that budesonide does not accumulate in the human body after 4 weeks of treatment, and mean plasma cortisol values did not change during this period of time. In a second study[11], a low-viscosity formulation of budesonide shows a better capacity to reach more proximal parts of the colon (up to splenic flexure, in 15 min) than a high-viscosity one. In the third of these studies[17], the dose of 2 mg/day shows the same efficacy results as the 4 mg/day, but with less plasma cortisol suppression than the latter. It also demonstrates that budesonide enemas given twice weekly are not enough to maintain remission, and prevent relapses in patients with quiescent disease. However, in CD, a recent report[18] shows that oral budesonide (6 mg/day) is effective for prolonging time to relapse and rates of relapse at 3 and 6 months (but not 12 months) in CD patients with medically induced remission.

## Topical budesonide compared with placebo

In the first of the two studies[19], shown in Table 2 budesonide is significantly more effective than placebo in achieving improvement (endoscopic, histological and clinical) in UC patients and does not decrease plasma cortisol levels. The second study[20] which, apart from comparing budesonide with placebo evaluates three different dosages (0.5, 2 and 8 mg), proves that budesonide is significantly superior to placebo in UC patients with distal active UC and proctitis. The 2 mg dose enema is recommended.

## Topical budesonide compared with topical corticosteroids

The majority of the studies on budesonide for UC patients, compare it with classical corticosteroids (Table 3). Most of them use enemas, but two[21,22] use foam as the vehicle for the drug. In almost all of them budesonide shows similar efficacy as do classical topical steroids, with a better safety profile because budesonide does not decrease plasma cortisol levels. An important factor to take into account is that, when budesonide foams are compared with betamethasone enemas[22], in terms of quality of life, there were no significant differences between the two, although betamethasone reduced plasma cortisol levels and budesonide did not. There is sufficient evidence to conclude that budesonide should replace classical corticosteroids in the context of UC patients with left-sided or distal affection.

## Topical budesonide compared with topical aminosalicylate

In the two studies of budesonide revised and shown in Table 4, budesonide is compared to topical 5-ASA[30,31] and demonstrated similar results in terms of efficacy with an excellent safety profile.

## Topical budesonide compared with oral metronidazole

There is only one study in which topical budesonide is compared to oral metronidazole for the treatment of active pouchitis[32]. Budesonide is as efficacious as metronidazole but with a rather better profile of adverse effects. Although more clinical trials are needed on this topic, budesonide could be a good alternative to therapies accepted for the treatment of active pouchitis.

## Oral budesonide

Compared with the number of studies with oral budesonide for the treatment of CD, only three three clinical studies in UC patients treated with oral budesonide have been published (Table 5). In the first of them[3], oral budesonide (10 mg/day) shows similar efficacy to prednisolone (40 mg/day) in active extensive and left-sided UC, while the advantage of budesonide over prednisolone is that the former does not modify plasma cortisol levels. The second study[33] uses oral budesonide for steroid-dependent UC patients (with a broad spectrum of disease extension: from pancolitis to proctitis), in order to accomplish steroid withdrawal and clinical resolution of the active disease. In 11 of 14 patients clinical improvement was obtained, and ended systemic steroid treatment. The last of these studies[34] in patients with distal active UC, oral budesonide (Budenofalk®), showed encouraging clinical results, although the work was designed to study the pharmacokinetics and pharmacodynamics of this formulation. Significant levels of budesonide were found in the distal colon and rectum. This study suggests that this formulation of oral budesonide could be used for the treatment of distal disease. The microgranules of budesonide are designed to dissolve at a pH $>6.4$, and this would permit distribution of Budenofalk® to more distal segments of the intestine.

## FUTURE PERSPECTIVES

This review clearly shows that topical budesonide is a good alternative to topical 5-ASA for the treatment of distal active UC. Almost all the studies conclude that budesonide is as effective as topical 5-ASA, with a good safety profile. Budesonide does not decrease plasma cortisol levels, which differentiate it from classical glucocorticosteroids, indicating that budesonide should be the glucocorticoid of choice in the treatment of distal active UC. Evidence for the usefulness of oral budesonide is not as strong as that for the rectal topical preparations. There are very few studies in this regard. We could suggest that Budenofalk®, which dissolves at pH $>6.4$, and is present in acceptable quantities in distal colon and rectum of UC patients treated with this drug[34], would be useful for the treatment of UC patients. Since Entocort® CD can reach transverse and descending colon[35] at least in controls and in CD patients, a comparative trial, as some authors have suggested[4], between these two oral formulation of budesonide, would be of interest (Figure 1). Further studies are needed on this topic, because UC patients would benefit from the potent action of steroids to obtain clinical, endoscopic and histological improvement of their disease, without the deleterious effects[36] associated with the use of classical glucocorticosteroids.

**Table 1** Pharmacokinetic studies of topical budesonide

| Year of publication | Reference | No. of patients | Ulcerative colitis characteristics | Medication (dose) | Time and evaluation parameters | Results/conclusions; cortisol depression |
|---|---|---|---|---|---|---|
| 1993 | Danielsson et al.[16] | 28 | Distal active UC and proctitis | Budesonide ENE (2 mg) | 4 weeks Pharmacokinetic assessment E + H | Improvement of E + H Budesonide did not accumulate Mean plasma cortisol values did not change during treatment |
| 1994 | Nyman-Pantelidis et al.[11] | 5 | Distal active UC and proctitis | Budesonide ENE (two different formulations: low and high viscosity) | – Area of spread of enema | Low viscosity ENE gets splenic flexure in 15 min; high-viscosity ENE gets less far and in much greater time |
| 2002 | Lingren et al.[17] | 149 | Distal active UC | Budesonide ENE Acute phase: 2 mg (o.d. or t.i.d.) until 8 weeks/ remission Maintenance: 2 mg/twice weekly until 24 weeks or relapse | Acute phase: 8 weeks Maintenance: 24 weeks | Remission rates at week 4 and 8 the same in 2 and 4 mg groups 4 mg group much adrenal alteration Budesonide for maintenance at this interval is not effective to prevent relapse |

E: endoscopical evaluation; H: histological evaluation; Clin: clinical evaluation. ENE: enemas. FO: foam.

102

**Table 2** Studies comparing topical budesonide with placebo

| Year of publication | Reference | No. of patients | Ulcerative colitis characteristics | Medication (dose) | Time and evaluation parameters | Results/conclusions: cortisol depression |
|---|---|---|---|---|---|---|
| 1992 | Danielsson et al.[19] | 41 | Distal active UC and proctitis | Budesonide ENE (2 mg/100 ml) vs placebo ENE | 4 weeks E + H + Clin | Budesonide more effective than placebo. Budesonide did not decrease cortisol plasma levels |
| 1998 | Hanauer et al.[20] | 233 | Distal active UC and proctitis | Budesonide ENE (0.5, 2, 8 mg/100 ml) vs placebo ENE | 6 weeks E + H + Clin | Budesonide (dose: 2 and 8 mg) better than placebo in E, H and Clin 90% of patients on budesonide normal plasma cortisol levels |

E: endoscopical evaluation; H: histological evaluation; Clin: clinical evaluation. ENE: enemas. FO: foam.

**Table 3** Studies comparing topical budesonide with topical corticosteroids

| Year of publication | Reference | No. of patients | Ulcerative colitis characteristics | Medication (dose) | Time and evaluation parameters | Results/conclusions: cortisol depression |
|---|---|---|---|---|---|---|
| 1987 | Danielsson et al.[23] | 64 | Distal active UC | Budesonide ENE (2 mg/100 ml) vs prednisolone ENE(31.25 mg/100 ml) | 4 weeks E + H + Clin | Budesonide > prednisolone in E, H and Clin evaluations. Prednisolone reduces cortisol, but not budesonide |
| 1991 | Danish Budesonide Study Group[24] | 146 | Distal active UC | Budesonide ENE (1,2 or 4 mg/100 ml) vs prednisolone ENE (25 mg/100 ml) | 2 weeks E + H + Clin | All treatments improved E + Clin (lower improvement in the 1 mg budesonide group). Prednisolone reduces cortisol, but not budesonide |
| 1994 | Bianchi Porro et al.[25] | 88 | Distal active UC | Budesonide ENE (2 mg/100 ml) vs methylprednisolone ENE (20 mg/100 ml) | 4 weeks E + H + Clin | All treatments improved E, H, and Clin, without significant differences between them. Prednisolone reduces cortisol, but not budesonide |
| 1994 | Ostergaard et al.[26] | 26 | Distal active UC | Budesonide ENE (2 mg/100 ml) vs prednisolone ENE (25 mg/100 ml) | 8 weeks Adrenal gland suppression | Prednisolone reduces cortisol, but not budesonide |
| 1994 | Lofberg et al.[27] | 100 | Distal active UC | Budesonide ENE (2.3 mg/115 ml) vs prednisolone ENE (31.25 mg/125 ml) | 8 weeks E + H + Clin | All treatments improved E, H, and Clin, without significant differences between them. Prednisolone reduces cortisol, but not budesonide |

**Table 3** (continued)

| Year of publication | Reference | No. of patients | Ulcerative colitis characteristics | Medication (dose) | Time and evaluation parameters | Results/conclusions: Cortisol depression |
|---|---|---|---|---|---|---|
| 1994 | Tarpila et al.[28] | 72 | Proctitis | Budesonide ENE (2 mg/100 ml) vs hydrocortisone acetate FO (125 mg/125 ml) | 4 weeks E + H + Clin | All treatments improved E, H, and Clin, without significant differences between them. Prednisolone reduces cortisol, but not budesonide |
| 1995 | Bayless et al.[29]* | 184 | Distal active UC | Budesonide ENE (2 mg) vs hydrocortisone ENE (100 mg) vs placebo | 6 weeks E + H + Clin | E: budesonide similar to hydrocortisone (both better than placebo) H and Clin: non significant differences between budesonide, prednisolone and placebo. Prednisolone reduces cortisol significantly more than budesonide |
| 2003 | Bar-Meir et al.[21] | 251 | Proctosigmoiditis | Budesonide FO (2 mg) vs hydrocortisone acetate FO (100 mg) | 8 weeks E + H + Clin | All treatments improved E, H, and Clin, without significant differences between them. Prednisolone reduces cortisol, but not budesonide |
| 2004 | Hammond et al.[22] | 38 | Distal active UC | Budesonide FO (2 mg/50 ml) vs betamethasone ENE (5 mg/100 ml) | 4 weeks QOL + E + H + Clin | Similar efficacy and QOL with budesonide and betamethasone. Betamethasone reduces cortisol, but not budesonide |

E: endoscopical evaluation; H: histological evaluation; Clin: clinical evaluation. ENE: enemas. FO: foam. QOL: quality of life. * just published in an abstract form.

**Table 4** Studies comparing topical budesonide with topical aminosalicylates

| Year of publication | Reference | No. of patients | Ulcerative colitis characteristics | Medication (dose) | Time and evaluation parameters | Results/conclusions: cortisol depression |
|---|---|---|---|---|---|---|
| 1995 | Lemann et al.[30] | 97 | Distal active UC and proctosigmoiditis | Budesonide E NE (2 mg/100 ml) vs 5-ASA ENE (mesalazine 1 g/100 ml) | 4 weeks E + H + Clin | Similar efficacy in E + H + Clin No adverse effects in both groups |
| 2000 | Rufle et al.[31] | 33 | Distal active UC, proctosigmoiditis and proctitis | Budesonide FO (1 mg/50 ml) (b.i.d.) vs mesalazine ENE (4 g/60 ml o.d.) | 4 weeks E + H + Clin | Similar efficacy in E + H + Clin No influence of either treatment in cortisol plasma levels |

E: endoscopical evaluation; H: histological evaluation; Clin: clinical evaluation. ENE: enemas. FO: foam.

**Table 5** Studies with oral budesonide

| Treatment compared | Year of publication | Reference | No. of patients | Ulcerative colitis characteristics | Medication (dose) | Time and evaluation parameters | Results/conclusions: cortisol depression |
|---|---|---|---|---|---|---|---|
| Oral budesonide compared to predisolone | 1996 | Lofteberg et al.[3] | 72 | Active extensive and left-sided UC | Budesonide (10 mg) vs prednisolone (40 mg) | 9 weeks E and plasma cortisol levels | Same E results Prednisolone supresses cortisol, but not budesonide |
| Oral budesonide alone | 1997 | Keller et al.[33] | 14 | Steroid-dependent UC (7 pancolitis, 3 extensive colitis, 3 left sided colitis and 1 proctitis) | Budesonide 3 mg t.d.s. | 6 months Clin and reduction of systemic steroid dose | 11 out of 14 Clin Improvement and ended systemic steroid treatment |
| | 2004 | Kolkman et al.[34] | 15 | Distal active UC | Budesonide 9 mg o.d. vs budesonide 3 mg t.i.d | 8 weeks Pharmacokinetics, pharmacodynamics, safety and efficacy | Better results in 9 mg o.d. group Budesonide reaches the distal part of colon and the rectum |

N: number of patients; E: endoscopical evaluation; H: histological evaluation; Clin: clinical evaluation. ENE: enemas. FO: foam.

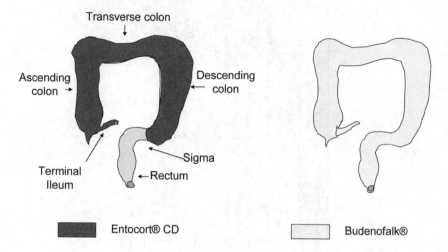

**Figure 1** Differences in ileocolonic distribution of Entocord$^{®}$ CD$^{35}$ and Budenofalk$^{®34}$ according to their pharmacokinetic oral profiles

## Acknowledgements

Dr Marín-Jiménez has a fellowship from the 'Fundación para la Investigación en Gastroenterología y Hepatología', from the Gastroenterology Department of Hospital General Universitario Gregorio Marañón, Madrid, Spain.

## References

1. Friend DR. Review article: issues in oral administration of locally acting glucocorticosteroids for treatment of inflammatory bowel disease. Aliment Pharmacol Ther. 1998;12:591–603.
2. Hamedani R, Feldman RD, Feagan BG. Review article: Drug development in inflammatory bowel disease: budesonide – a model of targeted therapy. Aliment Pharmacol Ther. 1997;11(Suppl. 3):98–107; discussion 107–8.
3. Lofberg R, Danielsson A, Suhr O et al. Oral budesonide versus prednisolone in patients with active extensive and left-sided ulcerative colitis. Gastroenterology. 1996;110:1713–18.
4. Fedorak RN, Bistritz L. Targeted delivery, safety, and efficacy of oral enteric-coated formulations of budesonide. Adv Drug Deliv Rev. 2005;57:303–16.
5. Klotz U, Schwab M. Topical delivery of therapeutic agents in the treatment of inflammatory bowel disease. Adv Drug Deliv Rev. 2005;57:267–79.
6. Ryrfeldt A, Edsbacker S, Pauwels R. Kinetics of the epimeric glucocorticoid budesonide. Clin Pharmacol Ther. 1984;35:525–30.
7. Jonsson G, Astrom A, Andersson P. Budesonide is metabolized by cytochrome P450 3A (CYP3A) enzymes in human liver. Drug Metab Dispos. 1995;23:137–42.
8. Spencer CM, McTavish D. Budesonide. A review of its pharmacological properties and therapeutic efficacy in inflammatory bowel disease. Drugs. 1995;50:854–72.
9. McKeage K, Goa KL. Budesonide (Entocort EC Capsules): a review of its therapeutic use in the management of active Crohn's disease in adults. Drugs. 2002;62:2263–82.

10. Edsbacker S, Andersson P, Lindberg C, Paulson J, Ryrfeldt A, Thalen A. Liver metabolism of budesonide in rat, mouse, and man. Comparative aspects. Drug Metab Dispos. 1987;15:403–11.

11. Nyman-Pantelidis M, Nilsson A, Wagner ZG, Borga O. Pharmacokinetics and retrograde colonic spread of budesonide enemas in patients with distal ulcerative colitis. Aliment Pharmacol Ther. 1994;8:617–22.

12. Miller-Larsson A, Gustafsson B, Persson CG, Brattsand R. Gut. mucosal uptake and retention characteristics contribute to the high intestinal selectivity of budesonide compared with prednisolone in the rat. Aliment Pharmacol Ther. 2001;15:2019–25.

13. Nugent SG, Kumar D, Rampton DS, Evans DF. Intestinal luminal pH in inflammatory bowel disease: possible determinants and implications for therapy with aminosalicylates and other drugs. Gut. 2001;48:571–7.

14. Cui N, Friend DR, Fedorak RN. A budesonide prodrug accelerates treatment of colitis in rats. Gut. 1994;35:1439–46.

15. Nolen H 3rd, Fedorak RN, Friend DR. Budesonide-beta-D-glucuronide: a potential prodrug for treatment of ulcerative colitis. J Pharm Sci. 1995;84:677–81.

16. Danielsson A, Edsbacker S, Lofberg R et al. Pharmacokinetics of budesonide enema in patients with distal ulcerative colitis or proctitis. Aliment Pharmacol Ther. 1993;7:401–7.

17. Lindgren S, Lofberg R, Bergholm L et al. Effect of budesonide enema on remission and relapse rate in distal ulcerative colitis and proctitis. Scand J Gastroenterol. 2002;37:705–10.

18. Sandborn WJ, Lofberg R, Feagan BG, Hanauer SB, Campieri M, Greenberg GR. Budesonide for maintenance of remission in patients with Crohn's disease in medically induced remission: a predetermined pooled analysis of four randomized, double-blind, placebo-controlled trials. Am J Gastroenterol. 2005;100:1780–7.

19. Danielsson A, Lofberg R, Persson T et al. A steroid enema, budesonide, lacking systemic effects for the treatment of distal ulcerative colitis or proctitis. Scand J Gastroenterol. 1992;27:9–12.

20. Hanauer SB, Robinson M, Pruitt R et al. Budesonide enema for the treatment of active, distal ulcerative colitis and proctitis: a dose-ranging study. U.S. Budesonide enema study group. Gastroenterology. 1998;115:525–32.

21. Bar-Meir S, Fidder HH, Faszczyk M et al. Budesonide foam vs. hydrocortisone acetate foam in the treatment of active ulcerative proctosigmoiditis. Dis Colon Rectum. 2003;46:929–36.

22. Hammond A, Andus T, Gierend M, Ecker KW, Scholmerich J, Herfarth H. Controlled, open, randomized multicenter trial comparing the effects of treatment on quality of life, safety and efficacy of budesonide foam and betamethasone enemas in patients with active distal ulcerative colitis. Hepatogastroenterology. 2004;51:1345–9.

23. Danielsson A, Hellers G, Lyrenas E et al. A controlled randomized trial of budesonide versus prednisolone retention enemas in active distal ulcerative colitis. Scand J Gastroenterol. 1987;22:987–92.

24. Group DBS. Budesonide enema in distal ulcerative colitis. A randomized dose–response trial with prednisolone enema as positive control. Danish Budesonide Study Group. Scand J Gastroenterol. 1991;26:1225–30.

25. Bianchi Porro G, Prantera C, Campieri M et al. Comparative trial of methylprednisolone and budesonide enemas in active distal ulcerative colitis. Eur J Gastroenterol Hepatol. 1994;6:125–30.

26. Ostergaard-Thomsen O, Andersen T, Langholz E et al. Lack of adrenal gland suppression with budesonide enema in active distal ulcerative colitis. Eur J Gastroenterol Hepatol. 1994;6:507–11.

27. Lofberg R, Ostergaard Thomsen O, Langholz E et al. Budesonide versus prednisolone retention enemas in active distal ulcerative colitis. Aliment Pharmacol Ther. 1994;8:623–9.

28. Tarpila S, Turunen U, Seppala K et al. Budesonide enema in active haemorrhagic proctitis – a controlled trial against hydrocortisone foam enema. Aliment Pharmacol Ther. 1994;8:591–5.

29. Bayless T, Sninsky C, for the US Budesonide Enema Study Group. Budesonide enema is an effective alternative to hydrocortisone enema in active distal ulcerative colitis. Gastroenterology. 1995;A778.

30. Lemann M, Galian A, Rutgeerts P et al. Comparison of budesonide and 5-aminosalicylic acid enemas in active distal ulcerative colitis. Aliment Pharmacol Ther. 1995;9:557–62.

31. Rufle W, Fruhmorgen P, Huber W, Kimmig JM. [Budesonide foam as a new therapeutic principle in distal ulcerative colitis in comparison with mesalazine enema. An open, controlled, randomized and prospective multicenter pilot study]. Z Gastroenterol. 2000;38:287–93.

32. Sambuelli A, Boerr L, Negreira S et al. Budesonide enema in pouchitis – a double-blind, double-dummy, controlled trial. Aliment Pharmacol Ther. 2002;16:27–34.

33. Keller R, Stoll R, Foerster EC, Gutsche N, Domschke W. Oral budesonide therapy for steroid-dependent ulcerative colitis: a pilot trial. Aliment Pharmacol Ther. 1997;11:1047–52.

34. Kolkman JJ, Mollmann HW, Mollmann AC et al. Evaluation of oral budesonide in the treatment of active distal ulcerative colitis. Drugs Today. (Barc) 2004;40:589–601.

35. Edsbacker S, Bengtsson B, Larsson P et al. A pharmacoscintigraphic evaluation of oral budesonide given as controlled-release (Entocort) capsules. Aliment Pharmacol Ther. 2003;17:525–36.

36. Buttgereit F, Burmester GR, Lipworth BJ. Optimised glucocorticoid therapy: the sharpening of an old spear. Lancet. 2005;365:801–3.

# 13
# How do I use steroids in Crohn's disease?

J. SCHÖLMERICH

## INTRODUCTION

Steroids are still widely used in the treatment of inflammatory bowel diseases; however, they are feared by patients and doctors alike[1]. This chapter deals exclusively with Crohn's disease (CD) and the use of steroids in different settings. After defining the aims of treatment a number of epidemiological data regarding steroid use will be discussed. Thereafter clinical studies available will be presented and possible alternatives will be analysed. This should lead to recommendations for daily practice.

## AIMS OF TREATMENT

At present the main target of treatment is the elimination or at least amelioration of complaints and symptoms of CD. A second aim is the prevention or reduction of flares when initial remission has been achieved (maintenance treatment). Other aims are mucosal healing and even 'causal treatment', although neither has really been achieved, with the exception of mucosal healing in some patients using potent immunosuppressants.

## EPIDEMIOLOGICAL CONSIDERATIONS

There is an impressive list of drugs currently used for CD and noteworthy glucocorticosteroids are on top of the list as in most textbooks and reviews (Table 1). However, when looking at the long-term follow-up of patients, it is apparent that most patients with CD at any given time-point are in remission with and without prior surgery or have a mild course. A minority only needs more aggressive treatment[2]. When looking at the use of steroids in the same cohort, the population-based patient group from Olmstead County, it turns out that less than half of the patients have been treated with steroids. Of those almost 60% obtained complete remission and 26% partial remission. At the end

111

**Table 1**  Drugs to be used for Crohn's disease

| | |
|---|---|
| Glucocorticoids | – Prednisolone<br>– Budesonide |
| 5-Aminosalicylates | – Large bowel release<br>– Small bowel release |
| Immunosuppressants | – Azathioprine/6-mercaptopurine<br>– Methotrexate<br>– Cyclosporin A<br>– Others |
| Antibiotics | – Metronidazole<br>– Ciprofloxazin |
| New substances | – Infliximab<br>– Others |

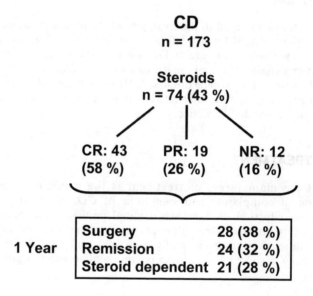

**Figure 1**  Population-related data from Olmstead County regarding the use of steroids for Crohn's disease[3]

of 1 year observation, 32% were in remission, 38% had surgery, and 28% were steroid-dependent (Figure 1)[3]. Those facts, the limited use in patients with CD and the limited success at least over a 1 year follow-up, raise the question on what data the recommendation of steroid use is based.

## AVAILABLE CLINICAL STUDIES

### Systemic steroids

A number of major trials in the 1970s and 1980s have proven that systemic steroids (prednisone, prednisolone and methylprednisolone) are effective in active CD[4,5] (Table 2). It is obvious from these studies that the combination of steroids with sulphasalazine is no better than steroids only, and steroids seem to be more effective than sulphasalazine. However, there are a number of patients who do not respond. Analysis of the large remission introduction run-in phase of a maintenance trial[6] indicates that patients with prior resection and patients with perianal disease are much less likely to respond to a course of steroids in order to achieve remission (Figure 2). This may be due to the fact that the 'activity' of the disease may be wrongly assessed in resected patients having chologenic diarrhoea as described in this study[6]. Furthermore an infectious complication such as perianal disease is not likely to respond to steroids, considering its biology.

**Table 2**   Treatment of active CD: ECCDS I[4]

|  | Remission (%) |
| --- | --- |
| Placebo | 37.9 |
| SASP (3 g/day) | 50.0 |
| M-prednisolone (48 → 8 mg) | 82.9 |
| SASP + M-prednisolone | 78.5 |

Systemic steroids are mainly used to achieve clinical remission, i.e. to eliminate or alleviate symptoms. As soon as this is achieved steroids can be tapered. The outcome after 18 months is not different if steroids are given for 5 more weeks in patients not showing endoscopic remission after standard treatment[7].

### Topical steroids

In the 1990s of the last century the non-systemic steroid budesonide was developed for CD patients. Initial small uncontrolled studies were performed in patients intolerant to conventional steroids[8,9]. A little later a series of controlled studies was published[10–13], all demonstrating that remission rates for 9 mg of budesonide were rather similar to those achieved with steroids, although always a little bit lower. In contrast side-effects were significantly less frequent with budesonide as compared to the systemic steroids (Table 3). Suppression of plasma cortisol was much lower with budesonide as compared to prednisolone[10]. Dose-finding studies using the time-dependent release preparation demonstrated that 9 mg was the optimal dose[11]. The largest trial thus far[14] using pH-dependent budesonide, 9 mg daily, showed an identical

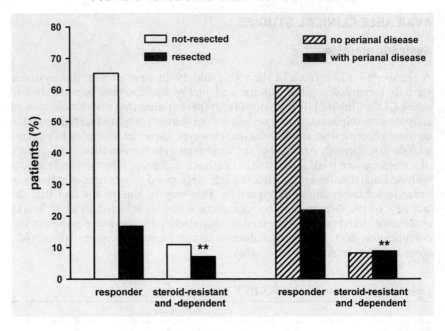

**Figure 2** Factors determining steroid refractoriness in Crohn's disease in a large group of patients treated with systemic steroids for induction of remission[6]

**Table 3** Remission rates and side-effects in several controlled trials with budesonide in active Crohn's disease

| Reference | Remission (%) | | Side-effects (%) | |
|-----------|---------------|---|------------------|---|
| | BUD (9 mg) | Steroids | BUD (9 mg) | Steroids |
| Rutgeerts et al.[10] | 53 | 66 | 33 | 55 |
| Greenberg et al.[11] | 51 | – | 26 | – |
| Gross et al.[12] | 56 | 73 | 29 | 70 |
| Campieri et al.[13] | 60/42 | 60 | 14/11 | 38* |

*Moon face only.

remission rate versus a tapered prednisone course. The remission rate without side-effects was significantly higher in the budesonide arm. In addition, for this pH-dependent release formulation a different dose response was obtained. While patients with mild to moderate activity (below 300 on the Crohn's Disease Activity Index) achieved the highest remission rate with 9 mg daily patients with a higher score more frequently achieved remission using 18 mg daily. This was also true for patients with colonic involvement as compared to those with only iliocolonic disease (Table 4)[15]. However, using 18 mg daily over more than 2 weeks resulted in a much more intense suppression of plasma cortisol as compared to 6 or 9 mg daily (Figure 3).

**Table 4** Dose response for budesonide (pH-dependent) in CD patients with different location and activity[15]

| 6 weeks | Remission (%) | | |
| --- | --- | --- | --- |
| | 6 mg | 9 mg | 18 mg |
| Initial CDAI | | | |
| <300 (n = 79) | 47 | 71 | 64 |
| ≥300 (n = 25) | 0 | 25 | 75* |
| Location | | | |
| Ileocolonic (n = 57) | 30 | 60 | 59 |
| Colonic distal (n = 4) | 31 | 46 | 73* |

*Significant.

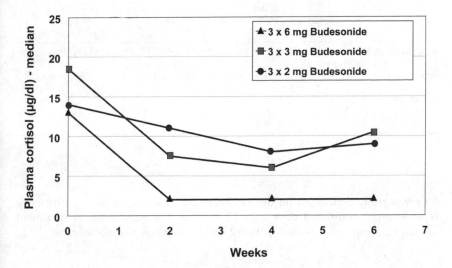

**Figure 3** Plasma cortisol – effects of different doses of pH-dependent budesonide over 6 weeks[15]

With regard to remission maintenance the early trials of systemic steroids showed that with initially inactive disease there was no advantage of methylprednisolone in a dose of 8 mg/day. Patients initially active seemed to have an advantage; this was however a *post-hoc* analysis[4].

More recently in this context budesonide orally at a dose of 3 mg/day did not show any difference compared to placebo in a very large study[16]. A number of other studies using the time-dependent release preparation[17–20] demonstrated a small shift to a later relapse, but no difference regarding overall relapse at the end of 1 year. A study of flexible budesonide use for remission maintenance comparing a patient group with a fixed dose of 6 mg/day with a group having 3,

**Table 5** Enteral nutrition vs drug treatment in active CD (ECCDS IV)[23]

|  | Enteral nutrition (n = 55) | Steroids (n = 52) |
|---|---|---|
| Remission* (%), 6 weeks | 53 | 79[#] |
| Time to remission (median, days) | 30.7 | 8.2[#] |

*CDAI 40% $\geqslant$ 100 points ↓.
[#]$p < 0.01$.

**Table 6** Mesalamine (pH-dependent) for mild to moderate active Crohn's disease[25]

|  | 5-ASA | | 6-Methylprednisolone |
|---|---|---|---|
|  | 4 g/day (tablets) (n = 35) | 4 g/day (microgranular) (n = 35) | 40 mg (n = 31) |
| Δ CDAI (median) | −113 (33–149) | −123 (77–155) | −154 (99–197) |
| Remission (%) | 60 | 79 | 61 |
| Withdrawn | | | |
| Failure (%) | 31 | 9 | 13 |
| AE (%) | 0 | 4 | 16 |

6 or 9 mg/day dependent on disease behaviour, did not show any difference regarding the consumed dose over 12 months, the percentage of treatment failures, and side-effects. Postoperative budesonide was also not effective[21,22].

## ALTERNATIVE OPTIONS

A number of alternatives to glucocorticosteroid treatment in active disease have been tested. In particular enteral nutrition has been advocated earlier. However, the data demonstrate that enteral nutrition is less effective than glucocorticosteroids with respect to time to response and remission rates (Table 5)[23]. This has also been shown in a meta-analysis[24]. Another alternative would be 5-aminosalicylic-acid (5-ASA) and its different galenic forms. A rather large study comparing 40 mg 6-methylprednisolone with 4 g/day 5-ASA, either as tablets or in a microgranular form, found no differences, but also did not prove equivalence (Table 6)[25]. A number of studies have compared steroids and 5-ASA in different doses, and mostly found that steroids were superior, but this may depend on the dose of 5-ASA used[26–29]. A comparison of budesonide 9 mg/day with 4 g 5-ASA as Pentasa demonstrated significantly better effects of budesonide[30].

**Table 7**  Azathioprine in active Crohn's disease – short- and long-term effects[31]

|  | Prednisolone (12 weeks, tapered) | |
| --- | --- | --- |
|  | + Placebo (n = 30) | + Azathioprine, 2.5 mg/kg (n = 33) |
| Remission 12 weeks (%) | 63 | 73 |
| Remission 15 months (%) | 7 | 42* |

*Significant.

From 12 weeks on only azathioprine.

However, 5-ASA may be a good alternative in a significant number of patients, as seems to be evident from the epidemiological data and from some of the studies available. Nutrition is probably useful only in a minority of patients. Regarding maintenance treatment the only effective alternative, according to available studies, is azathioprine, which significantly increased the remission rate after 15 months in patients initially treated with steroids and then continued with azathioprine or placebo (Table 7)[31].

When considering the aims of treatment defined initially it is obvious that glucocorticosteroids are able to rapidly eliminate or ameliorate complaints and symptoms in the majority of patients. They do not seem to be very effective in the prevention or reduction of flares, at least not in doses used or usable. It is obvious that applying those doses which are effective in remission induction will probably be suitable to maintain such remission, but at an unacceptable price, i.e. side-effects of high-dose glucocorticosteroids. With respect to mucosal healing, or even causal treatment, the aims have certainly not been fulfilled using glucocorticosteroids.

## RECOMMENDATION FOR DAILY PRACTICE

I would suggest the use of glucocorticosteroids for rapid relief of symptoms in patients with active inflammation. For moderate disease I prefer the topical forms while for severe flares the systemic preparations should be used. I would strongly argue against the use of glucocorticosteroids in maintenance – as discussed, it works, but at an unacceptable price. Steroids need to be substituted by immunosuppression (or surgery) when tapering/weaning is not possible after the initial induction of remission.

# References

1. Schölmerich J. Systemic and topical steroids in inflammatory bowel disease. Aliment Pharmacol Ther. 2004;20(Suppl. 4):66–74.
2. Silverstein MD, Loftus EV, Sandborn WJ et al. Clinical course and costs of care for Crohn's disease: Markov model analysis of a population-based cohort. Gastroenterology. 1999;117: 49–57.
3. Faubion WA Jr, Loftus EV Jr, Harmsen WS, Zinsmeister AR, Sandborn WJ. The natural history of corticosteroid therapy for inflammatory bowel disease: a population-based study. Gastroenterology. 2001;121:255–60.
4. Malchow H, Ewe K, Brandes JW et al. European Cooperative Crohn's Disease Study (ECCDS): results of drug treatment. Gastroenterology. 1984;86:249–66.
5. Summers RW, Switz DM, Sessions JT Jr, et al. National Cooperative Crohn's Disease Study: results of drug treatment. Gastroenterology. 1979;77:847–69.
6. Gelbmann C, Rogler G, Gross V et al. Prior bowel resections, perianal disease, and a high initial Crohn's disease activity index are associated with corticosteroid resistance in active Crohn's disease. Am J Gastroenterol. 1992;97:1438–45.
7. Landi B, Anh TN, Cortot A et al. Endoscopic monitoring of Crohn's disease treatment: a prospective, randomized clinical trial. The Group d'Études Thérapeutiques des Affections Inflammatoires Digestives. Gastroenterology. 1992;102:1647–53.
8. Roth M, Gross V, Schölmerich J, Ueberschaer B, Ewe K. Treatment of active Crohn's disease with an oral slow-release budesonide formulation. Am J Gastroenterol. 1993;88: 968–9.
9. Wolman SL, Greenberg GR. Oral budesonide in active Crohn's disease: an initial experience. Gastroenterology. 1991;100:A263.
10. Rutgeerts P, Löfberg R, Malchow H et al. A comparison of budesonide with prednisolone for active Crohn's disease. N Eng J Med. 1994;331:842–5.
11. Greenberg GR, Feagan BG, Martin F et al. Oral budesonide for active Crohn's disease. Canadian Inflammatory Bowel Disease Study Group. N Engl J Med. 1994;331:836–41.
12. Gross V, Andus T, Caesar I et al. Oral pH-modified release budesonide versus 6-methylprednisolone in active Crohn's disease. German/Austrian Budesonide Study Group. Eur J Gastroenterol Hepatol. 1996;8:905–9.
13. Campieri M, Ferguson A, Doe W, Persson T, Nilsson LG. Oral budesonide is as effective as oral prednisolone in active Crohn's disease. Global Budesonide Study Group. Gut. 1997; 41:209–14.
14. Bar-Meir S, Chowers Y, Lavy A et al. The Israeli Budesonide Study Group. Budesonide versus prednisone in the treatment of active Crohn's disease. Gastroenterology. 1998;115: 835–40.
15. Herfarth H, Gross V, Andus T et al. Analysis of the therapeutic efficacy of different doses of budesonide in patients with active Crohn's ileocolitis depending on disease activity and localization. Int J Colorectal Dis. 2004;19:147–52.
16. Gross V, Andus T, Ecker KW et al. Low dose oral pH modified release budesonide for maintenance of steroid induced remission in Crohn's disease. Gut. 1998;42:493–6.
17. Löfberg R, Rutgeerts P, Malchow H et al. Budesonide prolongs time to relapse in ileal and ileocaecal Crohn's disease. A placebo controlled one year study. Gut. 1996;39:82–6.
18. Greenberg GR, Feagan BG, Martin F et al. Oral budesonide as maintenance treatment for Crohn's disease: a placebo-controlled, dose-ranging study. Canadian Inflammatory Bowel Disease Study Group. Gastroenterology. 1996;110:45–51.
19. Ferguson A, Campieri M, Doe W, Persson T, Nygard G. Oral budesonide as maintenance therapy in Crohn's disease – results of a 12-month study. Global Budesonide Study Group. Aliment Pharmacol Ther. 1998;12:175–83.
20. Hanauer S, Sandborn WJ, Persson A, Persson T. Budesonide as maintenance treatment in Crohn's disease: a placebo-controlled trial. Aliment Pharmacol Ther. 2005;21:363–71.
21. Ewe K, Bottger T, Buhr HJ, Ecker KW, Otto HF. Low-dose budesonide treatment for prevention of postoperative recurrence of Crohn's disease: a multicenter randomized placebo-controlled trial. German Budesonide Study Group. Eur J Gastroenterol Hepatol. 1999;11:277–82.

22. Hellers G, Cortot A, Jewell D, Leijonmarck CE, Lofberg R, Malchow H. Oral budesonide for prevention of postsurgical recurrence in Crohn's disease. The IOIBD Budesonide Study Group. Gastroenterology. 1999;116:294–300.
23. Lochs H, Steinhardt HJ, Klaus-Wentz B et al. Comparison of enteral nutrition and drug treatment in active Crohn's disease. Results of the European Cooperative Crohn's Disease Study. IV. Gastroenterology. 1991;101:881–8.
24. Griffiths AM, Ohlsson A, Sherman PM, Sutherland LR. Meta-analysis of enteral nutrition as a primary treatment of active Crohn's disease. Gastroenterology. 1995;108:1056–67.
25. Prantera C, Cottone M, Pallone F et al. Mesalamine in the treatment of mild to moderate active Crohn's ileitis: results of a randomized, multicenter trial. Gastroenterology. 1999; 116:521–6.
26. Gross V, Andus T, Fischbach W et al. and the German 5-ASA Study Group. Comparison between high dose 5-aminosalicylic acid and 6-methylprednisolone in active Crohn's ileocolitis. A multicentre randomized double-blind study. German 5-ASA Study Group. Z Gastroenterol. 1995;33:581–4.
27. Mahida YR, Jewell DP. Slow-release 5-amino-salicylic acid (Pentasa) for the treatment of active Crohn's disease. Digestion. 1990;45:88–92.
28. Rasmussen SN, Lauritsen K, Tage-Jensen U et al. 5-Aminosalicylic acid in the treatment of Crohn's disease. A 16-week double-blind, placebo-controlled, multicentre study with Pentasa. Scand J Gastroenterol. 1987;22:877–83.
29. Schölmerich J, Jenss H, Hartmann F, Döpfer H and the German 5-ASA Study Group. Oral 5-aminosalicylic acid versus 6-methylprednisolone in active Crohn's disease. Can J Gastoenterol. 1990;4:446–51.
30. Ostergaard-Thomsen O, Cortot A, Jewell D et al. A comparison of budesonide and mesalamine for active Crohn's disease. International Budesonide-Mesalamine Study Group. N Engl J Med. 1998;399:370–4.
31. Candy S, Wright J, Gerber M, Adams G, Gerig M, Goodman R. A controlled double blind study of azathioprine in the management of Crohn's disease. Gut. 1995;37:674–8.

# 14
# Why corticosteroids should not be used as first-line therapy for Crohn's disease

J. M. RHODES

## UNDERSTANDING CROHN'S DISEASE (CD) PATHOGENESIS

The identification of NOD2/CARD15 as a CD-associated gene has given us a substantial clue towards understanding its pathogenesis. Although the functional implications of the Crohn's-related NOD2/CARD15 mutations are not fully understood, it is known that the NOD2 protein is expressed in the cytoplasm of macrophages and Paneth cells, that the Crohn's-related mutation is within the leucine-rich region of NOD2 that interacts with bacterial cell wall peptidoglycan, and that epithelial cells transfected with mutant NOD2 are unable to kill phagocytosed *Salmonella* whereas the same cells transfected with wild-type NOD2 are able to do so[1]. NOD2-defective CD patients also express lower levels of mucosal defensins, the bactericidal peptides that are secreted by Paneth cells[2], suggesting that the Crohn's-related NOD2 defect may be causing problems with mucosal defence against bacteria on at least two levels – at the mucosal surface and within macrophages. Moreover, NOD2-defective mice are susceptible to orally acquired infection with organisms such as *Listeria* which replicate within the cytoplasm of macrophages[3].

These findings suggest that CD may occur as a result of an inability of macrophages to kill intracellular bacteria that have invaded the mucosa. Further support for this comes from the rare inherited diseases chronic granulomatous disease[4] and glycogen storage disease type 1b[5], both of which are associated with phagocyte defects in killing of intracellular bacteria and both of which are associated with intestinal disease that closely mimics CD (Figure 1).

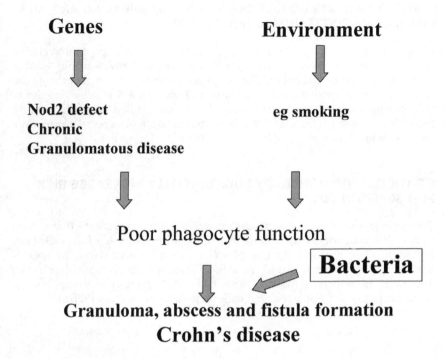

**Genes**

**Environment**

**Nod2 defect
Chronic
Granulomatous disease**

**eg smoking**

Poor phagocyte function

**Bacteria**

**Granuloma, abscess and fistula formation
Crohn's disease**

**Figure 1**    Crohn's disease viewed as a disorder of phagocyte function

## EVIDENCE FOR MUCOSA-ASSOCIATED AND INTRAMUCOSAL BACTERIA IN CD

Recent studies by three groups, including our own, have shown an increase in mucosa-associated bacteria in CD, particularly *Escherichia coli*[6–8], and have shown that these *E. coli* are able to live and proliferate within macrophages *in vitro*[9]. Immunohistochemical studies of CD tissue have shown macrophages containing intracellular bacteria, particularly *E. coli*, *Listeria* and Group F Streptococci[10]. The best-characterized environmental agent for CD – smoking – has been shown to be associated with an inability of pulmonary macrophages to kill *Listeria*[11] – an obligate intracytoplasmic organism that replicates within macrophages.

These findings are all in keeping with CD occurring as a result of defective defence against the gut microbiota due to either genetic or acquired problems with macrophage and/or defensin function[12]. The result is chronic bacterial infection within CD tissue, particularly within macrophages, with resulting granuloma formation, and septic complications including abscess and fistula formation.

## CORTICOSTEROIDS DO NOT CAUSE MUCOSAL HEALING AND ARE INEFFECTIVE FOR MAINTENANCE THERAPY

If CD is a consequence of ineffective clearance by macrophages of intracellular (and probably intracytoplasmic) bacteria then corticosteroids would seem a highly inappropriate treatment. There is good evidence to show that this is the case. Although corticosteroids are a cheap and effective way of achieving short-term symptomatic relief they only beat placebo for the first 3 months, and by the end of 1 year's treatment there is no benefit over placebo[13,14]; moreover there is no impact on mucosal healing[15] (Figure 2).

## CORTICOSTEROID THERAPY SUBSTANTIALLY INCREASES RISK FOR SEPSIS IN CD

The general side-effects of steroids are well known, but recent studies have shown that their use is particularly associated with severe sepsis in CD. They greatly increase not only the risk of serious postoperative sepsis, by over 5-fold[16], but also increase 9-fold the risk of serious intra-abdominal or pelvic abscess in non-operated patients with CD[17]. Interestingly azathioprine and mercaptopurine are not associated with these risks for bacterial sepsis[16,17] and

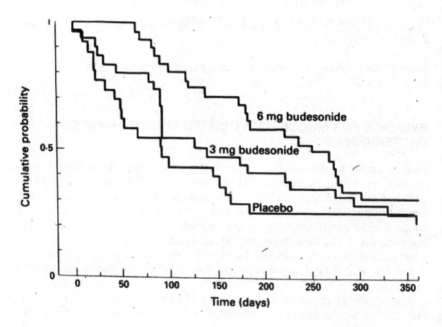

**Figure 2** Corticosteroids are no better than placebo for long-term maintenance in Crohn's disease; moreover the symptomatic benefit is confined to the first 3 months. From ref. 13 with permission

their use has been shown to heal mucosal ulceration[18]; moreover they have been shown to be effective in the absence of corticosteroids[19]. Azathioprine and mercaptopurine should therefore no longer be thought of as steroid-sparing but as effective therapies in their own right.

## EVEN VERY LOW DOSES OF CORTICOSTEROID INCREASE RISK FOR FRACTURE

Even though there is agreement that maintenance corticosteroids are ineffective in CD, it is often difficult for patients to stop them completely, and many patients are maintained on low-dose corticosteroids in the expectation that this is at least safe. There is now evidence that any regular dose of more than 2.5 mg prednisolone per day increases risk for fracture[20].

## WHAT ALTERNATIVES ARE THERE FOR CORTICOSTEROIDS?

Alternative therapies include the immunosuppressives, azathioprine, 6-mercaptopurine and methotrexate; enteral feeding as replacement for normal food; surgery if disease is limited, e.g. short stricture of terminal ileum; infliximab; and antibiotics[21,22].

### Enteral feeding

Enteral feeding probably has the best evidence base of any alternative to corticosteroids as initial therapy for CD. Meta-analyses suggest that this approach is less effective than corticosteroids[23], but it can be argued that the meta-analyses have grouped together the results with different enteral feeds, some of which may be genuinely less effective or even ineffective. Moreover there is some evidence that isolated colonic CD may be less responsive to enteral feeding and inclusion of these cases may also give a misleading result on meta-analysis. In children with CD meta-analyses have shown that enteral feeding is as effective as corticosteroids[24]; moreover it is associated with better growth[25]. In adults with CD, treatment with enteral feeding has been shown to maintain bone mineral density better than corticosteroid therapy[26].

### Immunosuppressives

The arguments against primary use of immunosuppressives are 2-fold. First they are perceived to have a high rate of associated side-effects. A strong case can be made, however, that their side-effect profile may actually be safer than for corticosteroids. It has already been mentioned that at least two studies have now shown that systemic corticosteroid therapy increases risk for serious sepsis in patients with CD, whereas immunosuppressives do not. The second argument concerns their relatively slow onset of action, probably around 3 months. This can be dealt with by using an alternative initial therapy such as enteral feeding, antibiotics or even infliximab.

COLITIS: DIAGNOSIS AND THERAPEUTIC STRATEGIES

## Antibiotics

Trials of antibiotics in CD suffer from the problems that afflict all trials that are attempted with drugs or indications for which there is little likelihood of commercial profit. As a result they have all been small, usually uncontrolled and underpowered. There is some evidence to support combinations such as ciprofloxacin and metronidazole[27-28]. It may be that some of the confusion surrounding the efficacy of antibiotics in CD results from the localization of bacteria within macrophages that might necessitate use of an antibiotic that has not only appropriate bactericidal properties but good intracellular penetration. Clarithromycin certainly has the latter property and shows some promise[29]. Further studies are needed to identify antibiotics that have the most appropriate properties, e.g. perhaps for killing *E. coli* and *Listeria* within macrophages.

## SHOULD A SPECIAL CASE BE MADE FOR ISOLATED COLONIC CD?

A strong case can be made that isolated colonic CD is a separate condition from 'typical' ileal or ileocaecal CD. Isolated colonic CD has been shown not to be associated with mutations of NOD2/CARD15[30]; moreover it tends to occur in members of the same family as ulcerative colitis (UC) but with smokers being at risk for colonic CD and non-smokers at risk for UC[31]. Isolated colonic CD and UC share similar HLA class 2 antigen associations[30,32], and are both associated with pANCA positivity and ASCA negativity. It is therefore looking increasingly likely that isolated colonic CD and 'typical' UC are phenotypic variants of the same condition as part of a spectrum, with indeterminate colitis at the midpoint. Isolated colonic CD tends to respond to antibiotics such as metronidazole[33], whereas UC does not, but this discrepancy might perhaps result from the impairment of phagocyte function related to smoking that has been discussed earlier. If isolated colonic CD and UC are phenotypic variants of the same condition, characterized by similar associations with HLA class 2 antigenicity and a similar tendency for autoantibody formation, then it may be reasonable to view both as autoimmune conditions that can be appropriately settled with a short course of corticosteroids. Based on this hypothesis, I feel that there is better justification for using systemic corticosteroids in isolated colonic CD than in ileal or ileocolonic disease.

## Surgery

It may sometimes be appropriate to consider surgery as initial therapy even in the absence of an absolute indication such as perforation or obstruction. In a patient who has recently presented with a short, tight, terminal ileal stricture and with no past history of previous resection a right hemicolectomy, particularly if this is laparoscope-assisted, may be a very reasonable first option. Comparison of this approach with initial medical therapy should ideally be subjected to randomized study. Such a study, albeit very challenging, is in progress in Scandinavia, and its results are awaited with interest. Patient preference should of course play an important part in the choice of initial therapy, particularly as there will often be several reasonable alternatives with no clear best choice.

## WHATEVER OPTION MIGHT EVENTUALLY PROVE TO BE THE BEST FOR PATIENTS WITH CD IT WILL NOT INCLUDE CORTICOSTEROIDS!

CD is the only condition for which physicians commonly prescribe high-dose corticosteroids with no expectation of having any useful effect on the long-term course of the disease. Although they 'buy a quick fix' for the first 3 months, from then on their use is nearly always detrimental yet, once started, they are often hard to stop. Better not to start, then!

## References

1. Hisamatsu T, Suzuki M, Reinecker HC, Nadeau WJ, McCormick BA, Podolsky DK. CARD15/NOD2 functions as an antibacterial factor in human intestinal epithelial cells. Gastroenterology. 2003;124:993–1000.
2. Wehkamp J, Harder J, Weichenthal M et al. NOD2 (CARD15) mutations in Crohn's disease are associated with diminished mucosal alpha-defensin expression. Gut. 2004;53: 1658–64.
3. Kobayashi KS, Chamaillard M, Ogura Y et al. Nod2-dependent regulation of innate and adaptive immunity in the intestinal tract. Science. 2005;307:731–4.
4. Huang JS, Noack D, Rae J et al..Chronic granulomatous disease caused by a deficiency in p47(phox) mimicking Crohn's disease. Clin Gastroenterol Hepatol. 2004;2:690–5.
5. Sanderson IR, Bisset WM, Milla PJ, Leonard JV. Chronic inflammatory bowel disease in glycogen storage disease type 1B. J Inher Metab Dis. 1991;14:771–6.
6. Swidsinski A, Ladhoff A, Pernthaler A et al. Mucosal flora in inflammatory bowel disease. Gastroenterology. 2002;122:44–54.
7. Martin HM, Campbell BJ, Hart CA et al. Enhanced *Escherichia coli* adherence and invasion in Crohn's disease and colon cancer. Gastroenterology. 2004;127:80–93.
8. Darfeuille-Michaud A, Boudeau J, Bulois P et al. High prevalence of adherent-invasive *Escherichia coli* associated with ileal mucosa in Crohn's disease. Gastroenterology. 2004;127:412–21.
9. Glasser AL, Boudeau J, Barnich N, Perruchot MH, Colombel JF, Darfeuille-Michaud A. Adherent invasive *Escherichia coli* strains from patients with Crohn's disease survive and replicate within macrophages without inducing host cell death. Infect Immun. 2001;69: 5529–37.
10. Liu Y, van Kruiningen HJ, West AB, Cartun RW, Cortot A, Colombel JF. Immunocytochemical evidence of *Listeria, Escherichia coli*, and *Streptococcus* antigens in Crohn's disease. Gastroenterology. 1995;108:1396–404.
11. King TE Jr, Savici D, Campbell PA. Phagocytosis and killing of *Listeria monocytogenes* by alveolar macrophages: smokers versus nonsmokers. J Infect Dis. 1988;158:1309–16.
12. Rhodes JM. Advances in inflammatory bowel disease. In: Weber E, editor. Horizons in Medicine. London: Royal College of Physicians, 2003:249–57.
13. Lofberg R, Rutgeerts P, Malchow H et al. Budesonide prolongs time to relapse in ileal and ileocaecal Crohn's disease. A placebo controlled one year study. Gut. 1996;39:82–6.
14. Steinhart AH, Ewe K, Griffiths AM, Modigliani R, Thomsen OO. Corticosteroids for maintenance of remission in Crohn's disease. Cochrane Database Syst Rev. 2003(4): CD000301.
15. Rutgeerts PJ. Review article: The limitations of corticosteroid therapy in Crohn's disease. Aliment Pharmacol Ther. 2001;15:1515–25.

16. Aberra FN, Lewi JD, Hass D, Rombeau JL, Osborne B, Lichtenstein GR. Corticosteroids and immunomodulators: postoperative infectious complication risk in inflammatory bowel disease patients. Gastroenterology. 2003;125:320–7.
17. Agrawal A, Durrani S, Kennedy S et al. Corticosteroid therapy as a risk factor for serious abscess in non-operated Crohn's disease. Gut. 2004;53:A96 and Clin Gastroenterol Hepatol. (2005, in press).
18. D'Haens G, Geboes K, Rutgeerts P. Endoscopic and histologic healing of Crohn's (ileo-) colitis with azathioprine. Gastrointest Endosc. 1999;50:667–71.
19. Goldstein ES, Marion JF, Present DH. 6-Mercaptopurine is effective in Crohn's disease without concomitant steroids. Inflamm Bowel Dis. 2004;10:79–84.
20. Vestergaard P, Rejnmark L, Mosekilde L. Fracture risk associated with systemic and topical corticosteroids. J Intern Med. 2005;257:374–84.
21. Nayar M, Rhodes JM. Management of inflammatory bowel disease. Postgrad Med J. 2004; 80:206–13.
22. Present DH. How to do without steroids in inflammatory bowel disease. Inflamm Bowel Dis. 2000;6:48–57; discussion 58.
23. Griffiths AM, Ohlsson A, Sherman PM, Sutherland LR. Meta-analysis of enteral nutrition as a primary treatment of active Crohn's disease. Gastroenterology. 1995;108:1056–67.
24. Heuschkel RB, Menache CC, Megerian JT, Baird AE. Enteral nutrition and corticosteroids in the treatment of acute Crohn's disease in children. J Pediatr Gastroenterol Nutr. 2000;31: 8–15.
25. Azcue M, Rashid M, Griffiths A, Pencharz PB. Energy expenditure and body composition in children with Crohn's disease: effect of enteral nutrition and treatment with prednisolone. Gut. 1997;41:203–8.
26. Dear KL, Compston JE, Hunter JO. Treatments for Crohn's disease that minimise steroid doses are associated with a reduced risk of osteoporosis. Clin Nutr. 2001;20:541–6.
27. Prantera C, Zannoni F, Scribano ML et al. An antibiotic regimen for the treatment of active Crohn's disease: a randomized, controlled clinical trial of metronidazole plus ciprofloxacin. Am J Gastroenterol. 1996;91:328–32.
28. Greenberg GR. Antibiotics should be used as first-line therapy for Crohn's disease. Inflamm Bowel Dis. 2004;10:318–20.
29. Leiper K, Morris AI, Rhodes JM. Open label trial of oral clarithromycin in active Crohn's disease. Aliment Pharmacol Ther. 2000;14:801–6.
30. Newman B, Silverberg MS, Gu X et al. CARD15 and HLA DRB1 alleles influence susceptibility and disease localization in Crohn's disease. Am J Gastroenterol. 2004;99: 306–15.
31. Lee JC, Lennard-Jones JE. Inflammatory bowel disease in 67 families each with three or more affected first-degree relatives. Gastroenterology. 1996;111:587–96.31.
32. Ahmad T, Armuzzi A, Neville M et al. The contribution of human leucocyte antigen complex genes to disease phenotype in ulcerative colitis. Tiss Antig. 2003;62:527–35.
33. Sutherland L, Singleton J, Sessions J et al. Double blind, placebo controlled trial of metronidazole in Crohn's disease. Gut. 1991;32:1071–5.

# Section V
# Azathioprine

**Chair: S. GHOSH and A.S. PEÑA**

# 15
# Azathioprine: molecular mechanism of action

## M. F. NEURATH

## INTRODUCTION

Azathioprine and its metabolite 6-mercaptopurine (6-MP) were discovered by Elion and Hitchings[1]. These drugs have been used in numerous chronic inflammatory and autoimmune diseases such as multiple sclerosis, rheumatoid arthritis and primary biliary cirrhosis[2,3]. They have also been tested in patients with inflammatory bowel diseases (IBD). IBD in humans comprise ulcerative colitis (UC) and Crohn's disease (CD)[4]. Starting with the initial description of Bean in 1962[5] and the large controlled trial by Present et al. in 1980[6], numerous studies have addressed the role of 6-MP or azathioprine in IBD. It was found that azathioprine and 6-MP may induce clinical remission in IBD patients and, more importantly, are highly effective in maintaining remission[7–13].

In spite of the overwhelming clinical evidence for a therapeutic efficacy of azathioprine and 6-MP, little was known about the exact mechanism of action of these drugs. However, these drugs are considered as classical purine antimetabolite drugs that block T cell proliferation[3]. Specifically, it is believed that intracellular accumulation of 6-MP metabolites, so-called 6-thioguanine nucleotides (6-TGN), results in blockade of purine metabolism, DNA repair and cell division based on random incorporation into DNA. However, several lines of evidence suggest that this mechanism is unlikely to play a role for the therapeutic effects of azathioprine and 6-MP in IBD patients. First, azathioprine and 6-MP fail to block T cell proliferation in cell culture at therapeutically relevant doses (5 micromolar) (Tiede et al., unpublished data). Second, lamina propria T cells are poor proliferators as compared to blood T cells and thus unlikely to respond to a therapeutic agent that primarily blocks T cell proliferation[14,15]. Third, a therapeutic principle based on random incorporation would predict random side-effects and highly variable efficacy, which is against the clinical observations made in azathioprine-treated IBD patients[12,16]. Finally, the clinical observations in azathioprine-treated patients point towards a very specific mechanism of action that targets T lymphocytes.

Interestingly, Tiede and co-workers recently found evidence that lamina propria T cells are the key target of azathioprine therapy in IBD[17]. Such lamina propria T lymphocytes have emerged as key effector cells in the chronic phase of IBD where they produce proinflammatory cytokines leading to tissue damage. Furthermore, the survival of these lamina propria T cells is altered: whereas in the normal gut lamina propria T cells are more susceptible to undergo programmed cell death (apoptosis) as compared to peripheral T cells, T lymphocytes in IBD patients are resistant against apoptosis and survive in the inflamed gut for prolonged periods of time. This observation may contribute to an expansion of effector T cells in the lamina propria of IBD patients. Therefore, targeting of T lymphocytes emerges as an important strategy to treat IBD. As will be discussed below, it appears that the molecular mechanism of azathioprine induces selective T cell death in the inflamed gut of IBD patients by eliminating activated, costimulated T lymphocytes.

## AZATHIOPRINE TARGETS T CELLS IN IBD

Azathioprine and 6-MP exhibit therapeutic efficacy both in CD and UC. Lamina propria T cells in CD produce a Th1 type cytokine profile characterized by IFN-gamma and TNF production. At the molecular level these cells also express markers of Th1 cells such as IL-12R beta2 chain and the transcription factor T-beta. The cytokine profile in UC is characterized by the increased production of the Th2 cytokines IL-5 and IL-13[18], although the hallmark cytokine of Th2 cells, IL-4, is not produced at high levels[19]. Such CD4[+] Th1 or Th2 cells seem to play a key pathogenic role in IBD patients. As azathioprine is effective both in CD and in UC, it appears that azathioprine can target the activation and effector function of both Th1 and Th2 cells in the mucosa.

Tiede et al.[17] provided evidence that azathioprine induces T cell apoptosis of CD45RO memory T cells. Since CD45RO T lymphocytes are considered to be key effector cells in the lamina propria of IBD patients by producing Th1 and Th2 cytokines, it appears that the excellent therapeutic efficacy of azathioprine in IBD could be due to the induction of local T cell apoptosis. This hypothesis is supported by the finding that successful azathioprine treatment in IBD patients leads to an increased number of apoptotic T cells in the peripheral blood and the lamina propria, whereas no apoptosis is seen in patients unresponsive to azathioprine therapy[17]. Moreover, the clinical responsiveness to 6-MP therapy correlated with the presence of apoptotic mononuclear cells in the gut, while IBD patients who did not respond to azathioprine had no such apoptotic cells[17].

The induction of apoptosis by azathioprine was critically dependent on T cell co-stimulation via the costimulatory molecule CD28 that is known to inhibit TCR-induced apoptosis during a primary T cell response by activation of the antiapoptotic bcl-xL protein. Interestingly, azathioprine down-regulates bcl-xL expression at the mRNA and protein level, strongly suggesting that this drug blocks a key regulatory pathway in CD28 signalling. Therefore, by blocking bcl-xL, azathioprine is capable of inducing a mitochondrial pathway of T cell apoptosis that is dependent on caspase-9 rather than caspase-8. These findings would explain how azathioprine induces selective apoptosis of activated T lymphocytes.

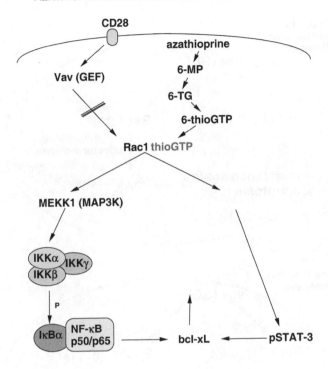

**Figure 1**   Azathioprine blocks Rac1 activation via 6-ThioGTP. For details see text below

The CD28 signalling pathway is important not only for the initial activation of T cells, but also for maintaining their viability and responsiveness during a persistent immune response. Additional studies by Tiede et al.[17] showed that azathioprine-induced suppression of CD28 signalling is due to suppression of the activation of Rac1; a Rac GTPase that is known to play a key role in CD28 signalling[20,21]. Rac proteins play a major role in T cell development, differentiation and proliferation. For instance, whereas dominant positive Rac mutations have been associated with increased cell proliferation and tumours, functionally inactive Rac mutations are associated with immunodeficiencies in humans. Azathioprine-mediated suppression of Rac1 activation in T cells was mediated by direct binding of an azathioprine metabolite (6-ThioGTP) to Rac1. The observed up-regulation of vav expression in azathioprine-treated T cells is most likely an insufficient compensatory mechanism to achieve Rac1 activation by up-regulation of the corresponding guanosine exchange factor. Thus, the molecular mechanism of action of azathioprine is based on the suppression of Rac1 activation via 6-ThioGTP (Figure 1). Azathioprine-induced suppression of Rac1 activation leads to suppression of bcl-xL expression (via blockade of NF-κB and STAT-3 activation) and a mitochondrial pathway of T cell apoptosis. These findings suggest that

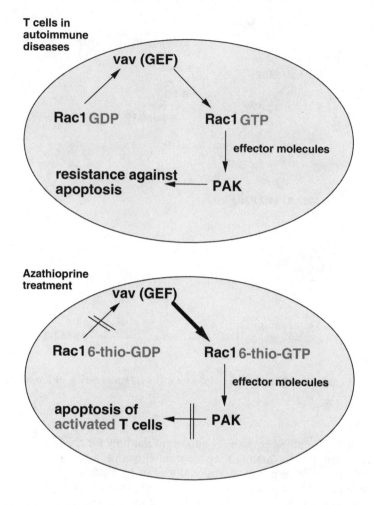

**Figure 2** A molecular mechanism of azathioprine action. Azathioprine blocks vav exchange activity on Rac proteins

azathioprine-induced immunosuppression is mediated by suppression of Rac1 activation and the consecutive induction of T cell apoptosis. It should be noted, however, that azathioprine-induced apoptosis affects mainly CD45RO effector T cells upon costimulation via CD28, suggesting that azathioprine may be particularly effective in eliminating pathogenic memory T cells in autoimmune and chronic inflammatory diseases (Figure 2).

Recent data from various groups suggest that deleting pathogenic T effector cells appears to be beneficial for therapy of IBD patients in general. For instance, antibodies to TNF that are successfully used in treating CD patients (e.g. infliximab) have been shown to induce rapid mucosal T cell apoptosis within several days indicating that the therapeutic efficacy of these antibodies could be due to the induction of T cell apoptosis[22]. Apparently, some anti-TNF antibodies have the capacity to bind to the membrane bound form of TNF on T cells, thereby inducing reverse signalling and induction of T cell death. There is also some evidence that methotrexate and cyclosporin exhibit beneficial effects in IBD patients by targeting T cell activation.

In summary, considerable progress has been made in understanding the immunopathogenesis of IBD in humans. Various studies point towards an important role of T cell apoptosis in experimental colitis and IBD patients. Recent data by Tiede and co-workers indicate that azathioprine induces T cell apoptosis in IBD patients by specifically blocking the Rac1 pathway[17,23]. These data provide a rationale for the design of novel therapeutic strategies in IBD in the near future that are based on the specific blockade of the Rac1 pathway.

# References

1. Elion GB. The George Hitchings and Gertrude Elion Lecture. The pharmacology of azathioprine. Ann NY Acad Sci. 1993;685:400–7.
2. Huglus G. Double-masked trial of azathioprine in multiple sclerosis. Lancet. 1988;2:179–86.
3. Lennard L. The clinical pharmacology of 6-mercaptopurine. Eur J Clin Pharmacol. 1992;43:329–35.
4. Shanahan F. Crohn's disease. Lancet. 2002;359:62–9.
5. Bean RHD. The treatment of chronic active ulcerative colitis with 6-mercaptopurine. Med J Aust. 1962;2:592–3.
6. Present DH, Korelitz BI, Wisch N, Glass JL, Sachar DB, Pasternack BS. Treatment of Crohn's disease with 6-mercaptopurine: a long-term randomized, double-blind study. N Engl J Med. 1980;302:981–7.
7. Ewe K, Press A, Singe CC, Stufler M, Hommel G, Büschenfelde KHM. Azathioprine combined with prednisolone or monotherapy with prednisone in active Crohn's disease. Gastroenterology. 1993;105:367–76.
8. Pearson DC, May GR, Fick GH, Sutherland LR. Azathioprine and 6-mercaptopurine in Crohn disease. A meta-analysis. Ann Intern Med. 1995;123:132–42.
9. Sandborn WJ, Tremaine WJ, Wolf DC et al. Lack of effect of intravenous administration on time to respond to azathioprine for steroid-treated Crohn's disease. Gastroenterology. 1999;117:527–35.
10. Hanauer SB, Korelitz BI, Rutgeerts P et al. Postoperative maintenance of Crohn's disease remission with 6-mercaptopurine, mesalamine, or placebo: A 2-year trial. Gastroenterology. 2004;127:723–9.
11. Hanauer SB. Medical therapy for ulcerative colitis 2004. Gastroenterology. 2004;126:1582–92.
12. Dubinsky MC. Azathioprine, 6-mercaptopurine in inflammatory bowel disease: pharmacology, efficacy, and safety. Clin Gastroenterol Hepatol. 2004;2:731–43.
13. Candy S, Wright J, Gerber M, Adams G, Gerig M, Goodman R. A controlled double blind study of azathioprine in the management of Crohn's disease. Gut. 1995;37:674–8.
14. Targan SR, Deem RL, Liu M, Wang S, Nel A. Definition of a lamina propria T cell responsive state. Enhanced cytokine responsiveness of T cells stimulated through the CD2 pathway. J Immunol. 1995;154:664–75.
15. Boirivant M, Marini M, Di-Felice G et al. Lamina propria T cells in Crohn's disease and other gastrointestinal inflammation show defective CD2 pathway-induced apoptosis. Gastroenterology. 1999;116:557–65.
16. Duchmann R, Zeitz M. Crohn's disease. In: Ogra P, Strober W, editors. Handbook of Mucosal Immunology. New York: Academic Press, 1998:118–34.

17. Tiede I, Fritz G, Strand S et al. CD28-dependent Rac1 activation is the molecular target of azathioprine in primary human CD4+ T lymphocytes. J Clin Invest. 2003;111:1133–45.
18. Fuss IJ, Heller F, Boirivant M et al. Nonclassical CD1d-restricted NK T cells that produce IL-13 characterize an atypical Th2 response in ulcerative colitis. J Clin Invest. 2004;113:1490–7.
19. Fuss I, Neurath MF, Boirivant M et al. Disparate CD4+ lamina propria (LP) lymphocyte secretion profiles in inflammatory bowel disease. J. Immunol. 1996;157:1261–70.
20. Tybulewicz VL, Ardouin L, Prisco A, Reynolds LF. Vav1: a key signal transducer downstream of the TCR. Immunol Rev. 2003;192:42–52.
21. Simon AR, Vikis HG, Stewart S, Fanburg BL, Cochran BH, Guan KL. Regulation of STAT3 by direct binding of the Rac1 GTPase. Science. 2000;290:144–7.
22. Peppelenbosch MP, van-Deventer SJ. T cell apoptosis and inflammatory bowel disease. Gut. 2004;53:1556–8.
23. Poppe D, Tiede I, Fritz G et al. Azathioprine suppresses ERM-dependent T cell-APC conjugation through inhibition of Vav guanosine exchange activity on Rac proteins. J Immunol. 2005 (In press).

# 16
# Pharmacogenetics of azathioprine – useful in clinical practice?

R. IACOB and J.-F. COLOMBEL

## INTRODUCTION

The thiopurines base 6-mercaptopurine (6-MP) and its prodrug azathioprine (AZA) are widely used in the treatment of inflammatory bowel diseases (IBD). Inherited differences in drug metabolism can significantly impact their safety and efficacy. This genetic regulation still provides the best example of pharmacogenetics in IBD even though translation to clinical practice remains controversial[1]. Excellent reviews on this topic have been recently published[2,3].

## CLINICAL PHARMACOLOGY (reviewed in ref 3) (Figure 1)

After absorption, AZA is converted rapidly to 6-MP by a non-enzymatic reaction. 6-MP undergoes a complex biotransformation to its inactive and active metabolites via competing catabolic and anabolic metabolic pathways. About 84% of 6-MP is quickly metabolized by xanthine oxidase (XO) found in high concentrations in enterocytes and hepatocytes. 6-MP also serves as a substrate for the thiopurine methyltransferase (TPMT) enzyme, which methylates 6-MP to the inactive methylated-mercaptopurine metabolite. 6-MP is metabolized to 6-thioinosine 5′-monophosphate (TIMP) by the enzyme hypoxanthine phosphoribyl transferase (HPRT). The three enzymes metabolizing 6-MP are in constant competition for substrate and the concentrations of the metabolites of MP are based on the concentrations of these enzymes. TIMP is eventually metabolized to 6-thioguanine (thioguanine) nucleotides (6-TGN). The cytotoxic and immunosuppressive effects of thiopurines were, until recently, presumed to be primarily mediated via the incorporation of 6-TGN into cellular nucleic acids, ultimately resulting in inhibition of lymphocyte proliferation. Recently, 6-thioguanine triphosphate (6-TGTP) has been shown to bind to Rac1 instead of guanine triphosphate and, with co-stimulation with CD28, leads to inhibition of Rac1 and apoptosis of T lymphocytes[4].

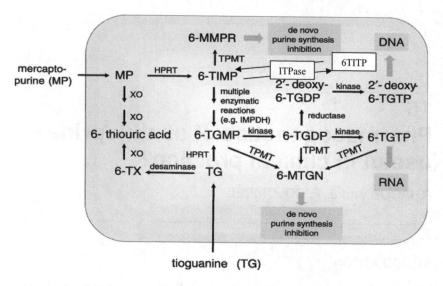

**Figure 1** Metabolic scheme of mercaptopurine and tioguanine. HPRT, hypoxanthine phosphoribosyltransferase; XO, xanthine oxidase; IMPH, inosine monophosphate dehydrogenase; TPMT, thiopurine *S*-methyltransferase; 6-TIMP, 6-thioinosine 5′-monophosphate; 6-MMPR, 6-methylmercaptopurine ribonucleotides; 6-TGMP, 6-thioguanosine 5′-monophosphate; 6-TGDP, 6-thioguanosine 5′-diphosphate; 6-TGTP, 6-thioguanosine 5′-triphosphate; 6-MTGN, 6-methylthioguanine nucleotides; 6-TX, 6 thioxanthine, ITPase, inosine triphosphate pyrophosphatase; 6-TITP, 6-thioinosine triphosphate

## GENETIC VARIATION OF METABOLISM (reviewed in ref 3)

It has been demonstrated that not all individuals methylate thiopurines equally, and that the genetic variability in TPMT enzyme activity is responsible for the majority of the individual differences observed in both the efficacy and toxicity of thiopurines. Approximately 5% of the white population carry one or more variant TPMT alleles. More than 10 variant alleles have been reported. These alleles lead to amino acid substitutions (TPMT*2, *3A, *3C, *3D, *5, *6, *7, *8), formation of a premature stop codon (TPMT*3D), or disruption of splice site (TPMT*4). The functional consequences of alleles *2, *2A, *3B, and *3C, which together account for more than 90% of mutant alleles, have been characterized extensively. The relative frequency of TPMT alleles varies between different ethnic groups: allele *3A accounts for more than 80% of mutant alleles in white populations in the United States and northern Europe, but only 17% of mutant alleles in blacks. Population studies have shown that the distribution of TPMT activity is trimodal: 0.3% of the population have low to absent activity (TPMTL/TPMTL), 11% have intermediate activity (TPMTL/TPMTH), and 89% inherit normal to high enzyme activity (TPMTH/TPMTH). Importantly, a correlation has been observed between TPMT genotype and enzyme activity, with possession of two variant alleles associated with deficient TPMT activity and heterozygosity associated with intermediate enzyme activity. TPMT methylation competes with the activation pathway and influences the relative proportion of intracellular active 6-TGN produced by a given individual. Patients with intermediate or absent TPMT activity can produce significantly higher concentrations of 6-TGN. This inverse relationship between TPMT and 6-TGN has important implications in both the efficacy and toxicity of thiopurines. Data from studies of 6-MP in paediatric patients with acute lymphoblastic leukaemia have shown that low peripheral red blood cell TPMT activity predicts high blood 6-TGN levels and a greater risk of myelotoxicity.

Another genetic variation in the metabolism of AZA has been ascribed to a polymorphism in the gene encoding inosine triphosphate pyrophosphatase (ITPase)[5]. The nucleotide 6-TIMP is a central intermediate in purine metabolism and is converted in guanine nucleotides in nucleated cells (Figure 1). 6-TIMP may also be phosphorylated to 6-TITP. ITPase converts back ITP to IMP so that ITP does not accumulate. Since the identification of the molecular basis of ITPase deficiency, a clinically benign condition characterized by abnormal accumulation of ITP in erythrocytes, the possibility of a correlation between thiopurine toxicity and ITPase deficiency has been raised. Complete ITPase deficiency was found to be associated with a homozygous missense 94C>A mutation that encodes a Pro32Thr exchange, whereas an intronic IVS2+21A>C polymorphism was shown to have a less severe effect, homozygotes retaining 60% ITPase activity. It was then postulated that, in ITPase-deficient patients treated with thiopurine drugs, a 6-thio-ITP metabolite could accumulate, resulting in toxicity[5]

## MONITORING SAFETY

The most commonly observed dose-dependent adverse event is myelosuppression. The relationship of leucopenia and various TPMT genotypes in the setting of AZA or 6-MP treatment has been the focus of several research studies. In a study by Colombel et al. of 41 patients with Crohn's disease (CD) who developed leucopenia while being treated with AZA or MP, 10% of patients were homozygous for TPMT mutant alleles and 17% were heterozygous for TPMT mutant alleles[6]. The median time to leucopenia was significantly shorter in those with homozygous TPMT mutations, 1 month (range 0–1.5) compared with 4 months (range 1–18) in those with one mutant allele, and 3 months (range 0.5–87) in those with normal TPMT. Seventy-three per cent had no known TPMT coding mutations, suggesting that predictive genotyping has a low negative predictive value. These data stress that other factors – both genetic and environmental – may influence TPMT activity and the risk of myelotoxicity, including patient age and renal function and transfusion within the previous 2 months. Other reports outside of the IBD literature also support the positive association between TPMT and leucopenia and have proposed screening patients for low TPMT activity before initiating thiopurine therapy to identify at-risk individuals and to modify dosing[2,3]. The prevalence (one of 300) of low TPMT enzyme is high enough, and the potential complications of myelosuppression severe enough, for some clinicians to recommend obtaining a TPMT enzyme activity level prior to starting therapy. For the majority of thiopurine recipients, clinicians can safely administer what is considered an optimal starting dose of 6-MP (1–1.5 mg · kg$^{-1}$ · day$^{-1}$) and AZA (2.0–2.5 mg · kg$^{-1}$ · day$^{-1}$) as a result of normal to high TPMT activity. It is not yet clear whether patients heterozygous for a TPMT mutation are more likely to develop leucopenia compared to those with normal TPMT. These patients can safely receive thiopurines at lower doses (30–50% of standard dose), and dose escalation can be successful while patients are monitored closely with regular blood counts. A few small studies have suggested that TPMT-deficient patients can safely use low doses of MP/AZA[7], but most often other immunomodulators should be considered. Despite the apparent safety advantage to using pharmacogenetics (TPMT)-based dosing over empiric or weight-based strategies, controversy still remains as to whether TPMT-based dosing really does maximize patient safety and is cost-effective. Whether it is empiric or TPMT-based dosing, patients require regular blood count and liver chemistry monitoring throughout the duration of thiopurine therapy. In patients who do not receive TPMT before dose initiation, clinicians need to consider weekly monitoring for the first month of therapy, because early leucopenia can occur in TPMT-deficient patients treated with standard doses.

In contrast to what we know about the influence of TPMT deficiency on myelosuppression, the safety implications of having high TPMT activity remain unclear[3] Elevated levels of 6-methylmercaptopurine (6-MMP) have been shown to be associated with an increased frequency of hepatotoxicity[8,9]. However, not all patients with AZA liver toxicity have high 6-MMP levels, and not all patients with high 6-MMP levels experience an elevation in transaminase levels.

It is not yet clear whether TPMT genotype or phenotype can also be used to predict other adverse effects of AZA such as nausea, vomiting, hepatitis and pancreatitis, because of conflicting data.

A recent study in 62 patients with IBD reported a significant association between the ITPase 94C>A polymorphism and AZA-related adverse effects, specifically flu-like symptoms, rash, and pancreatitis[10]. No correlation was observed with occurrence of neutropenia but only 11 patients were studied. This prompted us to investigate the occurrence of ITPase mutations in the series of 41 patients with CD patients who had experienced leucopenia during AZA/6-MP therapy in order to evaluate whether genotyping of the ITPase gene could improve the detection rate of patients at risk of thiopurine myelotoxicity[11]. Patients were genotyped for the ITPase 94C>A and IVS2 +21A>C mutations according to a previously described procedure based on endonuclease digestion of polymerase chain reaction products. Allele frequencies in the CD population were 0.085 for the 94C>A mutation and 0.12 for the IVS2+2 1A>C mutation, similar to frequencies observed in the control population (0.06 and 0.13, respectively) (Table 1). There was no significant difference in the genotype distribution between the two populations, which confirmed the lack of association between ITPase deficiency and myelosuppression during thiopurine therapy. Due to the retrospective nature of the study, no correlation with other side-effects could be investigated.

**Table 1** Distribution of ITPase genotypes in 41 Crohn's disease (CD) patients and 100 healthy Caucasians (after ref 11)

| ITPase genotype | CD patients (n = 41) | Control population (n = 100) |
|---|---|---|
| Wt/Wt | 26 (0.63)* | 64 (0.64) |
| Wt/94C>A | 6 (0.15) | 10 (0.10) |
| Wt/IVS2+21A>C | 7 (0.17) | 24 (0.24) |
| 94C>A/94C>A | 0 (0.00) | 0 (0.00) |
| IVS2+21A>C/IVS2+21A>C | 1 (0.02) | 0 (0.00) |
| 94C>A/IVS2+21A>C | 1 (0.02) | 2 (0.02) |

*Values in parentheses represent genotype frequencies.

## MONITORING EFFICACY

The metabolites 6-TGN and 6-MMP have been used to determine likelihood of therapeutic response[2,3]. Initial studies in children reported that 6-TGN was significantly and independently associated with therapeutic response[8]. Discriminant levels of 235–250 pmol/$8 \times 10^8$ have been considered predictive of response. Despite these initial results, there remain conflicting data on the clinical utility of monitoring in IBD. Several studies[2,12] have shown subjects who were in remission receiving MP or AZA with 6-TGN levels lower than 235–250 pmol/$8 \times 10^8$. The positive predictive value for remission of 6-TGN levels >230–250 range from 24% to 83%[2]. Perhaps the most significant role of metabolite monitoring is in defining therapeutic failures[3]. Non-compliance and underdosing remain the most common reasons for therapeutic failure. Both of these can be uncovered by measuring 6-MP metabolite levels. When both 6-TGN and 6-MMP levels are undetectable, there is a high likelihood that the patient is not adhering to therapy. However, a subgroup of patients continues to fail therapy despite dose escalation and receiving standard or even higher than standard doses of thiopurines. These patients can be divided into two distinct subgroups and are defined biochemically by their metabolite profiles. The most common subgroup is composed of patients resistant to thiopurines and biochemically characterized by the persistence of subtherapeutic 6-TGN (<235) and the preferential shunting towards excessive potentially hepatotoxic 6-MMP levels on 6-MP/AZA dose escalation. Individuals unmask this metabolic profile when they are challenged with higher doses of the drug. There is a small group of refractory patients who, despite therapeutic (>235) and often potentially toxic 6-TGN (>450) levels, are unable to benefit from the immunosuppressive properties of these therapies. The identification of these two subgroups early in the course of therapy can significantly improve patient outcomes by moving patients quickly to alternative immunomodulator therapy.

Therapeutic drug monitoring in IBD provides physicians with an alternative approach to thiopurine dose optimization. Levels can help differentiate between non-compliance, underdosing, drug resistance, and refractory states. In the former two case scenarios, clinicians might safely dose escalate or reintroduce drug. As with TPMT testing, metabolite monitoring is not considered standard of care. There are many clinicians who choose to follow the complete blood count and mean corpuscular volume as markers of compliance and toxicity, and use these tests to gauge decisions with regard to dosing. Regardless of what strategy is chosen, patients need to be carefully monitored and well informed about the potential risks but, most importantly, the clear benefits, associated with thiopurine therapy. Prospective randomized dose-optimization studies are currently under way to determine whether individualized (pharmacogenetic/TPMT and pharmacokinetic/6-TGN based) dosing is superior, in both safety and efficacy, to weight-based dosing. Recent advances in the understanding of the mechanism of action of thiopurines and the prominent role of the 6-thioguanine triphosphate nucleotide may offer some new therapeutic benefit of metabolite monitoring in the management of IBD.

## CONCLUSION

In summary, although there is consensus that measurement of TPMT activity or genotype may be useful for avoiding the use of AZA in individuals possessing two TPMT variant alleles (1/300 patients), the use of these tests in directing therapy for the overwhelming majority of individuals (heterozygotes or those possessing no variant alleles) remains highly controversial. Application of ITPase genotyping tests does not seem to improve the identification of patients at risk of myelosuppression with AZA/6-MP therapy. Therefore, continued monitoring of white and red blood cell counts remains mandatory for all patients. Further work is needed on the role of other candidate genes that may be involved in thiopurine haematotoxicity.

Therapeutic drug monitoring by measuring 6-TGN and 6-MMP levels in patients treated with AZA or 6-MP may be most useful, and can be considered in patients suspected of non-compliance and possibly patients who are failing to respond to standard doses of drug. The latter has yet to be proven in a prospective controlled fashion. Results of ongoing studies comparing the benefit of dosing based upon 6-TG levels vs weight-based dosing are eagerly waited.

## References

1.  Ahmad T, Tamboli CP, Jewell D, Colombel JF. Clinical relevance of advances in genetics and pharmacogenetics of IBD. Gastroenterology. 2004;126:1533–49.
2.  Aberra FN, Lichtenstein GR. Review article: Monitoring of immunomodulators in inflammatory bowel disease. Aliment Pharmacol Ther. 2005;21:307–19.
3.  Dubinsky MC. Azathioprine, 6-mercaptopurine in inflammatory bowel disease: pharmacology, efficacy, and safety. Clin Gastroenterol Hepatol. 2004;2:731–43.
4.  Tiede I, Fritz G, Strand S et al. CD28-dependent Rac1 activation is the molecular target of azathioprine in primary human CD4+ T lymphocytes. J Clin Invest. 2003;111:1133–45.
5.  Sumi S, Marinaki AM, Arenas M et al. Genetic basis of inosine triphosphate pyrophosphohydrolase deficiency. Hum Genet. 2002;111:360–7.

6. Colombel JF, Ferrari N, Debuysere H et al. Genotypic analysis of thiopurine *S*-methyltransferase in patients with Crohn's disease and severe myelosuppression during azathioprine therapy. Gastroenterology. 2000;118:1025–30.
7. Kaskas BA, Louis E, Hindorf U et al. Safe treatment of thiopurine *S*-methyltransferase deficient Crohn's disease patients with azathioprine. Gut. 2003;52:140–2.
8. Dubinsky MC, Lamothe S, Yang HY et al. Pharmacogenomics and metabolite measurement for 6-mercaptopurine therapy in inflammatory bowel disease. Gastroenterology. 2000;118:705–13.
9. Dubinsky MC, Yang H, Hassard PV et al. 6-MP metabolite profiles provide a biochemical explanation for 6-MP resistance in patients with inflammatory bowel disease. Gastroenterology. 2002;122:904–15.
10. Marinaki AM, Ansari A, Duley JA et al. Adverse drug reactions to azathioprine therapy are associated with polymorphism in the gene encoding inosine triphosphate pyrophosphatase (ITPase). Pharmacogenetics. 2004;14:181–7.
11. Allorge D, Hamdan R, Broly F, Libersa C, Colombel JF. ITPA genotyping test does not improve detection of Crohn's disease patients at risk of azathioprine/6-mercaptopurine induced myelosuppression. Gut. 2005;54:565.
12. Griffiths AM. Monitoring of azathioprine/6-mercaptopurine treatment in children is not necessary. Inflamm Bowel Dis. 2003;9:389–91.

# 17
# Azathioprine: long-term side-effects
### E. V. LOFTUS Jr

## REAL-WORLD EXPERIENCES WITH AZATHIOPRINE (AZA) AND 6-MERCAPTOPURINE (6-MP)

The experience of thiopurines in randomized controlled trials for Crohn's disease is generally favourable. In a 1995 meta-analysis, Pearson and colleagues estimated a pooled odds ratio (OR) of study withdrawal due to adverse events from thiopurines of 5.3 (95% CI 2.2–12.6)[1]. The prevalence of study withdrawals due to adverse events ranged from 0% to 15%, and the average rate was 9% (versus 2% in placebo-treated patients). In the past several years a number of observational studies suggest that the rate of withdrawal from thiopurines due to adverse events is higher in a 'real-world setting.' Five studies published between 2002 and 2004 suggest that the prevalence of stopping AZA or 6-MP due to adverse events ranged from 22% to 28% (Table 1)[2–6]. It remains to be seen whether different methods of administering AZA or 6-MP result in different rates of short-term adverse events. For example, nausea is a frequent cause for withdrawal in these observational studies. Perhaps administering AZA initially at a low dose and then gradually increasing the dose would result in fewer withdrawals due to nausea. Another point to remember is that approximately half of patients who discontinue AZA for reasons other than allergic-type reactions seem to tolerate 6-MP[3,7,8].

**Table 1** 'Real-world' experiences with azathioprine and 6-mercaptopurine in inflammatory bowel disease

| Setting (reference) | n | Withdrawal due to adverse events |
|---|---|---|
| Olmsted County, Minnesota[3] | 102 | 25 |
| Canterbury, New Zealand[4] | 216 | 26 |
| Oxford, UK[2] | 622 | 28 |
| Groningen, Netherlands[6] | 318 | 23 |
| Nijmegen, Netherlands[5] | 50 | 22 |

## WHAT IS THE ROLE OF INOSINE TRIPHOSPHATE PYROPHOSPHATASE POLYMORPHISMS?

The enzyme inosine triphosphate pyrophosphatase (ITPA) plays a role in thiopurine metabolism. ITPA dephosphorylates the phosphorylated derivatives of 6-thio-inosine monophosphate. It has been hypothesized that polymorphisms in the ITPA gene may explain some of the idiosyncratic reactions that are observed with the use of these agents (e.g. flu-like symptoms, rash, and pancreatitis). One study compared 62 inflammatory bowel disease (IBD) patients who had experienced adverse reactions to AZA to 68 patients who had tolerated the drug for at least 3 months[9]. The ITPA polymorphism 94C > A was significantly associated with adverse events overall. The allele frequency of this polymorphism was 17% in those patients who had experienced idiosyncratic reactions and only 4% in the patients who had tolerated the drug (OR 4.2; 95% CI 1.6–11.5)[9]. When individual adverse events were examined, the OR for flu-like symptoms was 4.7 (95% CI 1.2–18.1), for rash, 10.3 (95% CI 4.7–62.9), and for pancreatitis 6.2 (95% CI 1.1–32.6). However, other studies have not been able to confirm these findings[10].

Some have speculated that ITPA polymorphisms may explain in part leucopenia following AZA or 6-MP therapy[11,12]. In one study of 41 Crohn's disease patients with leucopenia and 100 controls the prevalence of the 94 C > A polymorphism was 15% in leucopenic patients versus only 10% in the controls[12]. In another study of 254 IBD patients and 129 healthy volunteers, leucopenia was identified in 11% of the IBD patients. The 94 C > A polymorphism was identified in 25% of the leucopenic patients but in only 10% of the controls. In this study, however, 94 C > A polymorphisms did not predict hepatotoxicity or pancreatitis[11]. At the present time it is hard to make definitive conclusions about the role of ITPA polymorphisms in the idiosyncratic reactions seen with thiopurines, and more studies are needed to confirm or refute these observations.

## HAEMATOLOGICAL ADVERSE EVENTS: ROLE OF DRUG INTERACTIONS

Variations in thiopurine methyltransferase (TPMT) activity may explain only a small proportion of leucopenic events in patients taking thiopurines. Typically, TPMT explains early leucopenic events but not late ones. In a French study, TPMT deficiency explained only 27% of all leucopenic events[13]. The role of ITPA polymorphisms in leucopenic events remains unclear. It is important to note that patients on thiopurines need to be monitored periodically for leucopenia indefinitely while on medication.

Interactions with other medications typically used in IBD may explain some delayed leucopenic events. In one study of 34 Crohn's disease patients who were in remission on stable doses of AZA or 6-MP, serial leucocyte counts and thioguanine nucleotide levels were obtained before and after the introduction of sulphasalazine, mesalamine, and balsalazide[14]. Significant leucopenia (WBC < 3500) occurred over the next 8 weeks in five patients receiving mesalamine

1000 mg q.i.d. (50%), six patients taking sulphasalazine 1000 mg q.i.d. (54%), and two patients taking balsalazide 2.25 g t.i.d. (20%). Serum thioguanine nucleotide levels rose significantly after the introduction of either mesalamine or sulphasalazine[14].

The influence of infliximab on thioguanine nucleotide levels and leucocyte counts was studied in 32 Crohn's disease patients on stable doses of AZA[15]. These patients were on a median AZA dose of 2.8 mg/kg body weight daily (range, 0.6–3.6). After infliximab infusions were begun, the mean serum thioguanine nucleotide level rose from 277 pmol/$8 \times 10^8$ erythrocytes to 442 pmol/$8 \times 10^8$ erythrocytes over the next 1–3 weeks, and the mean leucocyte count dropped from $4.3 \times 10^9$/L to $3.6 \times 10^9$/L in the same time frame ($p < 0.01$)[15].

## FERTILITY, TERATOGENICITY, AND PREGNANCY SAFETY

Few studies have examined the effects of AZA or 6-MP on fertility in men with IBD. Dejaco and colleagues studied 18 men with IBD who had been on AZA for at least 3 months[16]. They measured semen quality via a number of parameters, including total sperm count, density, motility, and morphology. By all measures, semen quality was normal in this group of men[16]. A group of 11 men with IBD who were started on AZA after their first semen analysis were analysed. At baseline the semen parameters were slightly diminished compared to what would have been expected in normals[16]. There was no worsening in these parameters after a mean of 11 months of AZA treatment. The authors also described six men who were on AZA who fathered seven healthy children[16].

There has been concern for many years about the potential teratogenicity of AZA or 6-MP. The active metabolites can cross the placenta. Data in the IBD literature are fairly limited. The biggest and best studies come from the transplant and rheumatology (systemic lupus erythematosus) literature. In one study of 146 kidney transplant recipients who were on either AZA plus corticosteroids or AZA alone, low birth weights occurred in 39% of the offspring, premature births were seen in 52%, and congenital anomalies were identified in 4% of offspring[17]. The background rate in the general population of congenital anomalies is approximately 3%.

In one study of AZA and 6-MP use during pregnancy in patients seen at a single private practice in New York City over a 40-year period, a total of 76 women were observed on 6-MP at some point during their pregnancy[18]. Among the 61 women who stopped 6-MP once they discovered they were pregnant, 72% achieved full term in their pregnancies, 5% had premature birth, 16% had spontaneous abortion, 3% had offspring with congenital anomalies, and 2% had offspring with neonatal or early childhood infections. Among the 15 pregnancies in which 6-MP was continued throughout the pregnancy, 67% went to full term, 27% were premature births, and 7% had spontaneous abortions[18]. The prevalences of congenital anomalies and neonatal infections were 7% and 13%, respectively. A multivariate analysis of all factors potentially associated with adverse pregnancy outcomes suggested that the odds ratio of a successful pregnancy outcome in women on 6-MP was 0.8 (95% CI 0.5–1.5)[18]. In a second paper from a different private practice in New York City, among 72 pregnancies in women on 6-MP, 71% had live births, 22% had spontaneous abortions, 3% had ectopic pregnancies, and fetal demise occurred in 29%. Congenital anomalies were observed in 6% of all offspring[19]. In a population-based study from North Jutland, Denmark, a total of 10 women who were on a purine analogue during their entire pregnancy were identified out of a total of 19 418 pregnancies[20]. Thirty per cent of these pregnancies were associated with low birth weight, 30% had pre-term birth, and 20% had congenital anomalies. The risk of perinatal death was 10%[20]. All three of these studies are hampered by very small sample sizes, and future studies of pregnancy safety with thiopurines in IBD patients are desperately needed.

## INFECTIOUS COMPLICATIONS OF AZATHIOPRINE

A study of 410 IBD patients on thiopurines from Lenox Hill Hospital in New York City over a 20-year period showed that infections occurred in up to 14% of patients[21]. Pneumonia was observed in 4%, and herpes zoster infections were seen in 3%. Cytomegalovirus infections occurred in less than 1%. Upper respiratory infections were seen in 7%. It is not well understood if combination therapy with anti-tumour necrosis factor agents and immunosuppressives will synergistically increase the risk of infection. Many centres currently advocate such combination therapy to reduce the risk of formation of antibodies to infliximab. One study of 217 IBD patients from Stockholm County, Sweden, who had received such combination therapy, observed severe infections in 18 patients (8%), including two patients who died of sepsis[22]. In an observational study from Mayo Clinic, among 500 Crohn's disease patients who received infliximab (the majority of whom were on combination therapy), infections were observed in 41 patients (8%)[23]. This included two deaths from sepsis and two deaths from pneumonia. Further studies are needed to compare the efficacy and safety of infliximab alone with azathioprine alone and with combination therapy.

## HEPATOTOXICITY OF THIOPURINES

The overall prevalence of hepatic biochemical abnormalities in patients receiving thiopurines is estimated to be 3–4%[24]. Most of these abnormalities are dose-dependent. It has been hypothesized that hepatotoxicity in many cases may be related to over-accumulation of 6-methylmercaptopurine ribonucleotides due to high TPMT activity[25]. Some hepatic biochemical abnormalities seem to resolve spontaneously or with dose reduction. Serious hepatotoxicity, including cholestatic liver injury[26], veno-occlusive disease of the liver[27] and nodular regenerative hyperplasia[28], have been uncommonly reported following treatment with AZA or 6-MP. The true incidence of serious hepatotoxicity with these agents is unknown.

Many researchers were encouraged by the initial results reported with 6-thioguanine as a primary treatment for IBD[29-32]. Fewer idiosyncratic reactions, such as fever and pancreatitis, occurred with this agent. However, serious hepatotoxicity in up to 26% of 6-thioguanine-treated treated patients has been reported[33]. This hepatotoxicity includes nodular regenerative hyperplasia, early hepatic fibrosis, acute sinusoidal obstruction, and veno-occlusive disease of the liver[34-36]. Many clinicians have concluded that the risk of serious hepatotoxicity outweighs the potential benefits of 6-thioguanine therapy in patients intolerant of AZA and 6-MP.

## LYMPHOMA RISK WITH THIOPURINES

In order to estimate the risk of lymphoma with purine analogue therapy in IBD one must understand the presence and magnitude of lymphoma risk in the IBD population as a whole. Studies from referral centres indicate a two-fold to six-fold increase in relative risk of lymphoma; however, the influence of referral bias with these studies is not entirely clear[37]. An alternative hypothesis to explain the increased risk in referral populations is that perhaps lymphoma is associated with more severe forms of IBD. The vast majority of population-based studies of lymphoma risk in IBD indicate little or no increased risk (Table 2)[38-45].

**Table 2** Population-based studies of lymphoma in inflammatory bowel disease

| Reference | Setting | Patients | Relative risk (95% CI) |
|---|---|---|---|
| Ekbom et al.[38] | Uppsala, Sweden | CD 1655 | 0.4 (0–2.4) |
| | | UC 3121 | 1.2 (0.5–2.4) |
| Persson et al.[58] | Stockholm, Sweden | CD 1251 | 1.4 (0.4–3.5) |
| Karlen et al.[40] | Stockholm, Sweden | UC 1547 | 1.2 (0.3–3.5) |
| Loftus et al.[41] | Olmsted County, USA | CD 216 | 2.4 (0.1–13) |
| | | UC 238 | 0 (0–6.4) |
| Palli et al.[42] | Florence, Italy | CD 231 | 2.5 (0.3–9) |
| | | UC 689 | 9.3 (2.5–24) |
| Bernstein et al.[43] | Manitoba, Canada | CD 2857 | 2.4 (1.2–5) |
| | | UC 2672 | 1.0 (0.5–2.2) |
| Lewis et al.[44] | GPRD, UK | CD 6605 | 1.4 (0.5–3.4) |
| | | UC 10 391 | 1.2 (0.7–2.1) |
| Askling et al.[45] | Multiple Swedish cohorts | CD 20 120 | 1.3 (1.0–1.6) |
| | | UC 27 559 | 1.0 (0.8–1.3) |

95% CI, 95% confidence intervals; CD, Crohn's disease; UC, ulcerative colitis; GPRD, General Practice Research Database.

**Table 3** Lymphoma risk in inflammatory bowel disease patients on thiopurines: meta-analysis

| Reference | Setting | N | Observed | Expected | SIR (95% CI) |
|---|---|---|---|---|---|
| Kinlen[46] | UK | 321 | 2 | 0.16 | 12.5 (1.2–46) |
| Connell et al.[47] | London | 755 | 0 | 0.52 | 0 |
| Farrell et al.[48] | Dublin, Ireland | 238 | 2 | 0.05 | 37.5 (3.5–138) |
| Fraser et al.[49] | Oxford, UK | 626 | 3 | 0.65 | 4.6 (0.9–13.7) |
| Korelitz et al.[50] | New York City, USA | 486 | 3 | 0.61 | 4.9 (0.9–14.5) |
| Lewis et al.[44] | GPRD, UK | 1465 | 1 | 0.64 | 1.6 (0.001–9) |
| Pooled analysis | | 3891 | 11 | 2.63 | 4.2 (2.1–7.5) |

Adapted from Kandiel et al.[51]
SIR, standardized incidence ratio (observed/expected); 95% CI, 95% confidence intervals; GPRD, General Practice Research Database.

Studies of lymphoma risk in IBD patients on AZA and 6-MP from several population-based and referral-based cohorts do not individually demonstrate an increased relative risk of lymphoma, with one exception (Table 3)[44,46–50]. In a recently published meta-analysis the pooled relative risk for lymphoma in IBD patients on 6-MP or AZA was increased roughly four-fold[51]. In a sensitivity analysis, where studies with the highest or lowest relative risk were excluded, the results remained significant.

It appears that many lymphomas occurring in IBD patients on thiopurines are positive for the Epstein–Barr virus (EBV). In a study from Mayo Clinic, six IBD patients with lymphoma were identified between 1985 and 1992, and only one of these patients was EBV-positive. In contrast, a total of 12 such patients were identified between 1993 and 2000, approximately half of these lymphomas were EBV-positive, and all but one of these patients were on thiopurine therapy[52]. Few studies have examined the effect of immunosuppressive medications on the viral load of EBV. One study of 138 Crohn's disease patients with serial EBV viral load measurements was only able to identify two patients with viral loads in a range that would be compatible with lymphoma risk[53]. There was no clear-cut relationship between immuno-suppressive therapy and viral loads in these two patients, however.

The increased relative risk of lymphoma looms large in many practitioners' decisions to prescribe thiopurines. In these settings of uncertainty, sometimes decision analysis models can help clarify the benefits and risks of such therapy. One Markov model examined the gain of quality-adjusted life-years in a theoretical 35-year-old Crohn's disease patient who was given AZA[54]. The base case assumed a three-fold increase of lymphoma, and a 50% reduction in Crohn's disease-related mortality, in a patient taking AZA. Ten years of AZA therapy resulted in a gain of 1.25 quality-adjusted life-months[54]. In the sensitivity analyses AZA was no longer beneficial if the risk of death from a severe flare of Crohn's disease was less than 0.06%, if the relative lymphoma risk was eight times normal, if the background risk of lymphoma in Crohn's disease was greater than four times normal, and if the fear of AZA-related lymphoma resulted in a greater than 1% decrease in overall utility. Thus, in most situations, it appears that the benefits of AZA therapy will outweigh the risks, even after factoring in the increased relative risk of lymphoma[54].

It is not clear if prolonged leucopenia increases the cancer risk in patients on 6-MP. One study of 600 IBD patients treated with 6-MP at Lenox Hill Hospital in New York tried to answer this question[55]. In this cohort of patients, 31 developed sustained leucopenia, defined as a leucocyte count of less than 4000 for at least $2\frac{1}{2}$ weeks. Three matched controls, without leucopenia, were identified for each case. Eight cancers were noted in the 31 leucopenic patients (26%), versus 8% in the controls ($p = 0.017$)[55]. These cancers included leucaemias in two patients and a non-Hodgkin lymphoma in one. No colorectal cancers were observed.

Other cancers may occur at an increased frequency in patients on AZA and 6-MP. Non-melanoma skin cancer, especially squamous cell cancer, has been described in the transplant literature, with cumulative risks of up to 34% at 5 years after transplantation[56,57]. This risk may increase further with the addition of cyclosporin to the immunosuppressive regimen. Although some IBD cohort studies do show an increased risk of colorectal cancer following AZA therapy[47], this is to be expected given the extent and duration of colonic inflammation among patients in these cohorts.

## CONCLUSIONS

1. The tolerance of AZA and 6-MP in 'real-world' experiences may not be as good as the data seen in randomized clinical trials, with withdrawal rates of up to 28%.

2. Inosine triphosphate pyrophosphatase polymorphisms may explain some toxicity such as fever and pancreatitis, but data are conflicting.

3. Drug interactions between thiopurines and 5-aminosalicylate agents or infliximab may result in leucopenia.

4. Data on the safety of thiopurines in pregnancy in the IBD literature are sparse. There may be a small but real risk of adverse outcome, but the benefit of keeping the mother in remission may outweigh this risk. This needs to be discussed extensively with the patient.

5. Most hepatotoxicity in AZA- and 6-MP-treated patients is mild and reversible, but rarely, more serious hepatic injury may occur.

6. Most population-based studies of lymphoma in IBD suggest little to no increased relative risk.

7. The relative risk of lymphoma with AZA and 6-MP use is probably increased, up to four-fold; however, the absolute risk of lymphoma remains low.

8. Epstein–Barr virus is typically found in the lymphomas of IBD patients who are on purine analogue therapy.

## References

1. Pearson DC, May GR, Fick GH, Sutherland LR. Azathioprine and 6-mercaptopurine in Crohn disease. A meta-analysis. Ann Intern Med. 1995;123:132–42.
2. Fraser AG, Orchard TR, Jewell DP. The efficacy of azathioprine for the treatment of inflammatory bowel disease: a 30 year review. Gut. 2002;50:485–9.
3. Loftus CG, Loftus EV, Tremaine WJ, Sandborn WJ. The safety profile of azathioprine/6-mercaptopurine in the treatment of inflammatory bowel disease: a population-based study in Olmsted County, Minnesota. Am J Gastroenterol. 2003;98:S242 (Abstract).
4. Gearry RB, Barclay ML, Burt MJ, Collett JA, Chapman BA. Thiopurine drug adverse effects in a population of New Zealand patients with inflammatory bowel disease. Pharmacoepidemiol Drug Safety. 2004;13:563–7.
5. de Jong DJ, Goullet M, Naber TH. Side effects of azathioprine in patients with Crohn's disease. Eur J Gastroenterol Hepatol. 2004;16:207–12.
6. Weersma RK, Peters FT, Oostenbrug LE et al. Increased incidence of azathioprine-induced pancreatitis in Crohn's disease compared with other diseases. Aliment Pharmacol Ther. 2004;20:843–50.
7. Boulton-Jones JR, Pritchard K, Mahmoud AA. The use of 6-mercaptopurine in patients with inflammatory bowel disease after failure of azathioprine therapy. Aliment Pharmacol Ther. 2000;14:1561–5.
8. McGovern DP, Travis SP, Duley J, Shobowale-Bakre el M, Dalton HR. Azathioprine intolerance in patients with IBD may be imidazole-related and is independent of TPMT activity. Gastroenterology. 2002;122:838–9.
9. Marinaki AM, Ansari A, Duley JA et al. Adverse drug reactions to azathioprine therapy are associated with polymorphism in the gene encoding inosine triphosphate pyrophosphatase (ITPase). Pharmacogenetics. 2004;14:181–7.
10. Gearry RB, Roberts RL, Barclay ML, Kennedy MA. Lack of association between the ITPA 94C>A polymorphism and adverse effects from azathioprine. Pharmacogenetics. 2004;14:779–81.
11. Zelinkova Z, Derijks L, Stokkers P et al. Azathioprine induced myelosuppression is related to ITPA but not TPMT gene polymorphism in IBD patients. Gut. 2004;53:A49 (Abstract).
12. Allorge D, Hamdan R, Broly F, Libersa C, Colombel JF. ITPA genotyping test does not improve detection of Crohn's disease patients at risk of azathioprine/6-mercaptopurine induced myelosuppression. Gut. 2005;54:565.
13. Colombel JF, Ferrari N, Debuysere H et al. Genotypic analysis of thiopurine S-methyltransferase in patients with Crohn's disease and severe myelosuppression during azathioprine therapy. Gastroenterology. 2000;118:1025–30.
14. Lowry PW, Franklin CL, Weaver AL et al. Leucopenia resulting from a drug interaction between azathioprine or 6-mercaptopurine and mesalamine, sulphasalazine, or balsalazide. Gut. 2001;49:656–64.
15. Roblin X, Serre-Debeauvais F, Phelip JM, Bessard G, Bonaz B. Drug interaction between infliximab and azathioprine in patients with Crohn's disease. Aliment Pharmacol Ther. 2003;18:917–25.
16. Dejaco C, Mittermaier C, Reinisch W et al. Azathioprine treatment and male fertility in inflammatory bowel disease. Gastroenterology. 2001;121:1048–53.
17. Armenti VT, Ahlswede KM, Ahlswede BA, Jarrell BE, Moritz MJ, Burke JF. National Transplantation Pregnancy Registry – outcomes of 154 pregnancies in cyclosporine-treated female kidney transplant recipients. Transplantation. 1994;57:502–6.

18. Francella A, Dyan A, Bodian C, Rubin P, Chapman M, Present DH. The safety of 6-mercaptopurine for childbearing patients with inflammatory bowel disease: a retrospective cohort study. Gastroenterology. 2003;124:9–17.
19. Zlatanic J, Korelitz BI, Rajapakse R et al.. Complications of pregnancy and child development after cessation of treatment with 6-mercaptopurine for inflammatory bowel disease. J Clin Gastroenterol. 2003;36:303–9.
20. Norgard B, Pedersen L, Fonager K, Rasmussen SN, Sorensen HT. Azathioprine, mercaptopurine and birth outcome: a population-based cohort study. Aliment Pharmacol Ther. 2003;17:827–34.
21. Warman JI, Korelitz BI, Fleisher MR et al. Cumulative experience with short- and long-term toxicity to 6-mercaptopurine in the treatment of Crohn's disease and ulcerative colitis. J Clin Gastroenterol. 2003;37:220–5.
22. Ljung T, Karlen P, Schmidt D et al. Infliximab in inflammatory bowel disease: clinical outcome in a population based cohort from Stockholm County. Gut. 2004;53:849–53.
23. Colombel JF, Loftus EV Jr, Tremaine WJ et al. The safety profile of infliximab in patients with Crohn's disease: the Mayo clinic experience in 500 patients. Gastroenterology. 2004; 126:19–31.
24. Present DH, Meltzer SJ, Krumholz MP, Wolke A, Korelitz BI. 6-Mercaptopurine in the management of inflammatory bowel disease: short- and long-term toxicity. Ann Intern Med. 1989;111:641–9.
25. Dubinsky MC, Yang H, Hassard PV et al 6-MP metabolite profiles provide a biochemical explanation for 6-MP resistance in patients with inflammatory bowel disease. Gastroenterology. 2002;122:904–15.
26. Romagnuolo J, Sadowski DC, Lalor E, Jewell L, Thomson AB. Cholestatic hepatocellular injury with azathioprine: a case report and review of the mechanisms of hepatotoxicity. Can J Gastroenterol. 1998;12:479–83.
27. Holtmann M, Schreiner O, Kohler H et al. Veno-occlusive disease (VOD) in Crohn's disease (CD) treated with azathioprine. Dig Dis Sci. 2003;48:1503–5.
28. Daniel F, Cadranel JF, Seksik P et al. Azathioprine induced nodular regenerative hyperplasia in IBD patients. Gastroenterol Clin Biol. 2005;29:600–3.
29. Dubinsky MC, Hassard PV, Seidman EG et al. An open-label pilot study using thioguanine as a therapeutic alternative in Crohn's disease patients resistant to 6-mercaptopurine therapy. Inflamm Bowel Dis. 2001;7:181–9.
30. Bonaz B, Boitard J, Marteau P et al. Thioguanine in patients with Crohn's disease intolerant or resistant to azathioprine/mercaptopurine. Aliment Pharmacol Ther. 2003;18: 401–8.
31. Derijks LJ, de Jong DJ, Gilissen LP et al. 6-Thioguanine seems promising in azathioprine-or 6-mercaptopurine-intolerant inflammatory bowel disease patients: a short-term safety assessment. Eur J Gastroenterol Hepatol. 2003;15:63–7.
32. Herrlinger KR, Kreisel W, Schwab M et al. 6-thioguanine – efficacy and safety in chronic active Crohn's disease. Aliment Pharmacol Ther. 2003;17:503–8.
33. Dubinsky MC, Vasiliauskas EA, Singh H et al. 6-Thioguanine can cause serious liver injury in inflammatory bowel disease patients. Gastroenterology. 2003;125:298–303.
34. Geller SA, Dubinsky MC, Poordad FF et al. Early hepatic nodular hyperplasia and submicroscopic fibrosis associated with 6-thioguanine therapy in inflammatory bowel disease. Am J Surg Pathol. 2004;28:1204–11.
35. Kane S, Cohen SM, Hart J. Acute sinusoidal obstruction syndrome after 6-thioguanine therapy for Crohn's disease. Inflamm Bowel Dis. 2004;10:652–4.
36. Shastri S, Dubinsky MC, Fred Poordad F, Vasiliauskas EA, Geller SA. Early nodular hyperplasia of the liver occurring with inflammatory bowel diseases in association with thioguanine therapy. Arch Pathol Lab Med. 2004;128:49–53.
37. Loftus EV Jr, Sandborn WJ. Lymphoma risk in inflammatory bowel disease: influences of referral bias and therapy. Gastroenterology. 2001;121:1239–42.
38. Ekbom A, Helmick C, Zack M, Adami HO. Extracolonic malignancies in inflammatory bowel disease. Cancer. 1991;67:2015–19.
39. Persson PG, Karlen P, Bernell O et al. Crohn's disease and cancer: a population-based cohort study. Gastroenterology. 1994;107:1675–9.

40. Karlen P, Lofberg R, Brostrom O, Leijonmarck CE, Hellers G, Persson PG. Increased risk of cancer in ulcerative colitis: a population-based cohort study. Am J Gastroenterol. 1999; 94:1047–52.
41. Loftus EV Jr, Tremaine WJ, Habermann TM, Harmsen WS, Zinsmeister AR, Sandborn WJ. Risk of lymphoma in inflammatory bowel disease. Am J Gastroenterol. 2000;95:2308–12.
42. Palli D, Trallori G, Bagnoli S et al. Hodgkin's disease risk is increased in patients with ulcerative colitis. Gastroenterology. 2000;119:647–53.
43. Bernstein CN, Blanchard JF, Kliewer E, Wajda A. Cancer risk in patients with inflammatory bowel disease: a population-based study. Cancer. 2001;91:854–62.
44. Lewis JD, Bilker WB, Brensinger C, Deren JJ, Vaughn DJ, Strom BL. Inflammatory bowel disease is not associated with an increased risk of lymphoma. Gastroenterology. 2001;121: 1080–7.
45. Askling J, Brandt L, Lapidus A et al. Risk of haematopoietic cancer in patients with inflammatory bowel disease. Gut. 2005;54:617–22.
46. Kinlen LJ. Incidence of cancer in rheumatoid arthritis and other disorders after immunosuppressive treatment. Am J Med. 1985;78:44–9.
47. Connell WR, Kamm MA, Dickson M, Balkwill AM, Ritchie JK, Lennard-Jones JE. Long-term neoplasia risk after azathioprine treatment in inflammatory bowel disease. Lancet. 1994;343:1249–52.
48. Farrell RJ, Ang Y, Kileen P et al. Increased incidence of non-Hodgkin's lymphoma in inflammatory bowel disease patients on immunosuppressive therapy but overall risk is low. Gut. 2000;47:514–9.
49. Fraser AG, Orchard TR, Robinson EM, Jewell DP. Long-term risk of malignancy after treatment of inflammatory bowel disease with azathioprine. Aliment Pharmacol Ther. 2002;16:1225–32.
50. Korelitz BI, Mirsky FJ, Fleisher MR, Warman JI, Wisch N, Gleim GW. Malignant neoplasms subsequent to treatment of inflammatory bowel disease with 6-mercaptopurine. Am J Gastroenterol. 1999;94:3248–53.
51. Kandiel A, Fraser AG, Korelitz BI, Brensinger C, Lewis JD. Increased risk of lymphoma among inflammatory bowel disease patients treated with azathioprine and 6-mercaptopurine. Gut. 2005;54:1121–5.
52. Dayharsh GA, Loftus EV Jr, Sandborn WJ et al. Epstein-Barr virus-positive lymphoma in patients with inflammatory bowel disease treated with azathioprine or 6-mercaptopurine. Gastroenterology. 2002;122:72–7.
53. Reijasse D, Le Pendeven C, Cosnes J et al. Epstein-Barr virus viral load in Crohn's disease: effect of immunosuppressive therapy. Inflamm Bowel Dis. 2004;10:85–90.
54. Lewis JD, Schwartz JS, Lichtenstein GR. Azathioprine for maintenance of remission in Crohn's disease: benefits outweigh the risk of lymphoma. Gastroenterology. 2000;118: 1018–24.
55. DiSanti WD, Rajapakse R, Korelitz BI, Panagopoulos G, Furer S, Janamillo-Nieves L. Increased incidence of neoplasms in patients who develop sustained leukopenia during or after treatment with 6MP for inflammatory bowel disease. Am J Gastroenterol. 2004;99: S252 (Abstract).
56. Austin AS, Spiller RC. Inflammatory bowel disease, azathioprine and skin cancer: case report and literature review. Eur J Gastroenterol Hepatol. 2001;13:193–4.
57. Ulrich C, Schmook T, Sachse MM, Sterry W, Stockfleth E. Comparative epidemiology and pathogenic factors for nonmelanoma skin cancer in organ transplant patients. Dermatol Surg. 2004;30:622–7.

# 18
# State-of-the-Art Lecture: Trials and complications of ileal pouch surgery

S. P. BACH and N. J. McC. MORTENSEN

## INTRODUCTION

Proctocolectomy and ileostomy has historically been the conventional treatment for ulcerative colitis (UC) and it is against this standard that new procedures are judged. This technique is considered safe, benefiting from a relatively simple operative strategy that can be performed without exposing a patient to the risk of anastomotic breakdown. Nonetheless it is evident that a permanent stoma remains an unpalatable proposition for most patients. Attempts to avoid stoma formation utilizing a straight ileoanal anastomosis following proctocolectomy were first recorded by Ravitch and Sabiston in 1947[1], but this technique produced poor functional results with symptoms of urgency, frequency and incontinence in the majority of patients[2]. Parks and Nichols developed this work further by combining elements of Kock's pouch[3,4] with a rectal mucosal resection previously employed for removal of adenomas and haemangiomas[5,6]. They created an ileal pouch reservoir that was sutured to the dentate line using a per-anal anastomotic technique[7]. This procedure was well suited to the treatment of both UC and familial adenomatous polyposis coli (FAP) as all diseased tissue could be removed while retaining intestinal continuity. Ileal pouch–anal anastomosis (IPAA) is now considered to be the procedure of choice for patients with UC who ultimately require surgery. The widespread use of stapling techniques has brought IPAA surgery within the scope of many practising colorectal surgeons; however, this remains a complex operation with appreciable morbidity[8]. A wealth of data is now available detailing the technical advancements in IPAA surgery and the management of its complications. This chapter will present the evidence upon which key elements of ileo-anal pouch surgery are currently based.

## PATIENT SELECTION

### IPAA in those over 50 years of age

Due to the complexity of IPAA surgery its use was initially limited to young patients in good health, while enthusiasm for trials in older patients was tempered by concerns that anal dilation, mucosectomy and a per-anal hand-sewn IPAA would induce appreciable rates of incontinence. Sphincter damage might arise through excessive dilation of the anus or stripping of the internal anal sphincter (IAS) during mucosectomy. The 'elderly sphincter' with little functional reserve was deemed a poor candidate for this intervention. As the surgical community collectively moved towards stapled IPAA with preservation of the anal transition zone (ATZ), motivated by reports of improved faecal continence and ease of construction, several institutions reported results in patients in the 50–70-year age group. Complications and pouch preservation rates appear to be independent of age at operation whereas continence and quality of life are generally slightly worse with advancing years. In the largest study to date Delaney et al. determined that daytime stool frequency after a median of 4.6 years did not significantly differ according to age[9]. This varied from five to six stools per day in 1410 patients less than 45 years and 485 who were older than this. Nocturnal frequency was slightly worse during the first year in the older group (mean 1.93 vs 1.4). At 1 year, episodes of incontinence were reported by one-quarter of those below 45 and one-half of those over 55 years while night-time seepage occurred in one-third and one-half of patients respectively. These differences were maintained to 5 years but became less apparent at 10, although the proportion of patients experiencing symptoms gradually increased over time independent of age at the time of surgery. Farouk et al. determined that nocturnal stool frequency, faecal incontinence, protective pad usage and constipating medication requirements were all higher in patients aged 45 or older at the time of IPAA[10]. In general pouch function deteriorated over time in this older group while no similar variation was discernible in the remaining population. Nonetheless very high levels of satisfaction have been achieved in this population, and with adequate explanation of these risks it would appear that the procedure is appropriate for well-motivated elderly individuals without symptomatic disturbance of the anal sphincters.

### Indeterminate colitis

Patients with a clinical picture identical to that of UC, but who fall short of demonstrating the histological hallmarks of this disease, are classified as having indeterminate colitis (IndC) and constitute approximately 10–15% of all cases[11,12]. Uncertainty may follow an episode of fulminant colitis when the true histological diagnosis can be obscured or in some cases the colon may exhibit features common to both UC and Crohn's disease (CD). Patient's who clinically resemble Crohn's in whom a histological diagnosis of UC is made, are additionally labelled as indeterminate. The outcome of IPAA surgery in this subgroup has been studied, demonstrating key differences that should be clearly set out before a patient embarks upon pouch surgery. Of 82 patients treated at the Mayo Clinic with IPAA for IndC (from a total of 1437 IPAA cases) 15% were converted to a diagnosis of CD with median follow-up approaching 7 years[13]. Atypical distribution of disease, including skip lesions and rectal sparing, were the pre-operative features most associated with subsequent diagnosis of Crohn's; however, statistical significance was not reached.

Rates of pouch failure were significantly higher for IndC at 27% as compared to UC at 11% ($p < 0.001$). Outcome in those patients with IndC who did not convert to CD was statistically no different to patients with UC, 85% with functional pouches at 10 years. More non-CD IndC patients did, however, manifest pouch fistulas.

The Cleveland Clinic has reported more encouraging results with respect to IPAA and IndC but over a shorter period of 3 years[14]. In 171 of 1911 patients (9%) a post-operative pathological diagnosis of IndC was recorded, while in 1399 the diagnosis was UC. The rate of pouch failure was 3% for both UC and IndC; 4% of IndC patients converted to a diagnosis of CD during the study period while only 0.4% of matched controls with UC did likewise. Daytime stool frequency was six for both groups, night-time frequency was increased from one to two with comparatively more soiling, 28% versus 36%, for those with IndC. Rates of incontinence did not differ (25% moderate, 1% severe). There was less overall satisfaction with pouch surgery among those with IndC, although 93% declared that they would have surgery again.

The consensus among most surgeons is that patients with *bona-fide* IndC are suitable candidates for pouch surgery as long as they are fully informed and accept the risks involved. In our view patients with a suspicious history of pelvic sepsis or perineal fistula should not be considered for IPAA surgery.

## CD colitis

The postoperative diagnosis changed to CD in 20 of 551 patients followed for a minimum of 2.5 years following IPAA for a pre-operative diagnosis of UC. Eleven of these patients (55%) experienced pouch failure[15]. Others have replicated the finding that unsuspected CD is a leading cause of pouch failure[16,17]. Univariate analysis of outcome in 74 patients diagnosed with CD from a series of 1965 revealed a 9-fold increase in the likelihood of pouch failure over a median period of 4 years with baseline failure rates in the order of 4%[18]. Patients tend to lose their pouches due to unacceptable function or complex fistulas; however, in the remainder performance can be satisfactory. Ten-year follow-up of 41 patients treated for colonic CD with no pre-operative history of perianal or small bowel disease reported more favourable results[19], yet this disease remains an absolute contraindication to ileal pouch surgery in most people's eyes.

## Dysplasia and cancer

The presence of dysplasia or potentially curable cancer, either within the colon or high in the rectum, does not preclude IPAA, although in locally advanced cases it would seem prudent to defer pouch formation until adjuvant therapy has been administered[20,21]. We would consider mucosectomy and a hand-sewn pouch–anal anastomosis in patients with multiple tumours, widespread dysplasia or where these lesions are situated in close proximity to the anal canal.

## TECHNIQUE

### Pouch configuration

Parks and Nicholls originally devised a triple limb 'S'-shaped pouch[7]. Emptying difficulties secondary to a long efferent limb and relatively complicated construction currently limit its use. We prefer the modified J pouch of Utsunomiya, as it is simpler to construct, uses less intestine and can be performed more rapidly[22]. The functional results are equal to those of the other reservoir designs as the J pouch will ultimately accommodate up to 400 ml of faeces and empty spontaneously[23–25]. The pouch is formed from the terminal 30–40 cm of ileum using several applications of a linear, cutting stapler to appose the antimesenteric border of two 15–20 cm limbs.

### Mucosectomy versus double-stapling

Early in the natural history of the IPAA procedure mucosectomy was advocated to remove all columnar epithelium from the upper anal canal and prevent recurrence of UC at this site. The technique of mucosectomy is combined with a per-anal hand-sewn anastomosis, allowing precise placement of the pouch–anal anastomosis at the level of the dentate line. The anal canal must remain dilated for an average of 20 min (range 14–44) in expert hands[26], possibly longer for others, in order to complete this procedure. Some were concerned that this anal manipulation damaged the sphincter complex, leading to faecal incontinence in a proportion of patients. This was the conclusion of a study from the Cleveland Clinic[27]. Separate studies confirmed the relatively high incidence of minor faecal soiling, especially at night and in the order of 50%, following mucosectomy[23,28,29].

Mucosectomy and hand-sewn pouch–anal anastomosis also lead, in most cases, to removal of the ATZ. This is an area of cuboidal transitional epithelium, some four to 10 cells deep, richly innervated by sensory nerve endings that mediate anal sensory sampling reflexes and are implicated in the maintenance of continence[30].

A simpler, much quicker alternative to mucosectomy and hand-sewn pouch–anal anastomosis is to employ a double-stapling technique. A transverse stapler is placed across the anorectal junction from above, preserving the entire anal canal. A circular stapler is then introduced through the anus for construction of the pouch–anal anastomosis. An early report supported the view that the stapled anastomosis was less traumatic, with improved postoperative resting sphincter pressures and improved continence[31]. Retention of the ATZ significantly enhanced preservation of the sampling reflex in patients undergoing stapled anastomosis[32]. Several personal series were subsequently reported that also favoured this double-stapled technique with preservation of the ATZ[33–36]. One randomized controlled trial (RCT) comparing high versus low stapling of the anal canal demonstrated improved daytime and night-time continence when the anastomosis was placed high[37]. However, four RCT and one case–control study revealed no great difference between these techniques with respect to complication rate, anal physiology or pouch function[26,38–41]. Closer examination of the Hallgren et al. paper[39] reveals that marked functional differences did indeed exist between treatment groups; however, these did not reach statistical significance as the study was undoubtedly underpowered. Physiological data from Reilly et al.[41] point towards more robust sphincter function when the ATZ is preserved with a tendency towards better continence at night; an outcome also seen in the study of McIntyre et al.[40] Failure to prove clinical benefit may simply reflect the small number of patients randomized within each of these trials, and the complex nature of defecation. The small numbers examined may also hinder adequate assessment of the relative complication rates of stapled versus hand-sewn anastomosis. Ziv et al. reported the Cleveland Clinic's experience of these two techniques in 692 colitics[42]. They concluded that there was a significantly higher rate of anastomotic disruption and para-pouch abscess following formation of a hand-sewn anastomosis, culminating in more pouch excisions within this group. Complications of hand-sewn anastomosis did not equate to the surgeons' learning curve. As the trial was not prospectively randomized it remains unknown as to whether case selection may have skewed these findings somewhat. This group have subsequently devised a Cleveland Clinic pouch failure model and used this to determine that the anastomotic technique does not in fact influence the rate of pouch failure in 1965 patients who had pouch surgery for all indications between 1983 and 2001[18]. This is slightly puzzling as, in the same model, both anastomotic disruption and perianal sepsis were strongly associated with pouch failure. By 'controlling' for the putative risk factors of anastomotic leakage and sepsis, are important associations between failure and technique missed when the distribution of these factors will clearly be different between groups?

Two large series have evaluated the benefit of ATZ preservation in different ways. Gemlo et al. reported functional results (mean follow-up 70 months) of 235 pouch procedures of which a small minority were for FAP[43]. They essentially audited a change in practice from S pouch combined with mucosectomy to J pouch with double stapled anastomosis. The double-staple technique was associated with a significant reduction in both night-time incontinence (major and minor) and minor daytime incontinence. Choi et al. histologically subclassified 138 patients undergoing stapled anastomosis on the basis of the epithelial composition of the distal doughnut[44]. Those with predominantly squamous epithelium in the doughnut had significantly lower postoperative maximal resting pressure (MxRP) when compared to others with columnar epithelium. These lower values did not stray outside of the normal range, sphincter length was preserved and no difference in the proportion of patients with an intact recto-anal inhibitory reflex was noted between groups. Rates of continence, however, were not reported.

It seems that hand-sewn and stapling techniques both give rise to deterioration in the MxRP postoperatively, a phenomenon that has been variably attributed to autonomic denervation or direct trauma to the sphincter mechanism. Interestingly Winter et al. have reported results of a RCT comparing perianal application of 0.2% glyceryl trinitrate (GTN) ointment with placebo in 60 patients prior to circular stapler insertion[45]. Use of the active agent significantly reduced intraoperative mean resting pressure (MRP) and the need for anal digitation prior to insertion of the circular stapling device. Postoperative MRP did not deviate from preoperative values and function was excellent at 3 and 12 months. In contrast, following placebo, MRP was significantly reduced and function was poorer, even at 12 months. These findings suggest that local trauma may cause sphincter damage during stapling and that this outcome may be amenable to pharmacological modification.

## The columnar cuff

In the debate as to whether or not to retain the ATZ when forming a pouch–anal anastomosis, it must be remembered that, although the amount of columnar epithelium in the ATZ is very small, the ATZ itself is also much smaller than commonly thought[46]. This importantly leaves a 1.5–2.0-cm cuff of residual columnar epithelium above the ATZ after a double-stapled restorative proctocolectomy. Recurrent UC in the columnar cuff epithelium, termed 'cuffitis' produces symptoms that include discomfort, urgency, bloody discharge and stool frequency. In a retrospective study of 217 patients who had undergone a stapled IPAA, anal canal inflammation was evident both endoscopically and histologically in 48 patients (22%) of whom 32 were symptomatic[47]. There was evidence of associated pouchitis in 30 patients (14%) and of these 23 declared symptoms. Mesalazine suppositories 500 mg have been employed in this group of patients to reduce symptoms, and to improve endoscopic appearance and histopathology, although this was a small, uncontrolled study with a high rate of drop-out[48].

There is a theoretical risk of dysplasia and carcinoma within the retained anal cuff, and a small number of reports detailing adenocarcinoma below the IPAA anastomosis exist[49–51]. These cases have occurred in patients following resection of a colorectal malignancy. Coull et al. reported median 5-year follow-up of 135 UC patients who had undergone stapled IPAA and subsequent annual endoscopic surveillance of the columnar cuff[52]. None of the original specimens had shown evidence of dysplasia or carcinoma. While 94% of cuff biopsies revealed evidence of chronic inflammation, and in one-third of cases this was severe, none showed evidence of either dysplasia or carcinoma. Two separate reports of over 100 patients, each with a median 30-month follow-up, have corroborated these findings[53,54]. The Cleveland Clinic's experience is slightly different: of 289 patients undergoing transition zone sparing IPAA, 178 were followed by surveillance endoscopy and serial biopsy for more than 10 years[55]. No patient developed carcinoma of the ATZ but eight patients (4.5%) did develop dysplasias, of which six were considered low-grade and two high-grade. These histological features were not associated with any symptoms, and only one high-grade lesion showed signs of concomitant mucosal irregularity. Surveillance of patients with low-grade dysplasia revealed no further problems in four of the six. In the remaining two patients low-grade dysplasia persisted over a 2–3-year period, eventually being managed by mucosectomy and endo-anal pouch advancement. Low-grade dysplasia alone was evident within the resected specimens in each case. The two patients with high-grade dysplasia both had a history of colonic dysplasia/ cancer. In each case a second severely dysplastic biopsy arose. One came from the ATZ and this patient was treated by mucosectomy, while the second came from the ileal pouch in a patient also suffering from pouchitis. Subsequent biopsies from the pouch were not dysplastic, and the patient remained under observation. As no cancers developed, nor were any pouches lost, the investigators maintained that routine mucosectomy was unnecessary in the absence of rectal carcinoma or proven dysplasia within 8 cm of the anal verge. They recommend 3–6-monthly sampling of severe dysplasia with excision of the anal canal if an abnormality persists. For low-grade dysplasia mucosectomy is performed when three positive samples have been collected. It is interesting to note that risk of persistent dysplastic change may not be completely addressed following mucosectomy as small islands of rectal mucosa may survive in the denuded rectal muscular tube of up to 20% of patients[56,57].

In conclusion many surgeons, including ourselves, favour the double-staple technique as this is the simpler operation, and may indeed have a lower risk of failure, especially in the hands of those without very extensive experience[58]. This technique may also facilitate the performance of surgery in difficult circumstances such as those encountered in an obese patient, or when adequate mesenteric length becomes an issue. Comparison with the hand-sewn technique suggests a physiological benefit with regard to the sphincter mechanism, although is more difficult to be certain of definite clinical improvement. Although the randomized trials reveal no difference in complication rates they undoubtedly lack power. In a large institutional series double-stapling was associated with significantly less postoperative pelvic sepsis. The risk of dysplasia within the columnar cuff following double-stapling seems small, and is not a contraindication to this procedure. The anal canal is amenable to endoscopic inspection if desired. Nonetheless it would seem prudent to perform mucosectomy where a patient is demonstrated to harbour rectal dysplasia or is suffering from rectal malignancy. As a final note, care should be taken when stapling across the anorectal junction to avoid an error of judgement that results in a pouch–rectal anastomosis. The transverse stapling instrument should be positioned 2–3 cm beyond the dentate line, a distance roughly equivalent to the length of the distal metacarpal of the index finger.

## One-stage IPAA

Most surgeons have favoured creation of a temporary defunctioning loop ileostomy following IPAA surgery, as this avoids catastrophic pelvic contamination in the event of anastomotic dehiscence. It should be remembered that ileostomy formation demonstrates its own range of complications. This fact has prompted some surgeons to question its use for all patients, believing that a significant proportion may be safely treated by a one-stage procedure[59–67]. The argument is essentially one of risk management. Data from the Cleveland Clinic demonstrated that anastomotic separation occurred in 5.3% of 1965 IPAA patients[18], although leak rates of up to 14% are described for the one-stage IPAA[68,69]. In comparison the overall complication rate for 1504 ileostomy closures following IPAA was 11.4% and comprised 6.4% small bowel obstruction (one quarter required surgery), 1.5% wound infection, 1% abdominal sepsis and 0.6% enterocutaneous fistulas[70]. Other published complication rates for ileostomy closure range from 10% to 30%[71–78]. The Cleveland data would therefore suggest that ileostomy closure is likely to result in less major morbidity than one-stage IPAA.

Where studies have favoured one-stage surgery the results are not always compelling and additionally tend to lack the statistical power to detect changes in the incidence of pelvic sepsis. For instance Heuschen et al. produced a case-controlled study of 57 one-stage procedures versus 114 matched controls[79]. They concluded that the incidence of complications was greater following the two-stage procedure. This amounted to a significant difference in anastomotic stricture rate, a problem that was presumably dealt with at the time of ileostomy closure by gentle dilation in the majority of patients. Patients subject to the two-stage procedure were deemed equally suitable for a one-stage operation, but in an institution favouring the latter approach this was for some reason not undertaken. Lastly controls were taken from a period that began 5 years prior to one-stage surgery commencing at this unit. Several large series have now demonstrated that complication rates from pouch surgery within a unit decline significantly over time[15,18,80].

Contrasting results have been obtained from similar studies with an increase in the incidence of serious complications attributable to anastomotic leakage arising in patients in whom IPAA was performed without a covering ileostomy. Williamson et al. examined results of 100 consecutive patients with an equal proportion subject to one- and two-stage IPAA surgery[59]. Pelvic sepsis occurred in 11 and seven patients respectively, with faecal peritonitis in three of the former. While 7/11 one-stage patients required reoperation for sepsis, all two-stage patients were treated conservatively. This study describes what in reality should be obvious from the start; i.e. that the implications of anastomotic failure are potentially much greater where no covering ileostomy exists. At the time of IPAA we are unable to accurately predict whether a patient will subsequently leak. As these patients are generally young, often with children, we feel that unnecessary escalation of risk is not warranted.

One-stage surgery has also been shown to increase the relative risk of pouch failure from 8% to 15% compared to the two-stage approach in a group of 634 patients treated at St Marks[80]. However, in another series from Toronto only one of 117 pouches without ileostomy failed, compared to 14 of 234 that were defunctioned[15]. This result may simply reflect astuteness on the part of the operating surgeons at this institution rather than a cause-and-effect relationship.

While it is our belief that patients should routinely be offered two- or three-stage surgery, those who hold a firm preference for one-stage surgery may be treated accordingly if the risks are known/accepted and they are otherwise suitable candidates for this approach.

## Laparoscopic IPAA

The aims of laparoscopic colorectal surgery are to avoid wound pain that may impair mobility or breathing, encourage early restoration of intestinal function, reduce formation of intra-abdominal adhesions and subsequently the incidence of small bowel obstruction whilst also improving cosmetic appearance postoperatively. The procedure should be safe and economically viable. One can see that this approach may potentially transform proctocolectomy and ileoanal pouch surgery if these objectives were to be met; however, some difficulties exist. First it is no simple task to complete an operation of this magnitude laparoscopically. This issue gives rise to problems accruing clinical trials of sufficient power to appreciate whether laparoscopic surgery actually improves outcome. There are also some fairly obvious and immediate downsides to this type of surgery in terms of cost, complexity, and time spent operating in addition to that spent training. These issues do not always sit comfortably within the framework of our current health-care system. The surgical learning curve also has implications for patient morbidity that must be reconciled with current complication rates for open surgery.

Reports in the literature that currently outline early experience with this technique, focus upon the issue of feasibility utilizing relatively small numbers. A case-controlled study of 20 laparoscopic restorative proctocolectomies and 20 open procedures[13] for UC and seven for FAP in each group, with all but one UC patient defunctioned) demonstrated that patients in the laparoscopic group left hospital at a median of 6 versus 8 days as intestinal function returned sooner[81]. There was no difference in complication rates between groups. Other studies have confirmed that this operation is technically feasible[82,83] although not all have demonstrated a benefit in comparison to conventional surgery[84-86]. In a series of 32 selected one-stage laparoscopic restorative proctocolectomies there were two intraoperative complications, a rectal perforation during mobilization and one staple line misfire[87]. There were also 11 postoperative complications; three obstruction or ileus, two pouchitis, two wound infections, two strictures, one pelvic abscess, and one pouch leak. Re-operation was required in three patients for defunctioning ileostomy, adhesionolysis and peranal drainage of para-pouch sepsis.

In a prospectively randomized controlled trial of hand-assisted laparoscopic colonic mobilization combined with open pelvic dissection through an 8 cm Pfannenstiel incision versus open surgery through the midline in a total of 60 patients the laparoscopic approach offered no discernible benefit to quality of life[88]. Performance of open pelvic dissection would be expected to facilitate this procedure in terms of speed and ease of distal stapling; however, it may also negate some of the benefits of the laparoscopic approach.

## COMPLICATIONS

### Haemorrhage

Primary intraluminal haemorrhage may follow formation of a sutured or stapled pouch and it is therefore important to carefully inspect the mucosal surface before the pouch–anal anastomosis is constructed. Bleeding points are sutured. Reactionary intraluminal haemorrhage, within 24 h of surgery, is also likely to originate from the suture/staple lines. Initially the patient is resuscitated, coagulation checked while a saline solution containing 1:200 000 adrenaline can be employed to irrigate the pouch. This manoeuvre may control up to 80% of clinically significant haemorrhages[8]. If bleeding continues then the patient is returned to the operating room and the pouch inspected using an Eisenhammer anal speculum (Seward, London, UK), proctoscope or sigmoidoscope using suction and irrigation to accurately locate the bleeding point. This should then be amenable to a suture or injection with a solution containing 1:10 000 adrenaline. Secondary haemorrhage is less common and usually heralds pelvic sepsis. The pouch should be inspected in theatre with special attention to the ileoanal anastomosis. Bleeding points should be under-run with a search made for concomitant pelvic collections arising as a consequence of localized anastomotic breakdown. Such collections should be drained preferably via the original defect with the option to place a per-anal Foley catheter into the cavity.

Intra-abdominal haemorrhage occurs most frequently from mesenteric vessels, the pelvic side wall or the rectal stump in cases where a hand-sewn pouch–anal anastomosis has been constructed. Careful examination should allow treatment of the first two causes without undue difficulty. Inspection of the lower pelvis is usually best achieved if the pouch is detached and subsequent examination of the stump may be best achieved endoanally using a Lone Star retractor (Lone Star Medical Products Inc., Houston, TX). The pouch may be reattached using the hand-sewn technique once bleeding has ceased, or in a haemo-compromised patient the better approach is to exteriorize the pouch as a left iliac fossa mucous fistula. Reanastomosis can be entertained after several months. In cases where it is not possible to control pelvic haemorrhage at laparotomy, simply packing the cavity with a re-look within 48 h offers the best solution. Bleeding from the pouch is estimated to complicate 3.5% of cases[8].

### Small bowel obstruction

This is unfortunately a common complication, reflecting the extensive nature of pouch surgery, with multiple operations and appreciable rates of sepsis. In a series of 1178 patients from Toronto, prospective evaluation over a median of 8.7 years yielded 351 episodes of small bowel obstruction (SBO) in 272 (23%) patients[89]. The cumulative risk of SBO was 9% at 30 days, 18% at 1 year, 26% at 5 years and 31% at 10 years with re-operation rates of 0.8%, 2.7%, 6.7% and 7.5%, respectively. No deaths were attributable to SBO. Early SBO, defined as a postoperative stay of 14 days or more after IPAA or 10 days following closure of ileostomy or re-admission within 30 days of surgery, involved 145 patients

(15%) and accounted for 44% of all episodes. This figure undoubtedly incorporates cases of protracted ileus. Only eight (5%) patients required laparotomy; six for adhesions and two for internal herniation, the remainder settling with conservative measures. Early SBO did not predispose to late SBO. There were 197 episodes of late SBO, occurring more than 30 days after either IPAA surgery or closure of ileostomy in 149 patients. Seventy-two (36%) patients required laparotomy, with adhesions being the most frequent finding in 90% of cases (commonly between the small bowel and pelvis or previous stoma site). The risk of late SBO alone was 6% at 1 year, 14% at 5 years and 19% at 10 years with one-quarter of patients experiencing more than one episode and 5% requiring surgery. Twenty per cent of patients who underwent laparotomy and adhesionolysis developed further episodes of SBO, and in 5% a further laparotomy was necessary. Factors predisposing to late SBO were revisional pouch surgery (hazard ratio 2.1) and formation of a defunctioning stoma (hazard ratio 1.5). It would appear that aggressive conservative management does create unacceptable morbidity in these circumstances, as only four of the 80 patients who required laparotomy also had ischaemic bowel resected. This is an important fact as re-operation, especially in the acute setting, is fraught with danger due to fibrinous adhesions, and carries with it a risk of inadvertent enterotomy with subsequent enterocutaneous fistulas. Where no signs of ischaemia exist it is wise to pursue a non-operative strategy, allied to parenteral nutrition when indicated, for as long as possible.

Separate reports from the Cleveland[8], Mayo[90] and Lahey[91] clinics, detailing cohorts of 1005, 626 and 460 patients respectively, with follow-up in the order of 2–3 years, denote the risk of SBO to be 25%, 17% and 20% with operative intervention in 7% across the board. In a further report from the Lahey clinic 6/48 patients requiring re-operation for SBO were found to have acute angulation of the afferent small bowel limb running up to the pouch inlet[92]. Patients presented with recurrent bouts of obstruction. The loop was adherent to the posterior base of the pouch and mobilization was deemed hazardous to the pouch in 5/6 cases with the surgeons electing to fashion an enteroenterostomy, bypassing the loop instead. With median follow-up of 2 years four patients are symptom-free and one suffers from obstructed defecation.

Other recognized causes of SBO related to ileostomy formation include torsion of the loop, lateral space obstruction and a trephine that is too small. The latter will usually require digital dilation under general anaesthetic; however, in the remaining cases it may be desirable to aim for stoma closure if a contrast enema demonstrates healing of the pouch. In these cases intra-abdominal sepsis should first be excluded. Where the cause is not obvious a computed tomography with oral contrast may be helpful, or contrast studies via the stoma and by mouth.

In view of the considerable morbidity caused by adhesions several strategies have been devised to decrease their frequency. Dextran solutions have been used, but their efficacy in humans remains unproven[93] and concerns regarding safety remain. In a multicentre RCT the sodium hyaluronate bioresorbable barrier preparation, Seprafilm (Genzyme, Cambridge, MA) reduced the number of adhesions attached to the midline scar following IPAA[94].

Laparoscopic assessment at the time of stoma closure revealed that 43/85 (51%) patients receiving hyaluronate membrane as compared to 5/90 (6%) of control patients had no adhesions ($p < 0.001$), although no subsequent reduction in episodes of SBO occurred. Concerns have subsequently arisen regarding the incidence of anastomotic leak when Seprafilm is applied next to an anastomosis. A subgroup analysis of 1791 patients participating in an RCT of patients undergoing abdominopelvic surgery[95], the majority of whom had inflammatory bowel disease, revealed a significantly higher incidence of anastomotic leak in those who had received Seprafilm®. This finding in our view would currently preclude the use of this agent within the pelvis of pouch patients where adhesions commonly give rise to SBO.

## Pelvic sepsis

A febrile episode in a patient recovering from IPAA surgery should arouse the suspicion of pelvic sepsis, as this remains a relatively common acute complication and failure to react in a timely fashion is likely to compromise future function. Pouch-related septic complications follow anastomotic dehiscence or infection of a pelvic haematoma. In a series of 494 consecutive patients from Heidelberg undergoing a stapled J-pouch procedure followed by mucosectomy, preservation of a short rectal cuff and hand-sewn anastomosis for UC the rate of pouch-related sepsis was 15.6% at 1 year and 24.2% at 3 years[96]. No patients in this series were diagnosed with CD following pouch surgery. Fistulas accounted for 76% of all septic complications (56% pouch–anal anastomotic fistulas; 13% pouch–vaginal fistulas; 7% proximal pouch fistulas) while 16% were due to anastomotic separation and 8% were due to para-pouch abscess[97].

In a series of 1508 patients from the Mayo Clinic, of whom the majority underwent hand-sewn ileal J pouch–anal anastomosis for chronic UC, 73 (4.8%) were judged to have had a pelvic collection that complicated their recovery with only three of these documented to have a co-existing pouch fistula[98].

More recently the Cleveland Clinic evaluated 1965 IPAA procedures performed in patients with UC (60.7%), IndC (27.9%), CD (3.8%) and FAP (0.7%) to conclude that fistula formation occurred in 151 (7%), anastomotic separation in 104 (5%) and pelvic abscess in 109 (5%) cases[18].

Where pelvic sepsis is suspected a digital examination may demonstrate an anastomotic defect or alternatively localized tenderness associated with an indurated or fluctuant mass. CT or MRI determines the extent of sepsis and in most cases endoanal drainage into the bowel lumen is appropriate. Non-operative means were utilized to treat 24/131 (18%) cases of pelvic sepsis in the Heidelberg study[97]. Two patients (8%) experienced pouch failure in the long term. In the Mayo series 11/73 (15%) pelvic abscesses were considered 'early' and treated with antibiotics alone, with only three ultimately requiring surgery[98]. A further 16 patients (22%) had a pouch pelvic abscess localized and drained with the aid of CT. All but three settled without the need for surgery.

At examination under anaesthesia the vagina should be inspected for evidence of fistulation as a consequence of injury to the posterior wall during stapling of the IPAA. Any track should be probed to determine its configuration, associated areas of loculated sepsis are drained and a seton placed to facilitate the expulsion of infected material. The anus is inspected with an Eisenhammer retractor. Anastomotic breakdown can usually be visualized directly. The underlying area can then be probed to determine the extent of any associated abscess cavity, the contents of which are evacuated by suction. Larger defects may be amenable to digital examination followed by placement of a catheter to allow subsequent irrigation. In the presence of a pre-sacral collection and no obvious anastomotic defect then one is usually created in its posterior aspect. Regular re-examination under anaesthetic may be required for a period, to be confident that the cavity remains clean. While we would favour this approach for the majority of mild to moderate pouch-related sepsis other series appear to utilize this course of action less frequently, although it should be appreciated that standardization with regard to the patient population is not guaranteed. For instance in the series from Mayo Clinic dealing predominantly with isolated para-pouch abscesses, per-anal drainage was utilized in only 6/73 (8%)[98]. Heuschen et al. utilized per-anal drainage in 33/131 cases (33%) resulting in a pouch failure rate of 6.6%[97].

Re-laparotomy is reserved for severe cases either where minor surgery has failed to control sepsis or when the patient becomes profoundly compromised with evidence of generalized intraperitoneal contamination. In the series from Mayo Clinic 40/73 patients (55%) had an initial laparotomy for sepsis and in 14 the pouch was immediately excised, twice as a consequence of ischaemia and for 'extensive sepsis' in the remainder[98]. A total of 74/131 cases (56%) ultimately required laparotomy in the series from Heidelberg[97]. Where a major leak has occurred a proximal loop ileostomy should be performed if not already in place. Complete anastomotic disruption prompts consideration to mobilization and exteriorizing of the pouch. With evidence of gross ischaemia one should ideally resect and exteriorize the ileum.

Rates of pelvic sepsis are found to be substantially higher in those patients undergoing IPAA for UC versus FAP, leading us to conclude that factors specific to this disease, or indeed its treatment, play a role in the evolution of septic complications[96,99]. Risk factors for the development of pelvic sepsis have been evaluated by a number of institutions, with varying results. High-dose corticosteroid usage (systemic equivalent of >40 mg prednisolone per day) predisposed to sepsis in patients undergoing panproctocolectomy and IPAA when compared to use at lower levels or no steroid use at all[96]. Similar conclusions were drawn by the Toronto group from a review of 483 patients[100], whereas Ziv et al. found no association between prolonged high-dose corticosteroids (>20 mg) prior to surgery and the subsequent rate of acute septic complications, noted to be 6%, in 192 of 671 UC patients undergoing IPAA at the Cleveland Clinic[101]. Whether steroids impair healing of the anastomosis, decrease the ability to combat infection or simply mark a subgroup of patients who are in poor clinical condition remains unknown. Our approach is to avoid IPAA formation in those patients who are acutely unwell and receiving high-dose corticosteroids, undertaking subtotal colectomy first and IPAA at a later date, allowing corticosteroids to be reduced in dose if not discontinued completely.

Concerning the longer term in patients who have suffered from pelvic sepsis the Mayo series indicated that 4/73 patients progressed to form a chronic fistula, one pouch–vaginal (repaired) and three pouch perineal that required a long-term ileostomy[98]. Functional outcome was worse following pelvic sepsis with rates of frequent or major incontinence amounting to 16% vs 7%. In addition more patients relied upon constipating medication (72% vs 47%) and pads (41% vs 18%) although stool frequency remained unchanged at five per day. Quality-of-life measurements were adversely affected. From the 73 patients who experienced at least one episode of pelvic sepsis pouch failure occurred in 18 (27%) within 2 years. The corresponding failure rate of those who did not experience pelvic sepsis was 5.9%. A source of encouragement was the fact that the incidence of pouch-related sepsis declined markedly over the 15-year time frame of this study.

Overall pouch failure rates for patients experiencing septic complications from Heidelberg amounted to 29%, rising to 36% for those treated with laparotomy[97]. The major cause of failure was persistent pouch fistula (36%), followed by poor function secondary to a compromised anal sphincter (18%), outlet obstruction (13%), pelvic fibrosis (10%), pouchitis (10%) and finally unwillingness on the patients' part to undergo ileostomy closure (13%).

In a series of 628 patients mostly treated for UC at the Lahey Clinic pelvic sepsis was diagnosed with a frequency of 6.5% and associated positively with increased stool frequency and inability to discriminate the passage of stool from gas[102]. No difference in incontinence, medication or pad usage was found.

## Outflow obstruction

Anastomotic stricture may complicate leakage, tension or ischaemia at the IPAA[103]. It is estimated to occur with a frequency of 4–18%[8,102,104,105]. In a series of 982 patients treated at the Mayo Clinic, 42 (4%) strictures were diagnosed, of which 62% followed ileostomy closure[106]. For this reason a routine pouchogram would now be considered standard prior to restoration of intestinal continuity. Presenting symptoms consisted of straining (36%), diarrhoea (50%), anal pain (12%) or abdominal pain (12%). A single examination under anaesthesia with application of Hegar's dilators successfully treated 40% of cases; however, the rest either recurred or developed separate but related complications. Dilation was repeated for re-stenosis. Ultimately 6/42 (14%) cases required pouch excision for stenosis (three), fistulisation (two) or poor function (one), while one patient remained defunctioned at a median of 40 months and another was lost to follow-up. Of the 34 remaining patients with a functioning pouch, 11 were dependent upon periodic dilation. In 23 of these cases pouch function was deemed good or satisfactory.

In our experience it is often possible to attempt dilation at the time of pouchoscopy. Most strictures will respond to the use of Hegar's dilators and in some instances it may prove beneficial if the patient continues to use the dilator for several weeks while at home. In a few patients this approach may fail, especially if the stricture is particularly long or tight. In such cases further biopsies are taken to exclude CD. Once all sepsis has been eradicated, and the tissues have recovered, surgical revision by per-anal pouch advancement may be considered[107]. This technique can also be used to close fistula tracks situated at the level of the stricture. Partial dehiscence of the new suture line can occur, and is managed conservatively if possible with minimal debridement and drainage of any underlying cavity using a small catheter. If a per-anal approach is not feasible, as can occur when the stricture is particularly long, then laparotomy with pelvic mobilization is combined with per-anal anastomosis.

## Reoperation for pouch–vaginal fistulas

Fistulas arising between the vagina and IPAA occur relatively rarely, with an incidence variably estimated at 3–16%[29,108–111]. In a series of 68 patients from St Mark's pouch–vaginal fistulation originated from the IPAA in 76%, the pouch itself in 13% and a cryptoglandular or other source in 10%[112]. Causes are linked to operative trauma, surgical technique, postoperative pelvic sepsis or undiagnosed CD, and accordingly present either immediately postoperatively or several months later, with evidence to suggest the outcome is better in the former. In the St Mark's study associated early complications included pelvic sepsis in 29%, anastomotic separation in 24%, anastomotic stricture in 24%, small bowel obstruction in 25%, haemorrhage in 3% and pouchitis in 18%. Cases of unsuspected CD should be sought out as both fistula healing rates (25% vs 48%) and pouch failure rates (33% vs 14%) are much poorer than those for the group as a whole[111]. Indeed the St Mark's paper showed long-term healing rates of 0% in 12% of patients diagnosed with CD with all fistulas either persisting or recurring within 5 years of primary treatment.

Various surgical techniques can be used to treat this condition, including transanal ileal advancement flap, transabdominal advancement of the ileoanal anastomosis, transvaginal repair, a long-term seton or pouch excision. In a series of 60 cases reported from the Cleveland Clinic more than half of the fistulas were deemed to arise from below the anastomosis with a further 28% at that level[111]. A per-anal ileal advancement flap technique was used in 39 patients[107], preceded by seton drainage in a small proportion. Primary healing occurred in 17 cases (43%) with closure in a further four after a second procedure. The authors stress the need for careful haemostasis and a tension-free join when employing this technique; therefore the pouch must be mobile from the outset. Re-do IPAA was necessary in 16 patients, either as a primary procedure for high fistulation from the ileal pouch or in cases where transanal repair had failed or was deemed unsuitable as a consequence of tethering. Healing was achieved in 10 of these cases. Primary healing rates were better for fistulas that appeared within 6 months of surgery, although this is perhaps not surprising given that 40% of patients were eventually diagnosed with CD. Faecal diversion was not considered obligatory as part of the ileal advancement flap; indeed only 65% of all patients were defunctioned, including those whose stomas had not been reversed.

Per-anal access to fistulas arising within the anal canal may be difficult, especially where an anastomosis has been placed at the anorectal junction. For this reason transvaginal repair has gained popularity in some quarters. This technique may also avoid damage to the anal sphincters. It involves direct exposure of the internal anal opening through the posterior wall of the vagina, with mobilization of the pouch and primary closure of the defect followed by restitution of the vaginal wall and formation of a defunctioning stoma[113]. Successful closure was reported in 11/14 cases, although five patients required up to three operations with median follow-up of 18 months.

In cases where fistulation is demonstrated to stem from previously unrecognized CD, the antitumour necrosis factor monoclonal antibody infliximab may be effective in closing the defect[114,115].

## Pouchitis

This idiopathic inflammatory process constitutes the commonest cause of pouch dysfunction in UC patients. The mucosa of the ileal reservoir undergoes adaptive changes following prolonged exposure to the faecal stream. Commonly observed changes in up to 80% of pouches include mucosal villous atrophy, chronic inflammatory cell infiltrate and a degree of colonic metaplasia. Such changes are most evident in dependent portions of the pouch where contact with faecal residue is prolonged[116]. Pouchitis describes an acute-on-chronic relapsing inflammatory condition akin to UC with diarrhoea that may be bloody. This is variably accompanied by symptoms of urgency, abdominal bloating, pain and fever. Endoscopic appearances are again similar to those of UC with erythema, granularity, faded vascular markings and contact bleeding initially. Later punctate haemorrhages, mucus secretion, purulent discharge and superficial ulceration occur. The histological hallmarks of this disease are acute inflammation, that is polymorphonuclear leucocyte infiltration, with superficial ulceration on a background of chronic inflammatory changes[117,118]. Current evidence points to recurrence of UC in areas of colonic metaplasia as a potential cause of this condition, although alternative hypotheses abound.

Differential diagnoses include undiagnosed CD, especially in the presence of prominent ulceration, pre-pouch ileitis or fistula formation. Alternatively 'cuffitis' or 'strip colitis' describes recurrence of UC in the short cuff of ATZ mucosa that is preserved during stapled IPAA. Other causes of pouch dysfunction that should be excluded if symptoms are resistant to conventional treatments are infection with cytomegalovirus or *Clostridium difficile*, para-pouch pelvic sepsis, a low-volume reservoir, outlet obstruction including anastomotic stricture and incomplete emptying. In these instances stool examination, MRI and isotope or contrast pouchogram may help to elucidate the nature of malfunction. Alternatively, a non-inflammatory condition akin to irritable bowel syndrome, and termed irritable pouch syndrome (IPS), has been proposed to account for those patients with severe symptoms of pouch dysfunction, without gross endoscopic or histological changes[119].

The aetiology of pouch dysfunction in a cohort of 123 consecutive 'symptomatic' patients, thought to suffer from UC according to clinical, endoscopic and histological parameters, was pouchitis in 34%, unrecognized

CD in 15%, irritable pouch syndrome in 28% and cuffitis in 22%, of whom 6% had concomitant pouchitis[48]. The authors have utilized faecal lactoferrin levels, an iron-binding protein released by activated polymorphonuclear leucocytes, to accurately differentiate patients with inflammatory conditions requiring endoscopic evaluation from those with IPS in whom treatment with antidiarrhoeal, anticholinergic or antidepressant medications could commence without the need for this investigation[120].

Two tools have been created that standardize the diagnosis and reporting of pouchitis: the pouch disease activity index (PDAI) and the pouch activity score (PAS), each providing a numerical score based upon clinical, endoscopic and histological findings[121,122]. Neither index is currently deemed as accurate as the physician's assessment[123].

Lepisto et al. determined that, in a cohort of 468 patients followed up after IPAA, the cumulative probabilities of pouchitis, determined on the basis of symptomatology, endoscopic appearances and histology, were 20% at 1 year, 32% at 5 years and 40% at 10 years[124]. In cases where the indication for surgery had been FAP as opposed to UC (7% of patients) no pouchitis was seen. These rates are in general accordance with those from other centres. The incidence of pouchitis appears to be independent of surgical technique with respect to pouch construction, use of a defunctioning stoma and laparoscopy[25,79,125,126]. Patients with primary sclerosing cholangitis (PSC) are more prone to develop pouchitis, with a cumulative probability of 79% at 10 years[127]. Persistence of extraintestinal manifestations of UC has also been linked to an increased risk of developing pouchitis, and certain patients exhibit a temporal relationship between their pouchitis and extraintestinal symptoms akin to that described for UC, fuelling speculation that these two inflammatory processes represent variations of the same underlying condition[128]. Perpetuating this theme, smoking is considered to be protective against UC[129] and also reduces the incidence of pouchitis[130,131].

A genetic marker for pouchitis, allele 2 of the interleukin-1 receptor antagonist gene (IL-1ra), has been suggested following a study that associated the presence of this gene with the development of pouchitis[132]. IL-1ra is a competitive antagonist to the IL-1 receptor and therefore potentially anti-inflammatory. Allele 2 leads to reduced levels of IL-1ra, and this change is hypothesized to mediate inflammation within the pouch.

Use of preoperative serum perinuclear antineutrophil cytoplasmic antibody (pANCA) as a predictor of postoperative pouchitis was evaluated in 95 patient undergoing the IPAA procedure[133]. Sixty per cent of patients were pANCA-positive preoperatively, and pouchitis occurred in 42% of this group compared to 20% of pANCA-negative patients ($p = 0.09$). When patients were subclassified according to pANCA levels no significant difference was found in the incidence of acute pouchitis between those with high, moderate or low levels, although rates for chronic pouchitis were 56%, 22% and 16% respectively, a significant finding. It is interesting to note that the majority of PSC subjects are pANCA-positive[134]. It must, however, be stressed that, while many investigators have examined whether pANCA measurement predicts for pouchitis, a significant proportion have failed to show any association. A recent study by Reumaux et al. illustrates this point[135].

Long-term pouch function has been studied in patients who develop pouchitis. Hurst et al. determined that even a single episode of pouchitis predisposed to worse long-term pouch function[136]. They hypothesized that pouchitis was in fact a chronic condition affecting daily pouch function, and suggested that we currently clinically recognize only the acute exacerbations. Other investigators have failed to corroborate these findings but have suggested that chronic pouchitis, arising with an incidence in the order of 5% at 10 years, substantially increases frequency of defecation[137]. In most large institutional series the incidence of pouch failure approaches 10% at 10 years with severe pouchitis contributing 10% of these failures. Therefore over the past 20 years pouchitis has probably accounted for failure in 1% of all IPAA. This is a relatively small figure considering that the majority of patients experience at least one episode of pouchitis in their lifetime; we can therefore conclude that pouchitis rarely results in pouch failure.

Patients with new symptoms suggestive of pouchitis have a 50% chance of eventually being diagnosed with this condition, so empiric therapy is not appropriate in the first instance; patients should instead be fully worked up with endoscopy and biopsy. Once the diagnosis is established then it would be reasonable to instigate empirical therapy, with the caveat that patients who do not promptly settle should return for further endoscopic evaluation.

Hurst et al. concluded that oral metronidazole or ciprofloxacin were effective in clinically improving 96% of pouchitis cases in an institutional series from Chicago[138]. A 7-day course of metronidazole 250 mg t.d.s. successfully treated 41/52 subjects, with a further eight responding to ciprofloxacin 500 mg b.d. Two-thirds of patients went on to have further attacks and 6% became chronic sufferers. The efficacy of metronidazole has been confirmed in three small prospectively randomized studies[139-141] with the latter study suggesting that ciprofloxacin 500 mg b.d. for 2 weeks may be more effective, as determined by PDAI, and additionally produced no side-effects, while metronidazole induced dysgeusia, vomiting and transient peripheral neuropathy in 3/9 patients.

If episodes of pouchitis promptly recur the probiotic preparation VSL-3 may be taken orally, with some evidence that relapse rates decrease. Two randomized trials have shown relapse rates in the order of 10–15% at 9–12 months with VSL-3 compared to 94–100% for those receiving placebo[142,143]. This therapeutic agent has also been trialled in a prophylactic capacity following IPAA surgery. At 1 year 10% of VSL-3 patients had experienced at least one episode of pouchitis in contrast to 40% of those receiving placebo[144].

## Pouch dysplasia

With a subgroup of pouch patients experiencing long-term problems with pouchitis the question arises of whether these patients are at risk of dysplastic changes within their pouch, as described by some investigators in the field[145,146]. Ileal pouch adenocarcinoma has also been rarely described[147-150]. Such lesions are hypothesized to arise from either residual islands of rectal mucosa left on the rectal cuff, or alternatively from evolution via dysplastic ileal mucosa, although this is not a universal finding in the ileal pouch[151]. Similarly 15-year follow-up of the Kock pouch indicates that dysplastic change within the ileal mucosa does not occur[152].

## Sexual dysfunction

Rates of mild and severe impairment of sexual activity before and after IPAA surgery were found to be 20% versus 16% and 16% versus 3% respectively[10]. Twenty-five per cent of patients reported that their sex lives had improved; for 56% there was no change. The incidence of sexual dysfunction at 1 and 12 years in men and women was 1% versus 2% and 8% versus 11%.

## Fecundity and pregnancy

UC commonly affects young females of reproductive age. Neither the disease itself nor the medical treatments currently available are thought to compromise fertility, although data from patients with predominantly active disease are lacking[153]. Johnson et al. examined fertility rates in married or cohabiting females aged 18–44 years with a history of UC[154]. Of 153 patients who fulfilled the criteria, and who had undergone IPAA, 59 (38%) were unable to conceive following 1 year of unprotected intercourse compared to eight of 60 patients (13%) who had non-operative management for their UC. Diagnosis of UC had no effect upon subsequent fertility; however, in marked contrast, IPAA surgery led to a 98% reduction. Strategies to deal with this problem include performing subtotal colectomy and delaying proctectomy, or perhaps using an anti-adhesion strategy to avoid tubal obstruction.

## Effect of vaginal delivery upon pouch function

Vaginal delivery is associated with an appreciable rate of occult sphincter injury in the order of 30%[155]. Particular risk factors included epidural analgesia and instrumental delivery. Clinicians have been concerned that rates of incontinence might rise dramatically in the years following childbirth, leading to dissatisfaction with the procedure and greater pouch failure within this subgroup. Farouk et al. determined that pouch function, in terms of incontinence, pad usage and constipating medication, remained unaffected in 85 of 692 females who completed one or more vaginal delivery when compared to those women of childbearing age who did not have children[10]. In addition women who experienced complicated deliveries were not more likely to suffer an adverse long-term outcome when compared to those who delivered normally.

## Pouch failure

Failure of IPAA is defined by the need for pouch excision or indefinite retention of a defunctioning stoma. Several centres have now reported mature follow-up data detailing experience with large cohorts of patients, in the process identifying factors that predispose to pouch failure. Institutional pouch failure rates have notably fallen over the past 20 years, presumably following improvements in both patient selection and surgical technique. Tulchinsky et al. showed that the rate of failure for two halves of a 22-year study were 16.5% and 8.3%[80]. Similarly Fazio et al. observed failure rates of almost 15% in each of the first 3 years of an 18-year period fall to 2.1% for each of the last 3 years[18]. This trend has been apparent in other major centres[15]. Inevitably a proportion of the more recently performed procedures are destined to fail, and the gap between these figures will undoubtedly close as patients are followed.

Experience plays a key role in both pouch construction and the treatment of post-operative complications. The Cleveland Clinic group examined how operator experience, determined by previous number of IPAA operations, influenced long-term pouch failure rates using a technique that sought to compensate for mixed case loads[58]. Surgeons were grouped according to experience with two seniors who had performed IPAA surgery since the mid-1980s and 10 juniors who were completing an average of 67 IPAA cases each. Fifty per cent of juniors demonstrated a learning curve of 23 cases for this procedure as determined by their pouch failure rate. The initial learning curve for senior staff had been in the order of 40 cases. Notably pouch failure following hand-sewn anastomosis was significantly higher for junior staff when compared to their senior colleagues, although the two groups performed stapled anastomosis equally well.

In general two types of pouch failure have been considered. Early failure arises from complications of the primary procedure or from technical difficulties experienced at this time. Late failure is more likely to reflect poor function of the pouch reservoir. A consistent theme that emerges from the large institutional series is that early pouch failure is closely associated with the occurrence of perioperative pelvic sepsis, while that occurring later is often secondary to poor function or following an unexpected diagnosis of CD[10,15,18,80,124]. The demographics of these study populations with failure rates and causes of failure are given in Table 1. Most failures occur beyond the first year and a steady rate of attrition is evident up to 10 years. Certain operative practices that may have increased the rate of pouch failure, such as widespread use of the S pouch design that was prone to efferent limb obstruction, are now redundant.

## SALVAGE SURGERY

Historically 10% of IPAA procedures fail, some secondary to the complications of surgery; others follow technical errors in pouch construction while poor function arising either as a result of inflammation within the pouch or inadequate sphincter tone account for the majority. Those in whom a belated diagnosis of CD is made may require removal of the ileal reservoir; however, in the remainder, attempts may be made to correct the underlying problem and salvage the pouch.

Early failure tends to arise as a consequence of acute surgical complications of which sepsis is the most frequent. One should evaluate the sphincters, assess pelvic soft tissue compliance, make a judgement regarding the likely diagnosis (CD or UC) and determine the patient's general health and wishes. Re-do pouch surgery for definite UC has success rates that have improved from 50% to nearer 90%[106,156-160]. Unfortunately with CD fewer that 50% of patients will manage to keep their pouch at 5 years.

**Table 1** Causes of ileoanal pouch failure

| Reference | No of patients | Follow-up | Failure | Main causes of failure | Pouch survival | Predictive of failure |
|---|---|---|---|---|---|---|
| MacRae et al.[15] | 551 | (>2.5 years) | 58/551 (10.5%) | Anastomotic leak (39%) <br> Poor function (23%) <br> Pouchitis (12%) <br> Pouch leak (12%) <br> Perianal disease (12%) (8.5% CD) | | Tension at IAA <br> Hand-sewn IAA <br> Defunctioning ileostomy <br> Leak <br> Δ Crohn's (19%) |
| Farouk et al.[10] | 1386 | (8 years) <br> UC 100% | 92/1386 (6.6%) | Pelvic sepsis 47% (fistula 29%) <br> Unrecognized CD (17%) <br> Poor function (15%) <br> Pouchitis (13%) <br> Anastomotic stricture (4%) | 5 years (95%) <br> 10 years (90%) | |
| Lepisto et al.[124] | 486 | (2–16 years) <br> UC (92.5%) <br> FAP (7.5%) | 24/484 (4.9%) <br> 2 peri-operative deaths | Persistent fistula (21%) <br> Incontinence (21%) <br> Unrecognized CD (17%) (all fistulas) <br> Pouchitis (12.5%) <br> Pouchitis + fistula (8%) <br> Major anastomotic leak (8%) <br> Others (12.5%) | 1 years (99%) <br> 5 years (95%) <br> 10 years (93%) | Fistula formation |
| Tulchinsky et al.[80] | 634 | (7 years) <br> UC (96.4%) <br> IC (1.6%) <br> CD (2%) | 61/631 (9.7%) <br> 3 peri-operative deaths | Pelvic sepsis (52%) <br> Poor function (30%) <br> Pouchitis (11%) <br> Technical (6%) | 5 years (91%) <br> 10 years (87%) | Female sex |
| Fazio et al.[18] | 1965 | (4 years) <br> UC (60.8%) <br> IC (27.8%) <br> CD (3.8%) <br> FAP (7.3%) | 77/1963 (3.9%) <br> 3 peri-operative deaths | Not stated | 3 years (96.5%) <br> 5 years (95.7%) <br> 10 years (93.4%) | Crohn's pre-operative <br> Comorbidity <br> Anal pathology pre-operative <br> Abnormal manometry <br> Anastomotic defect <br> Symptomatic stricture <br> Pelvic sepsis <br> Fistula (perineal/vaginal) |

# CONCLUSIONS

The introduction of IPAA has revolutionized treatment of ulcerative colitis. Over the past 30 years we have witnessed convergence of operative technique towards a stapled J pouch design with stapled ileoanal anastomosis. This is perhaps the fastest and easiest way to create the IPAA. Complication rates have fallen and the surgical community is eager to improve the technique further by exploring methods of one-stage and minimally invasive pouch surgery. Unappreciated CD causes substantial morbidity among a minority of patients. Pouchitis is a more common problem for which we have empirical treatments, even though the underlying cause remains unknown. Ileoanal pouch surgery has quickly become the standard of care for chronic UC, and must be considered a major success in the field of gastrointestinal surgery.

## References

1.  Ravitch MM, Sabiston DC. Anal ileostomy with preservation of the sphincter. Surg Gynecol Obstet. 1947;84:1095–109.
2.  Valiente MA, Bacon HE. Construction of pouch using pantaloon technic for pull-through of ileum following total colectomy; report of experimental work and results. Am J Surg. 1955;90:742–50.
3.  Kock NG. Intra-abdominal 'reservoir' in patients with permanent ileostomy. Preliminary observations on a procedure resulting in fecal 'continence' in five ileostomy patients. Arch Surg. 1969;99:223–31.
4.  Kock NG. Present status of the continent ileostomy: surgical revision of the malfunctioning ileostomy. Dis Colon Rectum. 1976;19:200–6.
5.  Jeffery PJ, Hawley PR, Parks AG. Colo-anal sleeve anastomosis in the treatment of diffuse cavernous haemangioma involving the rectum. Br J Surg. 1976;63:678–82.
6.  Parks AG. Transanal technique in low rectal anastomosis. Proc R Soc Med. 1972;65:975–6.
7.  Parks AG, Nicholls RJ. Proctocolectomy without ileostomy for ulcerative colitis. Br Med J. 1978;2:85–8.
8.  Fazio VW, Ziv Y, Church JM et al. Ileal pouch–anal anastomoses complications and function in 1005 patients. Ann Surg. 1995;222:120–7.
9.  Delaney CP, Fazio VW, Remzi FH et al. Prospective, age-related analysis of surgical results, functional outcome, and quality of life after ileal pouch–anal anastomosis. Ann Surg. 2003;238:221–8.
10. Farouk R, Pemberton JH, Wolff BG, Dozois RR, Browning S, Larson D. Functional outcomes after ileal pouch–anal anastomosis for chronic ulcerative colitis. Ann Surg. 2000; 231:919–26.
11. McIntyre PB, Pemberton JH, Wolff BG, Dozois RR, Beart RW Jr. Indeterminate colitis. Long-term outcome in patients after ileal pouch–anal anastomosis. Dis Colon Rectum. 1995;38:51–4.
12. Marcello PW, Schoetz DJ Jr, Roberts PL et al. Evolutionary changes in the pathologic diagnosis after the ileoanal pouch procedure. Dis Colon Rectum. 1997;40:263–9.
13. Yu CS, Pemberton JH, Larson D. Ileal pouch–anal anastomosis in patients with indeterminate colitis: long-term results. Dis Colon Rectum. 2000;43:1487–96.
14. Delaney CP, Remzi FH, Gramlich T, Dadvand B, Fazio VW. Equivalent function, quality of life and pouch survival rates after ileal pouch–anal anastomosis for indeterminate and ulcerative colitis. Ann Surg. 2002;236:43–8.
15. MacRae HM, McLeod RS, Cohen Z, O'Connor BI, Ton EN. Risk factors for pelvic pouch failure. Dis Colon Rectum. 1997;40(3):257–62.
16. Peyregne V, Francois Y, Gilly FN, Descos JL, Flourie B, Vignal J. Outcome of ileal pouch after secondary diagnosis of Crohn's disease. Int J Colorectal Dis. 2000;15:49–53.
17. Sagar PM, Dozois RR, Wolff BG. Long-term results of ileal pouch–anal anastomosis in patients with Crohn's disease. Dis Colon Rectum. 1996;39:893–8.

18. Fazio VW, Tekkis PP, Remzi F et al. Quantification of risk for pouch failure after ileal pouch–anal anastomosis surgery. Ann Surg. 2003;238:605–14; discussion 614–7.

19. Regimbeau JM, Panis Y, Pocard M et al. Long-term results of ileal pouch–anal anastomosis for colorectal Crohn's disease. Dis Colon Rectum. 2001;44:769–78.

20. Ziv Y, Fazio VW, Strong SA, Oakley JR, Milsom JW, Lavery IC. Ulcerative colitis and coexisting colorectal cancer: recurrence rate after restorative proctocolectomy. Ann Surg Oncol. 1994;1:512–15.

21. Taylor BA, Wolff BG, Dozois RR, Kelly KA, Pemberton JH, Beart RW Jr. Ileal pouch–anal anastomosis for chronic ulcerative colitis and familial polyposis coli complicated by adenocarcinoma. Dis Colon Rectum. 1988;31:358–62.

22. Utsunomiya J, Iwama T, Imajo M et al. Total colectomy, mucosal proctectomy, and ileoanal anastomosis. Dis Colon Rectum. 1980;23:459–66.

23. McHugh SM, Diamant NE, McLeod R, Cohen Z. S-pouches vs. J-pouches. A comparison of functional outcomes. Dis Colon Rectum. 1987;30:671–7.

24. Johnston D, Williamson ME, Lewis WG, Miller AS, Sagar PM, Holdsworth PJ. Prospective controlled trial of duplicated (J) versus quadruplicated (W) pelvic ileal reservoirs in restorative proctocolectomy for ulcerative colitis. Gut. 1996;39:242–7.

25. Oresland T, Fasth S, Nordgren S, Hallgren T, Hulten L. A prospective randomized comparison of two different pelvic pouch designs. Scand J Gastroenterol. 1990;25:986–96.

26. Choen S, Tsunoda A, Nicholls RJ. Prospective randomized trial comparing anal function after hand-sewn ileoanal anastomosis with mucosectomy versus stapled ileoanal anastomosis without mucosectomy in restorative proctocolectomy. Br J Surg. 1991;78:430–4.

27. Tuckson W, Lavery I, Fazio V, Oakley J, Church J, Milsom J. Manometric and functional comparison of ileal pouch–anal anastomosis with and without anal manipulation. Am J Surg. 1991;161:90–5; discussion 95–6.

28. Pemberton JH, Kelly KA, Beart RW Jr, Dozois RR, Wolff BG, Ilstrup DM. Ileal pouch–anal anastomosis for chronic ulcerative colitis. Long-term results. Ann Surg. 1987;206:504–13.

29. Wexner SD, Jensen L, Rothenberger DA, Wong WD, Goldberg SM. Long-term functional analysis of the ileoanal reservoir. Dis Colon Rectum. 1989;32:275–81.

30. Miller R, Bartolo DC, Orrom WJ, Mortensen NJ, Roe AM, Cervero F. Improvement of anal sensation with preservation of the anal transition zone after ileoanal anastomosis for ulcerative colitis. Dis Colon Rectum. 1990;33:414–18.

31. Johnston D, Holdsworth PJ, Nasmyth DG et al. Preservation of the entire anal canal in conservative proctocolectomy for ulcerative colitis: a pilot study comparing end-to-end ileo-anal anastomosis without mucosal resection with mucosal proctectomy and endo-anal anastomosis. Br J Surg. 1987;74:940–4.

32. Holdsworth PJ, Johnston D. Anal sensation after restorative proctocolectomy for ulcerative colitis. Br J Surg. 1988;75:993–6.

33. Heald RJ, Allen DR. Stapled ileo-anal anastomosis: a technique to avoid mucosal proctectomy in the ileal pouch operation. Br J Surg. 1986;73:571–2.

34. Sagar PM, Holdsworth PJ, Johnston D. Correlation between laboratory findings and clinical outcome after restorative proctocolectomy: serial studies in 20 patients with end-to-end pouch–anal anastomosis. Br J Surg. 1991;78:67–70.

35. Sugerman HJ, Newsome HH. Stapled ileoanal anastomosis without a temporary ileostomy. Am J Surg. 1994;167:58–65; discussion 65–6.

36. Sugerman HJ, Newsome HH, Decosta G, Zfass AM. Stapled ileoanal anastomosis for ulcerative colitis and familial polyposis without a temporary diverting ileostomy. Ann Surg. 1991;213:606–17; discussion 617–19.

37. Deen KI, Williams JG, Grant EA, Billingham C, Keighley MR. Randomized trial to determine the optimum level of pouch–anal anastomosis in stapled restorative proctocolectomy. Dis Colon Rectum. 1995;38:133–8.

38. Luukkonen P, Jarvinen H. Stapled vs hand-sutured ileoanal anastomosis in restorative proctocolectomy. A prospective, randomized study. Arch Surg. 1993;128:437–40.

39. Hallgren TA, Fasth SB, Oresland TO, Hulten LA. Ileal pouch–anal function after endoanal mucosectomy and handsewn ileoanal anastomosis compared with stapled anastomosis without mucosectomy. Eur J Surg. 1995;161:915–21.

40. McIntyre PB, Pemberton JH, Beart RW Jr, Devine RM, Nivatvongs S. Double-stapled vs. handsewn ileal pouch–anal anastomosis in patients with chronic ulcerative colitis. Dis Colon Rectum. 1994;37:430–3.

41. Reilly WT, Pemberton JH, Wolff BG et al. Randomized prospective trial comparing ileal pouch–anal anastomosis performed by excising the anal mucosa to ileal pouch–anal anastomosis performed by preserving the anal mucosa. Ann Surg. 1997;225:666–76; discussion 676–7.

42. Ziv Y, Fazio VW, Church JM, Lavery IC, King TM, Ambrosetti P. Stapled ileal pouch–anal anastomoses are safer than handsewn anastomoses in patients with ulcerative colitis. Am J Surg. 1996;171:320–3.

43. Gemlo BT, Belmonte C, Wiltz O, Madoff RD. Functional assessment of ileal pouch–anal anastomotic techniques. Am J Surg. 1995;169:137–41; discussion 141–2.

44. Choi HJ, Saigusa N, Choi JS et al. How consistent is the anal transitional zone in the double-stapled ileoanal reservoir? Int J Colorectal Dis. 2003;18:116–20.

45. Winter DC, Murphy A, Kell MR, Shields CJ, Redmond HP, Kirwan WO. Perioperative topical nitrate and sphincter function in patients undergoing transanal stapled anastomosis: a randomized, placebo-controlled, double-blinded trial. Dis Colon Rectum. 2004;47:697–703.

46. Thompson-Fawcett MW, Warren BF, Mortensen NJ. A new look at the anal transitional zone with reference to restorative proctocolectomy and the columnar cuff. Br J Surg. 1998; 85:1517–21.

47. Lavery IC, Sirimarco MT, Ziv Y, Fazio VW. Anal canal inflammation after ileal pouch–anal anastomosis. The need for treatment. Dis Colon Rectum. 1995;38:803–6.

48. Shen B, Lashner BA, Bennett AE et al. Treatment of rectal cuff inflammation (cuffitis) in patients with ulcerative colitis following restorative proctocolectomy and ileal pouch–anal anastomosis. Am J Gastroenterol. 2004;99:1527–31.

49. Baratsis S, Hadjidimitriou F, Christodoulou M, Lariou K. Adenocarcinoma in the anal canal after ileal pouch–anal anastomosis for ulcerative colitis using a double stapling technique: report of a case. Dis Colon Rectum. 2002;45:687–91; discussion 691–2.

50. Laureti S, Ugolini F, D'Errico A, Rago S, Poggioli G. Adenocarcinoma below ileoanal anastomosis for ulcerative colitis: report of a case and review of the literature. Dis Colon Rectum. 2002;45:418–21.

51. Sequens R. Cancer in the anal canal (transitional zone) after restorative proctocolectomy with stapled ileal pouch–anal anastomosis. Int J Colorectal Dis. 1997;12:254–5.

52. Coull DB, Lee FD, Henderson AP, Anderson JH, McKee RF, Finlay IG. Risk of dysplasia in the columnar cuff after stapled restorative proctocolectomy. Br J Surg. 2003;90:72–5.

53. Thompson-Fawcett MW, Mortensen NJ. Anal transitional zone and columnar cuff in restorative proctocolectomy. Br J Surg. 1996;83:1047–55.

54. Haray PN, Amarnath B, Weiss EG, Nogueras JJ, Wexner SD. Low malignant potential of the double-stapled ileal pouch–anal anastomosis. Br J Surg. 1996;83:1406.

55. Remzi FH, Fazio VW, Delaney CP et al. Dysplasia of the anal transitional zone after ileal pouch–anal anastomosis: results of prospective evaluation after a minimum of ten years. Dis Colon Rectum. 2003;46:6–13.

56. O'Connell PR, Pemberton JH, Weiland LH et al. Does rectal mucosa regenerate after ileoanal anastomosis? Dis Colon Rectum. 1987;30:1–5.

57. Heppell J, Weiland LH, Perrault J, Pemberton JH, Telander RL, Beart RW Jr. Fate of the rectal mucosa after rectal mucosectomy and ileoanal anastomosis. Dis Colon Rectum. 1983;26:768–71.

58. Tekkis PP, Fazio VW, Lavery IC et al. Evaluation of the learning curve in ileal pouch–anal anastomosis surgery. Ann Surg. 2005;241:262–8.

59. Williamson ME, Lewis WG, Sagar PM, Holdsworth PJ, Johnston D. One-stage restorative proctocolectomy without temporary ileostomy for ulcerative colitis: a note of caution. Dis Colon Rectum. 1997;40:1019–22.

60. Sugerman HJ, Sugerman EL, Meador JG, Newsome HH Jr, Kellum JM Jr, DeMaria EJ. Ileal pouch–anal anastomosis without ileal diversion. Ann Surg. 2000;232:530–41.

61. Mowschenson PM, Critchlow JF, Rosenberg SJ, Peppercorn MA. Factors favoring continence, the avoidance of a diverting ileostomy and small intestinal conservation in the ileoanal pouch operation. Surg Gynecol Obstet. 1993;177:17–26.

62. Mowschenson PM, Critchlow JF. Outcome of early surgical complications following ileoanal pouch operation without diverting ileostomy. Am J Surg. 1995;169:143–5; discussion 145–6.
63. Metcalf AM, Dozois RR, Kelly KA, Wolff BG. Ileal pouch–anal anastomosis without temporary, diverting ileostomy. Dis Colon Rectum. 1986;29:33–5.
64. Matikainen M, Santavirta J, Hiltunen KM. Ileoanal anastomosis without covering ileostomy. Dis Colon Rectum. 1990;33:384–8.
65. Jarvinen HJ, Luukkonen P. Comparison of restorative proctocolectomy with and without covering ileostomy in ulcerative colitis. Br J Surg. 1991;78:199–201.
66. Hainsworth PJ, Bartolo DC. Selective omission of loop ileostomy in restorative proctocolectomy. Int J Colorectal Dis. 1998;13:119–23.
67. Gorfine SR, Gelernt IM, Bauer JJ, Harris MT, Kreel I. Restorative proctocolectomy without diverting ileostomy. Dis Colon Rectum. 1995;38:188–94.
68. Tjandra JJ, Fazio VW, Milsom JW, Lavery IC, Oakley JR, Fabre JM. Omission of temporary diversion in restorative proctocolectomy – is it safe? Dis Colon Rectum. 1993; 36:1007–14.
69. Galandiuk S, Wolff BG, Dozois RR, Beart RW Jr. Ileal pouch–anal anastomosis without ileostomy. Dis Colon Rectum. 1991;34:870–3.
70. Wong KS, Remzi FH, Gorgun E et al. Loop ileostomy closure after restorative proctocolectomy: outcome in 1504 patients. Dis Colon Rectum. 2005;48:243–50.
71. Edwards DP, Chisholm EM, Donaldson DR. Closure of transverse loop colostomy and loop ileostomy. Ann R Coll Surg Engl. 1998;80:33–5.
72. Winslet MC, Barsoum G, Pringle W, Fox K, Keighley MR. Loop ileostomy after ileal pouch–anal anastomosis – is it necessary? Dis Colon Rectum. 1991;34:267–70.
73. Wexner SD, Taranow DA, Johansen OB et al. Loop ileostomy is a safe option for fecal diversion. Dis Colon Rectum. 1993;36:349–54.
74. Hosie KB, Grobler SP, Keighley MR. Temporary loop ileostomy following restorative proctocolectomy. Br J Surg. 1992;79:33–4.
75. Senapati A, Nicholls RJ, Ritchie JK, Tibbs CJ, Hawley PR. Temporary loop ileostomy for restorative proctocolectomy. Br J Surg. 1993;80:628–30.
76. Lewis P, Bartolo DC. Closure of loop ileostomy after restorative proctocolectomy. Ann R Coll Surg Engl. 1990;72:263–5.
77. Mann LJ, Stewart PJ, Goodwin RJ, Chapuis PH, Bokey EL. Complications following closure of loop ileostomy. Aust NZ J Surg 1991;61:493–6.
78. Phang PT, Hain JM, Perez-Ramirez JJ, Madoff RD, Gemlo BT. Techniques and complications of ileostomy takedown. Am J Surg. 1999;177:463–6.
79. Heuschen UA, Hinz U, Allemeyer EH, Lucas M, Heuschen G, Herfarth C. One- or two-stage procedure for restorative proctocolectomy: rationale for a surgical strategy in ulcerative colitis. Ann Surg. 2001;234:788–94.
80. Tulchinsky H, Hawley PR, Nicholls J. Long-term failure after restorative proctocolectomy for ulcerative colitis. Ann Surg. 2003;238:229–34.
81. Marcello PW, Milsom JW, Wong SK, Hammerhofer KA, Goormastic M, Church JM, et al. Laparoscopic restorative proctocolectomy: case-matched comparative study with open restorative proctocolectomy. Dis Colon Rectum. 2000;43:604–8.
82. Santoro E, Carlini M, Carboni F, Feroce A. Laparoscopic total proctocolectomy with ileal J pouch–anal anastomosis. Hepatogastroenterology. 1999;46:894–9.
83. Seshadri PA, Poulin EC, Schlachta CM, Cadeddu MO, Mamazza J. Does a laparoscopic approach to total abdominal colectomy and proctocolectomy offer advantages? Surg Endosc. 2001;15:837–42.
84. Schmitt SL, Cohen SM, Wexner SD, Nogueras JJ, Jagelman DG. Does laparoscopic-assisted ileal pouch–anal anastomosis reduce the length of hospitalization? Int J Colorectal Dis. 1994;9:134–7.
85. Brown SR, Eu KW, Seow-Choen F. Consecutive series of laparoscopic-assisted vs. minilaparotomy restorative proctocolectomies. Dis Colon Rectum. 2001;44:397–400.
86. Kienle P, Weitz J, Benner A, Herfarth C, Schmidt J. Laparoscopically assisted colectomy and ileoanal pouch procedure with and without protective ileostomy. Surg Endosc. 2003;17: 716–20.

87. Ky AJ, Sonoda T, Milsom JW. One-stage laparoscopic restorative proctocolectomy: an alternative to the conventional approach? Dis Colon Rectum. 2002;45:207–10; discussion 210–11.
88. Maartense S, Dunker MS, Slors JF et al. Hand-assisted laparoscopic versus open restorative proctocolectomy with ileal pouch–anal anastomosis: a randomized trial. Ann Surg. 2004;240:984–91; discussion 991–2.
89. MacLean AR, Cohen Z, MacRae HM et al. Risk of small bowel obstruction after the ileal pouch–anal anastomosis. Ann Surg. 2002;235:200–6.
90. Francois Y, Dozois RR, Kelly KA et al. Small intestinal obstruction complicating ileal pouch–anal anastomosis. Ann Surg. 1989;209:46–50.
91. Marcello PW, Roberts PL, Schoetz DJ Jr, Coller JA, Murray JJ, Veidenheimer MC. Obstruction after ileal pouch–anal anastomosis: a preventable complication? Dis Colon Rectum. 1993;36:1105–11.
92. Read TE, Schoetz DJ Jr, Marcello PW et al. Afferent limb obstruction complicating ileal pouch–anal anastomosis. Dis Colon Rectum. 1997;40:566–9.
93. Jansen RP. Failure of intraperitoneal adjuncts to improve the outcome of pelvic operations in young women. Am J Obstet Gynecol. 1985;153:363–71.
94. Becker JM, Dayton MT, Fazio VW et al. Prevention of postoperative abdominal adhesions by a sodium hyaluronate-based bioresorbable membrane: a prospective, randomized, double-blind multicenter study. J Am Coll Surg. 1996;183:297–306.
95. Beck DE, Cohen Z, Fleshman JW, Kaufman HS, van Goor H, Wolff BG. A prospective, randomized, multicenter, controlled study of the safety of Seprafilm adhesion barrier in abdominopelvic surgery of the intestine. Dis Colon Rectum. 2003;46:1310–19.
96. Heuschen UA, Hinz U, Allemeyer EH et al. Risk factors for ileoanal J pouch-related septic complications in ulcerative colitis and familial adenomatous polyposis. Ann Surg. 2002; 235:207–16.
97. Heuschen UA, Allemeyer EH, Hinz U, Lucas M, Herfarth C, Heuschen G. Outcome after septic complications in J pouch procedures. Br J Surg. 2002;89:194–200.
98. Farouk R, Dozois RR, Pemberton JH, Larson D. Incidence and subsequent impact of pelvic abscess after ileal pouch–anal anastomosis for chronic ulcerative colitis. Dis Colon Rectum. 1998;41:1239–43.
99. Dozois RR, Kelly KA, Welling DR et al. Ileal pouch–anal anastomosis: comparison of results in familial adenomatous polyposis and chronic ulcerative colitis. Ann Surg. 1989;210:268–71; discussion 272–3.
100. Cohen Z, McLeod RS, Stephen W, Stern HS, O'Connor B, Reznick R. Continuing evolution of the pelvic pouch procedure. Ann Surg. 1992;216:506–11; discussion 511–12.
101. Ziv Y, Church JM, Fazio VW, King TM, Lavery IC. Effect of systemic steroids on ileal pouch–anal anastomosis in patients with ulcerative colitis. Dis Colon Rectum. 1996;39: 504–8.
102. Breen EM, Schoetz DJ Jr, Marcello PW et al. Functional results after perineal complications of ileal pouch–anal anastomosis. Dis Colon Rectum. 1998;41:691–5.
103. Williams NS, Johnston D. The current status of mucosal proctectomy and ileo-anal anastomosis in the surgical treatment of ulcerative colitis and adenomatous polyposis. Br J Surg. 1985;72:159–68.
104. de Silva HJ, de Angelis CP, Soper N, Kettlewell MG, Mortensen NJ, Jewell DP. Clinical and functional outcome after restorative proctocolectomy. Br J Surg. 1991;78:1039–44.
105. Senapati A, Tibbs CJ, Ritchie JK, Nicholls RJ, Hawley PR. Stenosis of the pouch–anal anastomosis following restorative proctocolectomy. Int J Colorectal Dis. 1996;11:57–9.
106. Galandiuk S, Scott NA, Dozois RR et al. Ileal pouch–anal anastomosis. Reoperation for pouch-related complications. Ann Surg. 1990;212:446–52; discussion 452–4.
107. Fazio VW, Tjandra JJ. Pouch advancement and neoileoanal anastomosis for anastomotic stricture and anovaginal fistula complicating restorative proctocolectomy. Br J Surg. 1992; 79:694–6.
108. O'Kelly TJ, Merrett M, Mortensen NJ, Dehn TC, Kettlewell M. Pouch-vaginal fistula after restorative proctocolectomy: aetiology and management. Br J Surg. 1994;81:1374–5.
109. Keighley MR, Grobler SP. Fistula complicating restorative proctocolectomy. Br J Surg. 1993;80:1065–7.
110. Groom JS, Nicholls RJ, Hawley PR, Phillips RK. Pouch–vaginal fistula. Br J Surg. 1993; 80:936–40.

111. Shah NS, Remzi F, Massmann A, Baixauli J, Fazio VW. Management and treatment outcome of pouch-vaginal fistulas following restorative proctocolectomy. Dis Colon Rectum. 2003;46:911–17.
112. Heriot AG, Tekkis PP, Smith JJ, Bona R, Cohen RG, Nicholls RJ. Management and outcome of pouch–vaginal fistulas following restorative proctocolectomy. Dis Colon Rectum. 2005;48:451–8.
113. Burke D, van Laarhoven CJ, Herbst F, Nicholls RJ. Transvaginal repair of pouch–vaginal fistula. Br J Surg. 2001;88:241–5.
114. Ricart E, Panaccione R, Loftus EV, Tremaine WJ, Sandborn WJ. Successful management of Crohn's disease of the ileoanal pouch with infliximab. Gastroenterology. 1999;117:429–32.
115. Colombel JF, Ricart E, Loftus EV Jr et al. Management of Crohn's disease of the ileoanal pouch with infliximab. Am J Gastroenterol. 2003;98:2239–44.
116. Shepherd NA, Healey CJ, Warren BF, Richman PI, Thomson WH, Wilkinson SP. Distribution of mucosal pathology and an assessment of colonic phenotypic change in the pelvic ileal reservoir. Gut. 1993;34:101–5.
117. Shepherd NA, Hulten L, Tytgat GN et al. Pouchitis. Int J Colorectal Dis. 1989;4:205–29.
118. Madden MV, Farthing MJ, Nicholls RJ. Inflammation in ileal reservoirs: 'pouchitis'. Gut. 1990;31:247–9.
119. Shen B, Achkar JP, Lashner BA et al. Irritable pouch syndrome: a new category of diagnosis for symptomatic patients with ileal pouch–anal anastomosis. Am J Gastroenterol. 2002;97:972–7.
120. Parsi MA, Shen B, Achkar JP et al. Fecal lactoferrin for diagnosis of symptomatic patients with ileal pouch–anal anastomosis. Gastroenterology. 2004;126(5):1280–6.
121. Sandborn WJ, Tremaine WJ, Batts KP, Pemberton JH, Phillips SF. Pouchitis after ileal pouch–anal anastomosis: a Pouchitis Disease Activity Index. Mayo Clin Proc. 1994;69: 409–15.
122. Heuschen UA, Autschbach F, Allemeyer EH et al. Long-term follow-up after ileoanal pouch procedure: algorithm for diagnosis, classification, and management of pouchitis. Dis Colon Rectum. 2001;44:487–99.
123. Heuschen UA, Allemeyer EH, Hinz U et al. Diagnosing pouchitis: comparative validation of two scoring systems in routine follow-up. Dis Colon Rectum. 2002;45:776–86; discussion 786–8.
124. Lepisto A, Luukkonen P, Jarvinen HJ. Cumulative failure rate of ileal pouch–anal anastomosis and quality of life after failure. Dis Colon Rectum. 2002;45:1289–94.
125. Sagar PM, Godwin PG, Holdsworth PJ, Johnston D. Influence of myectomy, ileal valve, and ileal reservoir on the ecology of the ileum. Dis Colon Rectum. 1992;35:170–7.
126. Pace DE, Seshadri PA, Chiasson PM, Poulin EC, Schlachta CM, Mamazza J. Early experience with laparoscopic ileal pouch–anal anastomosis for ulcerative colitis. Surg Laparosc Endosc Percutan Tech. 2002;12:337–41.
127. Penna C, Dozois R, Tremaine W et al. Pouchitis after ileal pouch–anal anastomosis for ulcerative colitis occurs with increased frequency in patients with associated primary sclerosing cholangitis. Gut. 1996;38:234–9.
128. Lohmuller JL, Pemberton JH, Dozois RR, Ilstrup D, van Heerden J. Pouchitis and extraintestinal manifestations of inflammatory bowel disease after ileal pouch–anal anastomosis. Ann Surg. 1990;211:622–7; discussion 627–9.
129. Beaugerie L, Massot N, Carbonnel F, Cattan S, Gendre JP, Cosnes J. Impact of cessation of smoking on the course of ulcerative colitis. Am J Gastroenterol. 2001;96:2113–16.
130. Merrett MN, Mortensen N, Kettlewell M, Jewell DO. Smoking may prevent pouchitis in patients with restorative proctocolectomy for ulcerative colitis. Gut. 1996;38:362–4.
131. Stahlberg D, Gullberg K, Liljeqvist L, Hellers G, Lofberg R. Pouchitis following pelvic pouch operation for ulcerative colitis. Incidence, cumulative risk, and risk factors. Dis Colon Rectum. 1996;39:1012–18.
132. Carter MJ, Di Giovine FS, Cox A et al. The interleukin 1 receptor antagonist gene allele 2 as a predictor of pouchitis following colectomy and IPAA in ulcerative colitis. Gastroenterology. 2001;121:805–11.
133. Fleshner PR, Vasiliauskas EA, Kam LY et al. High level perinuclear antineutrophil cytoplasmic antibody (pANCA) in ulcerative colitis patients before colectomy predicts the development of chronic pouchitis after ileal pouch–anal anastomosis. Gut. 2001;49:671–7.

134. Duerr RH, Targan SR, Landers CJ et al. Neutrophil cytoplasmic antibodies: a link between primary sclerosing cholangitis and ulcerative colitis. Gastroenterology. 1991;100:1385–91.
135. Reumaux D, Colombel JF, Masy E et al. Anti-neutrophil cytoplasmic auto-antibodies (ANCA) in ulcerative colitis (UC): no relationship with disease activity. Inflamm Bowel Dis. 2000;6:270–4.
136. Hurst RD, Chung TP, Rubin M, Michelassi F. The implications of acute pouchitis on the long-term functional results after restorative proctocolectomy. Inflamm Bowel Dis. 1998;4:280–4.
137. Keranen U, Luukkonen P, Jarvinen H. Functional results after restorative proctocolectomy complicated by pouchitis. Dis Colon Rectum. 1997;40:764–9.
138. Hurst RD, Molinari M, Chung TP, Rubin M, Michelassi F. Prospective study of the incidence, timing and treatment of pouchitis in 104 consecutive patients after restorative proctocolectomy. Arch Surg. 1996;131:497–500; discussion 501–2.
139. Madden MV, McIntyre AS, Nicholls RJ. Double-blind crossover trial of metronidazole versus placebo in chronic unremitting pouchitis. Dig Dis Sci. 1994;39:1193–6.
140. McLeod RS, Taylor DW, Cohen Z, Cullen JB. Single-patient randomised clinical trial. Use in determining optimum treatment for patient with inflammation of Kock continent ileostomy reservoir. Lancet. 1986;1:726–8.
141. Shen B, Achkar JP, Lashner BA et al. A randomized clinical trial of ciprofloxacin and metronidazole to treat acute pouchitis. Inflamm Bowel Dis. 2001;7:301–5.
142. Gionchetti P, Rizzello F, Venturi A et al. Oral bacteriotherapy as maintenance treatment in patients with chronic pouchitis: a double-blind, placebo-controlled trial. Gastroenterology. 2000;119:305–9.
143. Mimura T, Rizzello F, Helwig U et al. Once daily high dose probiotic therapy (VSL#3) for maintaining remission in recurrent or refractory pouchitis. Gut. 2004;53:108–14.
144. Gionchetti P, Rizzello F, Helwig U et al. Prophylaxis of pouchitis onset with probiotic therapy: a double-blind, placebo-controlled trial. Gastroenterology. 2003;124:1202–9.
145. Veress B, Reinholt FP, Lindquist K, Lofberg R, Liljeqvist L. Long-term histomorphological surveillance of the pelvic ileal pouch: dysplasia develops in a subgroup of patients. Gastroenterology. 1995;109:1090–7.
146. Gullberg K, Stahlberg D, Liljeqvist L et al. Neoplastic transformation of the pelvic pouch mucosa in patients with ulcerative colitis. Gastroenterology. 1997;112:1487–92.
147. Stern H, Walfisch S, Mullen B, McLeod R, Cohen Z. Cancer in an ileoanal reservoir: a new late complication? Gut. 1990;31:473–5.
148. Ravitch MM. The reception of new operations. Ann Surg. 1984;200:231–46.
149. Puthu D, Rajan N, Rao R, Rao L, Venugopal P. Carcinoma of the rectal pouch following restorative proctocolectomy. Report of a case. Dis Colon Rectum. 1992;35:257–60.
150. Rodriguez-Sanjuan JC, Polavieja MG, Naranjo A, Castillo J. Adenocarcinoma in an ileal pouch for ulcerative colitis. Dis Colon Rectum. 1995;38:779–80.
151. de Silva HJ, Millard PR, Kettlewell M, Mortensen NJ, Prince C, Jewell DP. Mucosal characteristics of pelvic ileal pouches. Gut. 1991;32:61–5.
152. Ojerskog B, Kock NG, Nilsson LO, Philipson BM, Ahren C. Long-term follow-up of patients with continent ileostomies. Dis Colon Rectum. 1990;33:184–9.
153. Ording Olsen K, Juul S, Berndtsson I, Oresland T, Laurberg S. Ulcerative colitis: female fecundity before diagnosis, during disease, and after surgery compared with a population sample. Gastroenterology. 2002;122:15–19.
154. Johnson P, Richard C, Ravid A et al. Female infertility after ileal pouch–anal anastomosis for ulcerative colitis. Dis Colon Rectum. 2004;47:1119–26.
155. Sultan AH, Kamm MA, Hudson CN, Thomas JM, Bartram CI. Anal-sphincter disruption during vaginal delivery. N Engl J Med. 1993;329:1905–11.
156. Fonkalsrud EW, Bustorff-Silva J. Reconstruction for chronic dysfunction of ileoanal pouches. Ann Surg. 1999;229:197–204.
157. Fazio VW, Wu JS, Lavery IC. Repeat ileal pouch–anal anastomosis to salvage septic complications of pelvic pouches: clinical outcome and quality of life assessment. Ann Surg. 1998;228:588–97.
158. Cohen Z, Smith D, McLeod R. Reconstructive surgery for pelvic pouches. World J Surg. 1998;22:342–6.

159. MacLean AR, O'Connor B, Parkes R, Cohen Z, McLeod RS. Reconstructive surgery for failed ileal pouch–anal anastomosis: a viable surgical option with acceptable results. Dis Colon Rectum. 2002;45:880–6.
160. Ogunbiyi OA, Korsgen S, Keighley MR. Pouch salvage. Long-term outcome. Dis Colon Rectum. 1997;40:548–52.

# Section VI
# Immunomodulatory therapy

Chair: S.P.L. TRAVIS and A. TROMM

# 19
# Biologics in ulcerative colitis

T. J. CREED and C. S. J. PROBERT

## INTRODUCTION

There have been few trials of biological therapies in ulcerative colitis (UC). This is likely to reflect the perceived success of other treatments for UC: in the mid-late 1990s, cyclosporin therapy was at its most popular, while those patients who failed to respond to cyclosporin were cured by colectomy. Furthermore, ileoanal pouch surgery was becoming popular and offered a stoma-free solution for patients, making colectomy a less unattractive prospect. Consequently, although there have been numerous attempts to find novel agents to treat Crohn's disease (CD), the need to develop new approaches for UC has been less pressing.

CD and UC share many inflammatory mediators and, therefore, many agents that have been found to be effective for one condition have also been used for the other. Mesalazines are more effective in UC than CD, yet they are commonly prescribed for both conditions. Similarly, there is much more prospective trial data to support the use of azathioprine in CD than in UC, but azathioprine is used increasingly for both diseases. Recently, methotrexate, which has gained popularity in the management of CD, has been used in UC. In general terms, agents such as corticosteroids, mesalazine and azathioprine are considered to work in a broadly similar manner in both conditions.

However, basic scientific research targeted at understanding the immune response in inflammatory bowel disease (IBD) has focused on the differences between UC and CD. The interpretation of these findings was influenced by the Th1/Th2 paradigm popularized by the study of murine immunology. Furthermore, rodent models of IBD tended to support differences between the immune response in UC and CD. Such work polarized the immune response, and UC came to be considered a Th2 disease and CD a Th1 disease. Together these factors have led some investigators to believe that biological agents that target components of the immune response may not work equally well in both diseases. Some drugs, such as anti-interferon gamma antibodies, may work only for Th1 disorders, others for Th2 disorders. This may have delayed the evaluation of certain agents in conditions thought to be due to an immune response of the incorrect type.

However, other investigators have addressed the similarity between certain aspects of the immune response. The first similarity was, perhaps, tumour necrosis factor-α (TNF-α). The concentration of this proinflammatory cytokine was shown to be significantly increased in the blood and intestinal mucosa of patients with both active UC and CD when compared to healthy controls. It was reasonable, then, to expect biologics against this target to work equally well in both conditions.

## ANTI-TNF ANTIBODIES

CDP571 is a humanized mouse–human chimeric IgG4 antibody against human TNF-α. A study of CDP571, in 15 patients with ulcerative colitis, found that the disease activity quickly improved, but this was not sustained[1]. Further studies have not been reported with this agent.

The first reports of infliximab in the treatment of UC were also open-label series. Generally the results were positive, although such data should always be treated with caution. Chey et al.[2] reported eight patients all of whom appeared to respond dramatically to a single infusion of infliximab. The authors concluded that infliximab has a 'significant, major effect on active ulcerative colitis'.

Su et al.[3] reported their experience of infliximab therapy in 27 patients with active UC: most of the patients (89%) had severe disease activity and 20 (74%) had failed to respond to glucocorticoid therapy immediately before recruitment. Most (52%) patients had single infusions. Twelve patients (44%) achieved remission, six (22%) partial response, but nine (33%) did not respond, of whom five underwent colectomy. The median response time was 4 days. Interestingly, 11 of the 12 full responders had severe disease. The authors concluded that, whilst beneficial in treating patients with ulcerative colitis, the benefits were 'less in patients with steroid-refractory disease'.

Actis et al.[4] and Kohn et al.[5] published their open studies in 2002. Actis et al. reported that four of eight patients (50%) responded initially, but the sustained response rate was just 25%. Of the eight patients, six had not responded to glucocorticoid therapy. Kohn et al. reported 13 patients refractory to 7 days of parenteral methylprednisolone. Ten (77%) responded quickly, with a meaningful fall in their colitis activity index, but two underwent colectomy. Although the authors drew contrasting, though cautious, conclusions, they both urged that controlled studies be performed.

At present, five randomized controlled trails of infliximab in UC have been reported; three have been published in full, the others are in abstract form.

Sands et al.[6] reported eight patients who were randomized to receive single infliximab infusions, (three received 5 mg/kg, three 10 mg/kg and two 20 mg/kg), and three patients received placebo. Fifty per cent of the infliximab-treated patients responded by week 2. The authors were encouraged by the response rate.

We have reported a study in moderately severe steroid-resistant UC[7]; 23 received infliximab and 20 placebo. A single infusion of 5 mg/kg was administered, non-responders were offered open-label infliximab (10 mg/kg).

After 2 weeks the remission rate was 3/23 and 1/19 for active and placebo treatments respectively; by week 6 the rates were 9/23 (39%) and 6/20 (30%). We concluded the regimen did not support the widespread use of infliximab in the management of glucocorticoid-resistant moderately active UC.

Ochsenkuhn et al.[8] reported that five of six patients who were randomized to receive 5 mg/kg infliximab responded after 3 weeks; the benefit continued until follow-up at 13 weeks. Armuzzi et al.[9] performed a randomized open-label study of infliximab compared to methylprednisolone, in moderate to severe glucocorticoid-dependent UC. Three infliximab infusions were administered (0, 2 and 6 weeks). The reported remission rate was 9/10 with infliximab. However, 8/10 patients who received methylprednisolone also went into remission. This study appears encouraging; however the response to methylprednisolone in a group of patients dependent on glucocorticoid therapy is odd.

Finally, Jarnerot et al.[10] reported the outcome of a randomized trial of infliximab treatment in patients with moderate and severe UC. The rate of colectomy was significantly greater in patients who received placebo (14/21) than in those who received infliximab (7/24). The authors concluded that infliximab was a safe and effective rescue therapy.

Recently, two large randomized controlled trials of infliximab in UC have been completed. Act 1 and Act 2 used similar schedules to Accent 1 and Accent 2. The data will be presented at the forthcoming DDW (May 2005). Rumours abound that the response rate was significant, although the abstracts cannot be disseminated at this time.

## ANTI-CD3 ANTIBODIES

The results of a phase 1 study of humanized chimeric anti-CD3 monoclonal antibody, visilizumab, for the treatment of severe steroid-refractory UC have been reported in abstract form[11]. Data from 26 recruited patients were published in abstract form, eight patients received 15 μg/kg intravenously on days 1 and 2, 18 had 10 μg/kg intravenously on days 1 and 2. Of the 20 patients reported, 17 had a sustained response. Cytokine release syndrome was reported, and T-cell depletion lasting for up to 8 weeks was also seen. However, no significant opportunistic infections were reported, and an ongoing phase 1/2 trial is continuing to recruit patients with evidence of previous exposure to cytomegalovirus. Further evaluation of this compound in UC is warranted.

## ANTI-α4 ANTIBODIES

Natalizumab is a humanized chimeric antibody against the α4 subunit of an integrin, α4β7, that is associated with gut homing of lymphocytes. Natalizumab has been found to be useful in CD and in multiple sclerosis[12,13]. One open-label study has been reported in UC[14]; its design was similar to that of the study of natalizumab in CD. In the UC study 10 patients received a single infusion of natalizumab (3 mg/kg), five patients showed a good response by week 2, and six patients by week 4. Quality-of-life measures also improved. The drug was well tolerated. Unfortunately, recent concerns over the safety of natalizumab in multiple sclerosis patients, who were also receiving interferon-beta therapy, have led to its withdrawal pending further review.

## INTERFERONS

Studies have suggested that the interferons might have a role in the treatment of UC through the induction of anti-inflammatory cytokines such as the soluble TNF receptor p55, and the reduction of proinflammatory Th2 cytokines such as IL-5 and IL-13. An open-label study of 32 patients randomized to receive interferon-2α or prednisolone enemas in left-sided UC showed significant improvements in disease activity and histology in both groups, with no significant differences between the two groups[15]. However, in a randomized placebo-controlled trial of pegylated interferon-α in 60 patients with moderately active UC, no improvement over placebo was seen[16].

Interferon-β1a (IFN-B1a) has also been studied in a randomized controlled trial in moderately active UC[17]. Ten patients received IFN-β1a and seven received placebo. Clinical response (defined by a fall in UCSS of three or more points) was achieved in five patients (50%) in the IFN-β1a group and in one (14%) in the placebo group ($p = 0.14$). Endoscopic remission was achieved in three patients in the IFN-β1a group and in none in the placebo group ($p = 0.02$).

The interferons are associated with dose-limiting side-effects, and while the authors of the above studies advocate higher doses to achieve greater efficacy, this may be at the expense of tolerability.

## EPIDERMAL GROWTH FACTOR (EGF)

Interest in the use of recombinant growth factors initially focused upon the healing of peptic ulceration rather than colonic ulceration because of the difficulties in delivering these agents to the colon. Systemic administration of epidermal growth factor in necrotizing enterocolitis has been reported[18], but there are real concerns regarding the mitogenic potential of such treatments. Sinha et al.[19] treated patients with left-sided UC or proctitis with EGF enemas or placebo in addition to oral mesalazine. Ten of 12 patients were in remission at 2 weeks in the treatment group as compared to just one of 12 patients in the control group. While dysplasia was not seen in any of the rectal biopsies, caution must be exercised because these agents promote not only repair, but also proliferation.

## IL-2 RECEPTOR ANTIBODIES

Basiliximab is a chimeric monoclonal antibody against the α-subunit of the IL-2 receptor (CD25). It has been found to reduce the incidence of steroid-resistant graft rejection of allogenic renal transplants, although the mechanism of its action was not fully understood. Investigation in our laboratory suggests its action is to potentiate the effect of glucocorticoids upon activated T cells, thereby overcoming steroid resistance. We have reported a pilot study in 10 patients with steroid-refractory UC; a single 40 mg bolus was administered in addition to standard steroid therapy. Nine patients achieved clinical remission within 8 weeks[20]. Since this study further work has been undertaken and this was presented to DDW in 2004. In the second, open study in UC, 30 patients received a single dose of basiliximab; 10 patients had severe UC and 20 moderate UC. By 8 weeks 50% of the patients with severe UC had gone into remission, while 95% of patients with moderate UC had improved, 70% achieving full remission. These data suggest that basiliximab may be a valuable adjunct to glucocorticoid therapy in patients with UC.

Similar excitement followed a pilot study of a different, humanized IL-2 receptor antibody, daclizumab; 1 mg/kg was administered twice-weekly for 4 weeks. Eight of 10 patients who received open-label treatment for chronically active UC showed significant benefit at 8 weeks and five of 10 patients achieved remission[21]. However, a randomized controlled trial of daclizumab in 159 patients (unpublished) failed to meet the primary endpoint of significant difference in remission rates. The difference between the basiliximab and daclizumab results may lie in study design: dacluzimab was not used as a steroid enhancer. However, a randomized controlled trial of basiliximab is necessary to address this point, as well as its true efficacy in UC patients.

## CONCLUSION

Biological agents have revolutionized our management of difficult CD. It is evident from studies in CD that agents designed in different ways to respond to the same target have different clinical efficacies. In addition, drugs designed against a particular target that are effective in one condition may not necessarily work in another condition for which other, similar, agents may work.

Recently, Accent 1 and Accent 2 have highlighted the impact of repeated treatment and scheduling on clinical outcome. Treatment regimens have developed greatly from the earliest studies undertaken at a time when it was not certain that biological agents could be given more than once to an individual, because of concerns about their potential immunogenicity. Experience and the careful co-prescription of hydrocortisone and immunosuppressive agents have largely quelled such anxieties.

The data in UC suggest that particular biological agents may have a role in specific subgroups of patients. The data suggest that 'induction' therapy with infliximab may reduce the colectomy rate in patients. Whether this is relevant to patients with less severe disease remains to be seen. Natalizumab and visilizumab may also have a role, but further trials are necessary. The interferons may be effective at high doses, but will probably be limited by their side-effect profile. Basiliximab looks promising, although the experience with daclizumab underlines the importance of patient selection and the need for proper trial design.

Present data in UC give us a tantalizing glimpse into the future: not all biologics will work for all patients. As is so often the case, the devil will be in the detail of study design and patient selection.

## References

1. Evans R, Clarke L, Heath P, Stephens S, Morris A, Rhodes J. Treatment of ulcerative colitis with an engineered human anti-TNFalpha antibody CDP571. Aliment Pharmacol Therapeut. 1997;11:1031–5.

2. Chey WY, Kunze GY, Shah AN. Observations on therapeutic effect of infliximab on ulcerative colitis. Am J Gastroenterol. 2001;96:S288.

3. Su C, Salzberg BA, Lewis JD et al. Efficacy of anti-tumor necrosis factor therapy in patients with ulcerative colitis. Am J Gastroenterol. 2002;97:2577–84.

4. Actis GC, Bruno M, Pinna-Pintor M, Rossini FP, Rizzetto M. Infliximab for treatment of steroid-refractory ulcerative colitis. Dig Liver Dis. 2002;34:631–4.

5. Kohn A, Prantera C, Pera A, Cosintino R, Sostegni R, Daperno M. Anti-tumour necrosis factor alpha (infliximab) in the treatment of severe ulcerative colitis: result of an open study on 13 patients. Dig Liver Dis. 2002;34:626–30.

6. Sands BE, Tremaine WJ, Sandborn WJ et al. Infliximab in the treatment of severe, steroid-refractory ulcerative colitis: a pilot study. Inflamm Bowel Dis. 2001;7:83–8.

7. Probert CSJ, Hearing SD, Schreiber S et al. Infliximab in moderately severe glucocorticoid resistant ulcerative colitis: a randomised controlled trial. Gut. 2003;52:998–1002.

8. Ochsenkuhn T, Sackmann M, Goke B. Infliximab for acute, not steroid-refractory ulcerative colitis: a randomized pilot study. Aliment Pharmacol Ther. 2004;16;1167–71.

9. Armuzzi A, De Pascalis B, Lupasco A et al. Infliximab in the treatment of steroid-dependent ulcerative colitis. Gastroenterology. 2004;126(Suppl. 2):A464.

10. Järnerot G, Hertervig E, Friis-Liby I et al. Infliximab as rescue therapy in severe to moderately severe ulcerative colitis. A randomised placebo controlled study. Gastroenterology. 2005 (in press).

11. Plevy S, Salzberg B, van Assche G et al. A humanized anti-CD3 monoclonal antibody, visilizumab, for treatment of severe steroid-refractory ulcerative colitis: Results of a phase I study. Gastroenterology. 2004;126(Suppl. 2):A75.

12. Ghosh S, Goldin E, Gordon FH et al. and the Natalizumab Pan-European Study Group. Natalizumab for active Crohn's disease. N Engl J Med. 2003;348:24–32.

13. O'Connor PW, Goodman A, Willmer-Hulme AJ et al. and the Natalizumab Multiple Sclerosis Trial Group. Randomized multicenter trial of natalizumab in acute MS relapses: clinical and MRI effects. Neurology. 2004;62:2038–43.

14. Gordon FH, Hamilton MI, Donoghue S et al. A pilot study of treatment of active ulcerative colitis with natalizumab, a humanized monoclonal antibody to alpha-4 integrin. Aliment Pharmacol Ther. 2002;16:699–705.

15. Madsen SM, Schlichting P, Davidsen B et al. An open-labeled, randomized study comparing systemic interferon-[alpha]-2A and prednisolone enemas in the treatment of left-sided ulcerative colitis. Am J Gastroenterol. 2001;96:1807–15.

16. Tilg H, Vogelsang H, Ludwiczek O et al. A randomised placebo controlled trial of pegylated interferon (alpha) in active ulcerative colitis. Gut. 2003;52:1728–33.

17. Nikolaus S, Rutgeerts P, Fedorak R et al. Interferon (beta)-1a in ulcerative colitis: a placebo controlled, randomised, dose escalating study. Gut. 2003;52:1286–90.

18. Sullivan P, Brueton M, Tabara Z, Goodlad R, Lee C, Wright N. Epidermal growth factor in necrotising enteritis. Lancet. 1991;338:53–4.

19. Sinha A, Nightingale JMD, West KP, Berlanga-Acosta J, Playford RJ. Epidermal growth factor enemas with oral mesalamine for mild-to-moderate left-sided ulcerative colitis or proctitis. N Engl J Med. 2003;349:350–7.
20. Creed TJ, Norman MR, Probert CSJ et al. Basiliximab (anti-CD25) in combination with steroids may be an effective new treatment for steroid-resistant ulcerative colitis. Aliment Pharmacol Ther. 2003;18:65–75.
21. Assche G, Dalle I, Noman M et al. A pilot study on the use of the humanized anti-interleukin-2 receptor antibody daclizumab in active ulcerative colitis. Am J Gastroenterol. 2003;98:369–76.

BIBLIOGRAPHICAL NOTES

# Section VII
# Cancer and inflammatory bowel disease

**Chair: S. PRANTERA and J. SATSANGI**

# 20
# Diagnosis of colitis associated dysplasia: new colonoscopic techniques

R. KIESSLICH and M. F. NEURATH

## CANCER RISK AND SURVEILLANCE

Patients with long-standing extensive ulcerative colitis (UC) are at increased risk of developing colorectal cancer[1]. Colonoscopic surveillance is recommended to reduce associated mortality[2]. Surveillance relies on the detection of premalignant dysplastic tissue and, where multifocal dysplasia is detected, proctocolectomy remains the management of choice, although there is increasing evidence that adenoma-like dysplastic lesions may safely be resected endoscopically[3–5].

## DETECTION OF PREMALIGNANT LESIONS IN UC

In patients without UC the premalignant dysplastic lesion, the adenoma, usually occurs as a clearly delineated macroscopically visible abnormality. However, in UC there is no clear-cut adenoma–carcinoma sequence. Colitis-associated neoplasias can occur in addition to adenomas in patients with long-lasting UC. These lesions are triggered by inflammation and the macroscopic appearances are often flat and multifocal[6]. There are no clear-cut endoscopic, histological or immunohistochemical discriminators to permit accurate stratification of mass dysplasia in colitis, and no universally agreed definition. However, the term 'intraepithelial neoplasias', in accordance to the new Vienna classification, was established; this summarizes adenomas and colitis-associated neoplasias.

Currently multiple untargeted random biopsies are recommended to diagnose intraepithelial neoplasias. Four random biopsies per site over nine sites throughout the colon should be undertaken, with increased sampling from the rectosigmoid and with additional biopsies from raised or suspicious lesions[2]. However, this approach is time-consuming and dysplastic lesions might still be overlooked.

193

Chromoendoscopy can help to identify premalignant and malignant lesions. Magnifying endoscopy enables analysis of the surface structure, and confocal laser endomicroscopy enables *in-vivo* histology.

## CHROMOENDOSCOPY

Intravital staining is the oldest and simplest method used to improve the diagnosis of epithelial changes. Chromoendoscopy, vital staining and contrast endoscopy are synonyms for the same technique: dye solutions are applied to the mucosa of the gastrointestinal tract, enhancing the recognition of details in order to uncover mucosal changes not perceivable by purely optical methods prior to targeted biopsy and histology[7].

In general there are three classes of dyes which can be used for chromoendoscopy[7–8]: contrast, absorptive and reactive dyes.

### Contrast dyes

These simply coat the colonic mucosal surface, and neither react with nor are absorbed by it. An example is *indigo carmine*. Contrast dyes are effective because the colonic mucosa is covered with tiny pits and whorls of parallel 'innominate' grooves, similar to a fingerprint. When a dye is sprayed on the surface this pattern becomes evident, and disruption to these grooves caused by mucosal lesions (which have a different surface topography) is highlighted.

### Absorptive dyes

These are absorbed by different cells to different degrees, highlighting particular cell types. An example is *methylene blue* which, after a few minutes, avidly stains non-inflamed mucosa, but is poorly taken up by areas of active inflammation and of dysplasia.

### Reactive dyes

The binding of reactive colouring agents with certain mucosal areas is used to identify reactions. Their use is less common and their diagnostic relevance rather low.

In patients with UC the most common dyes are indigo carmine and methylene blue. Chromoendoscopy has two main goals. First, it improves the detection of subtle colonic lesions, raising the sensitivity of the endoscopic examination; this is important in UC, as flat dysplastic lesions can be difficult to detect. Secondly, once a lesion is detected, chromoendoscopy can improve lesion characterization, increasing the specificity of the examination. This can be further refined using a magnifying colonoscope. Surface analysis of colorectal lesions using magnifying endoscopes is a new optical impression for endoscopists. First, Kudo et al.[9] described that some of the regular staining patterns are often seen in hyperplastic polyps or normal mucosa, whereas

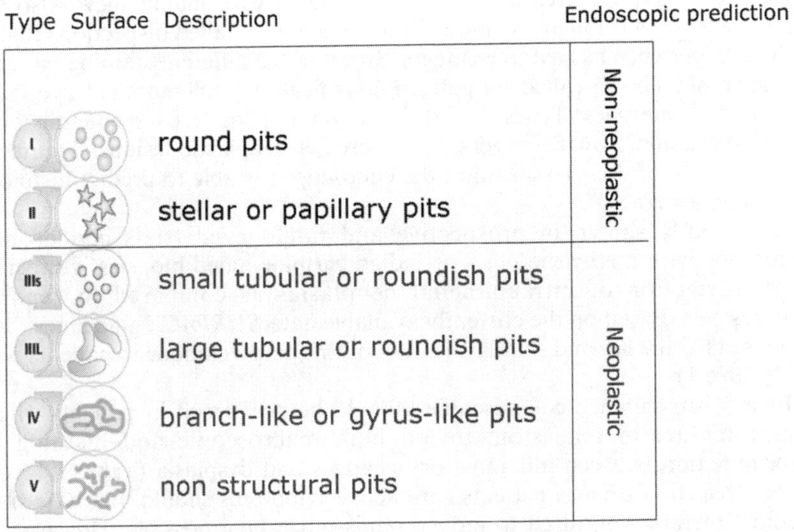

Type  Surface  Description

Endoscopic prediction

**Figure 2**  Pit pattern classification

**Table 1**  SURFACE – guidelines for chromoendoscopy in patients with ulcerative colitis

Strict patient selection
  Patients with histologically proven ulcerative colitis and at least 8 years' duration in clinical remission. Avoid patients with active disease

Unmask the mucosal surface
  Excellent bowel preparation is needed. Remove mucus and remaining fluid in the colon when necessary

Reduce peristaltic waves
  When drawing back the endoscope, a spasmolytic agent should be used (if necessary)

Full-length staining of the colon
  Perform full-length staining of the colon (panchromoendoscopy) in ulcerative colitis rather than local staining

Augmented detection with dyes
  Intravital staining with 0.4% indigo carmine or 0.1% methylene blue should be used to unmask flat lesions more frequently than with conventional colonoscopy

Crypt architecture analysis
  All lesions should be analysed according to the pit pattern classification. Whereas pit pattern types I–II suggest the presence of non-malignant lesions, staining patterns III–V suggest the presence of intraepithelial neoplasias and carcinomas

Endoscopic targeted biopsies
  Perform targeted biopsies of all mucosal alterations, particularly of circumscript lesions with staining patterns indicative of intraepithelial neoplasias and carcinomas (pit patterns III–V)

unstructured surface architecture was associated with malignancy. Also the kind of adenoma (tubular vs villous) can be seen by detailed inspection (Figure 1). This experience has led to a categorization of the different staining patterns in the colon. The so-called pit-pattern classification[9] differentiated five types and several subtypes. Types 1 and 2 are staining patterns predicting non-neoplastic lesions, whereas types 3 to 5 predict neoplastic lesions (Figure 2). With the help of this classification the endoscopist is able to predict histology with good accuracy[10].

As recently shown in prospective and randomized trials panchromo-endoscopy with methylene blue- or indigo carmine-aided biopsies is superior in the detection of intraepithelial neoplasias as compared to random biopsies[10–12]. Based on the currently available data *SURFACE* guidelines[13] are proposed for the use and standardization of this new technique in patients with UC (Table 1).

Ideally, surveillance colonoscopies should be performed in patients whose symptoms are in remission, to aid both macroscopic and histological discrimination between inflammatory changes and dysplasia (Table 1, 'Strict patient selection'). Thus, patients with active symptoms should first have their medical therapy optimized to induce remission, where possible. However, as patients with chronic active inflammation are at increased risk of colorectal neoplasia[14], the procedure should not be unduly delayed if they fail to respond to therapy.

## EXAMINATION TECHNIQUE[8]

A thorough bowel preparation is of crucial importance and prerequisite for chromoendoscopy. On insertion, all faecal fluid should be aspirated to ensure optimal mucosal views (Table 1, 'Unmask the mucosal surface'). When the caecal pole has been reached, meticulous inspection of the colonic mucosa is performed on withdrawal. To reduce spasm and haustral fold prominence (thus reducing blind spots), intravenous butyl-scopolamine 20 mg (or intravenous glucagon 1 mg) should be given when the caecal pole is reached. Further increments can be given as required (Table 1, 'Reduce peristaltic waves').

---

**Figure 1**   **A**: Chromoendoscopy and magnifying endoscopy of the terminal ileum. Single villi are clearly visible (black arrows). A small erosion (< 1 mm) is visible in the centre of the image. **B**: Magnification endoscopy after methylene blue-aided chromoendoscopy. Small inflammatory changes are visible (white arrow) surrounded by normal crypt architecture. Chromoendoscopy unmasks an aberrant crypt focus (black arrow). Pit pattern II. **C**: A tubular staining pattern (type IIIL) is clearly visible after intravital staining. Targeted biopsy revealed low-grade intraepithelial neoplasia. **D**: A flat-growing cancer with unstructured surface (pit pattern V; black arrow) with accompanying ulceration (white arrow) indicates malignancy

**Figure 3**   Scheme of endomicroscopy. **A**: Microarchitecture of the colonic wall. Topical acriflavine or systemic application of fluorescein is mandatory for confocal endomicroscopy. **B**: The confocal images are orientated in a horizontal fashion. The optical slice thickness is 7 μm with a lateral resolution of 0.7 μm. The field of view is 500 × 500 μm. The range of the z-axis is 0–250 μm below the surface layer

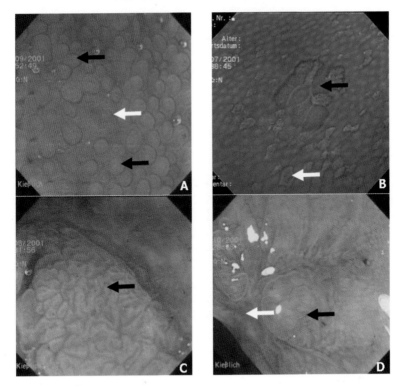

**Figure 1** (legend opposite)

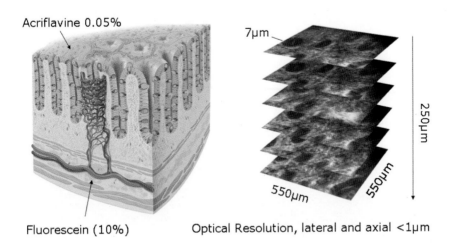

Acriflavine 0.05%

Fluorescein (10%)

7µm

250µm

550µm

550µm

Optical Resolution, lateral and axial <1µm

**Figure 3** (legend opposite)

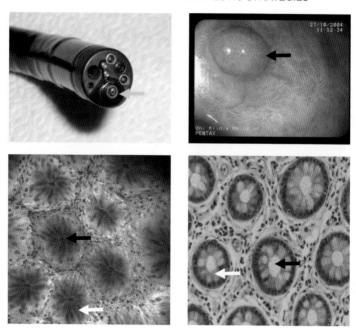

**Figure 4** (legend opposite)

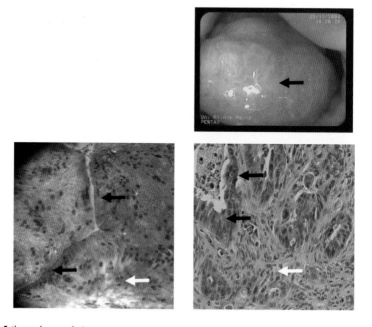

**Figure 5** (legend opposite)

Adequate air insufflation is necessary, and if the lumen remains collapsed the patient should be turned. Inspection is performed by scouring the mucosa in a spiral fashion. Dye-spraying of the entire colorectal mucosa (panchromoendoscopy) greatly reduces the risk of overlooking subtle abnormalities (Table 1, 'Full-length staining of the colon'), and adds little to the duration of the procedure. Before the procedure, 100 ml of 0.1% indigo carmine or 0.1% methylene blue is prepared, and drawn into 50-ml syringes. A dye-spray catheter is inserted down the instrumentation channel, and the tip protruded 2–3 cm. Under the direction of the endoscopist, an assistant firmly squeezes the syringe, generating a fine mist of dye, which is then painted onto the mucosa by withdrawing the colonoscope in a spiral fashion.

Spraying should be done in a segmental fashion (every 20–30 cm). Once a segment has been sprayed, excess dye is suctioned, and the colonoscope reinserted to the proximal extent of the segment. It is occasionally necessary to wait a few seconds for indigo carmine to settle into the mucosal contours; methylene blue takes about 60 s to be absorbed. Once that segment has been examined, the next segment is sprayed, and so on until the anal margin is reached. On average, 60–100 ml of solution is required to spray the entire colorectal mucosa.

Dye-spraying greatly aids the detection of intraepithelial neoplasias (Table 1, 'Augmented detection with dyes'). Areas of villiform (velvet-like) mucosa with clear borders (circumscript lesions) are of particular concern. Areas of nodularity or friable mucosa may also indicate intraepithelial neoplasia (Figure 1). Sessile (polypoid) lesions are easier to detect, but careful delineation of the edge of the lesion is required (aided by dye-spraying) and, if the lesion is endoscopically resectable, it is essential to take additional biopsies from the surrounding mucosa to ensure there is no residual neoplastic tissue, and to tattoo the site to permit re-inspection later.

The combination of chromoendoscopy and new-generation magnifying colonoscopes enables detailed mucosal analysis (Table 1, 'Crypt architecture analysis'). Neoplastic changes are characterized by an irregular, tubular or villous crypt architecture staining pattern. Non-neoplastic changes are

---

**Figure 4** Endomicroscopy in ulcerative colitis: non-neoplastic lesion. **A**: Confocal laser colonoscope: the confocal microscope is integrated in the distal tip. An additional microscopic window (arrow) enables the emission of blue laser light enabling *in-vivo* histology. **B**: A small polypoid lesion with regular staining pattern is clearly visible after methylene blue-aided chromoendoscopy. **C**: Targeted endomicroscopic imaging shows a normal contribution of crypts and crypt openings (black arrow). The goblet cells within the crypts are displayed black (white arrow). Connective tissue is arranged regularly in a hexagonal fashion. **D**: Corresponding histology confirms the endomicroscopic diagnosis. Normal crypts and round openings (black arrow) are visible. In addition mucin in the goblet cells is visible (white arrow). Note: due to shrinking artefacts the spaces in between the tissue are wider in conventional histology as compared with *in-vivo* histology

**Figure 5** Endomicroscopy in ulcerative colitis: neoplastic lesion. **A**: A large polypoid lesion is visible in the sigmoid. Chromoendoscopy is not necessary to recognize the lesion. **B**: Endomicroscopy shows neoplasia with tubular-arranged epithelium with loss of goblet cells (black arrows). In parts vessel and cell architecture is totally irregular (white arrow). **C**: Corresponding histology shows high-grade intraepithelial neoplasia with similar architecture

characterized by stellar or regular round pits. The different staining patterns are categorized using the 'pit pattern' classification[9].

By targeting biopsies towards mucosal abnormalities (Table 1, 'Endoscopic targeted biopsies'), the specificity of each biopsy for dysplasia is increased and the total number of biopsies taken per colonoscopic examination can be reduced in comparison to random biopsies with standard colonoscopy[10–12].

## EFFICIENCY OF CHROMOENDOSCOPY

The first randomized, controlled trial was published in 2003 to test whether chromoendoscopy and magnifying endoscopy might facilitate early detection of intraepithelial neoplasia in patients with UC by using magnifying chromoendoscopy[10]. One hundred and sixty-five patients with long-standing UC were randomized at a 1:1 ratio to undergo conventional colonoscopy or colonoscopy with chromoendoscopy using 0.1% methylene blue. Circumscript lesions in the colon were evaluated according to a modified pit pattern classification. In the chromoendoscopy group there was a significantly better correlation between the endoscopic assessment of degree and extent of colonic inflammation, and the histopathological findings compared with the conventional colonoscopy group. More targeted biopsies were possible, and significantly more intraepithelial neoplasias were detected in the chromoendoscopy group (32 vs 10). Using the modified pit pattern classification, both the sensitivity and specificity for differentiation between non-neoplastic and neoplastic lesions were 93%. The overall sensitivity of magnifying chromoendoscopy to predict neoplasia was 97% with a specificity of 93%. The ability of the dye technique to identify neoplastic from non-neoplastic lesions to enhance detection of more dysplastic lesions in flat mucosa is a potential major advance in dysplasia surveillance. These first promising data concerning chromoendoscopy in UC could be confirmed by Hurlstone[11]. In a prospective study, 162 patients with long-standing UC and established pancolitis underwent total colonoscopy by one endoscopist using a magnifying colonoscope. After detection of subtle mucosal changes such as fold convergence, air-induced deformation, interruption of innominate grooves or focal, discrete colour change, targeted intravital staining with indigo carmine was used. The macroscopic type and the staining pattern were defined. The control group consisted of 162 disease-matched patients, undergoing conventional colonoscopy. Chromoendoscopy with targeted biopsy significantly increased diagnostic yield for intraepithelial neoplasia and the number of flat neoplastic changes as opposed to conventional colonoscopy. Intraepithelial neoplasia in flat mucosal change was observed in 37 lesions, of which 31 were detected using chromoendoscopy.

Rutter and colleagues[12] investigated the third prospective trial in UC on 100 patients with back-to-back colonoscopy, starting with random and targeted biopsies followed by indigo carmine-aided panchromoendoscopy with targeted biopsies only. The diagnostic yield of dysplastic changes was increased in this study by the use of chromoendoscopy from two to seven patients (3.5-fold increase) and from two to nine dysplastic lesions (4.5-fold increase).

In conclusion, magnifying chromoendoscopy is a valid new tool for improving endoscopic detection of intraepithelial neoplasia in patients with long-standing UC. Chromoendoscopy increased the diagnostic yield of intraepithelial neoplasia as compared with conventional colonoscopy and biopsy techniques 3–4.5-fold, which further suggests that more patients with UC could be considered as candidates for colectomy. Differentiation of non-neoplastic from neoplastic lesions is possible with a high overall sensitivity and specificity.

## LIMITATIONS OF CHROMOENDOSCOPY AND MAGNIFYING ENDOSCOPY

Until now no severe side-effects have been reported regarding the local use of indigo carmine. However, Olliver and colleagues[15] recently raised some concerns about the intravital dye methylene blue despite a harmless transient discoloration of stool and urine. In patients with Barrett oesophagus they found oxidative DNA damage after chromoendoscopy (as measured by single-cell gel electrophoresis) and argued that methylene blue, together with white light, during endoscopy could also be a risk for patients, to drive carcinogenesis. Therefore, the question arises whether methylene blue-aided chromoendoscopy may contribute to the carcinogenic process in other diseases such as UC, and may lead to an increase of intraepithelial neoplasias in follow-up.

However, in a follow-up report (median follow-up 23 months) concerning the safety of methylene blue staining patients with previous chromoendoscopies showed fewer intraepithelial neoplasias as compared to patients who were screened by colonoscopy. These data suggest that chromoendoscopy with methylene blue is a safe and highly effective approach for the detection of flat colonic lesions in UC. The reported increase of DNA lesions upon methylene blue–light treatment is unlikely to have biological significance *in vivo*, and unwanted side-effects appear to be negligible in view of the advantages of the method[16].

The visual evaluation of minute detail allowed by magnification endoscopy is promising, but some points of criticism must be discussed. Inflammation can cause significant disturbance of the image seen when magnifying endoscopy is used to look for the minute changes indicative of neoplasia, and there is a danger of false-positive results. Inflamed epithelium should be treated prior to final endoscopic evaluation whenever possible. It is not useful or practical to permanently use the zoom mode when screening the lower gastrointestinal tract. The initial evaluation is performed in conventional mode and depends strictly on the knowledge and experience of the endoscopist. After the initial detection of discrete lesions, chromoendoscopy and magnification endoscopy are the tools used to enhance surface mucosal patterns. These techniques disclose a plethora of mucosal detail, the evaluation of which increases procedure time, at least when the endoscopist is learning the technique.

The proposed classification for colorectal lesions is too complex relative to its practical clinical value; a simplification is recommended. We are facing the same dilemma as our pathologist colleagues when evaluating dysplasias, with the difference that histological preparation is widely standardized, whereas standardized procedure recommendations are lacking for chromoendoscopy and magnification endoscopy. Another difficulty in the use of magnifying endoscopes is the high magnification levels. The newly developed systems allow enlargement of up to × 150. A sharp image is focused by manually adjusting the movable lens. Close examination can be difficult due to peristalsis and respiratory movements.

## PERSPECTIVES AND FUTURE TRENDS

The limits and concerns of magnifying chromoendoscopy are few and can be overcome by training and increased knowledge of endoscopists.

However, dream and goal of an ideal colonoscopy is virtual histology, which means 'online' *in-vivo* histology. Endoscopists can decide which is the area of interest and can remove the lesion in a targeted fashion without prior biopsy. Chromoendoscopy can illustrate the surface structure; but what is behind the surface? Cellular structure. Many new optical developments are aimed at further advancing early diagnosis of colorectal cancer. Raman spectroscopy, optical coherence tomography, light-scattering spectroscopy, confocal fluorescence endoscopy, and immunofluoresence endoscopy are some of the new methods with different advantages and disadvantages[17]. However, the closest step towards virtual histology is confocal laser endoscopy[18].

## CONFOCAL LASER ENDOMICROSCOPY

Confocal laser endomicroscopy allows subsurface analysis of the intestinal mucosa and *in-vivo* histology during ongoing endoscopy. The components of a confocal laser endoscope are based on integration of a confocal laser microscope in the distal tip of a conventional video endoscope (see Figure 3). During laser endoscopy a single-line laser delivers an excitation wavelength of 488 nm and the maximum laser power output is ≤ 1 mW at the surface of the tissue. Confocal image data are collected at a scan rate of 0.8 frames/s ($1024 \times 512$ pixels) or 1.6 frames/s ($1024 \times 1024$ pixels). The optical slice thickness is 7 μm with a lateral resolution of 0.7 μm. The field of view is $500 \times 500$ μm). The range of the $z$-axis was 0–200 μm below the surface layer. Confocal images can be generated simultaneously with endoscopic images (Figure 3).

## TECHNIQUE OF CONFOCAL LASER ENDOMICROSCOPY

A fluorescent contrast agent is used to achieve high-contrast images using confocal endomicroscopy. Potentially suitable agents are fluorescein, acriflavine, tetracycline or cresyl violet. The contrast agents can be applied systemically (fluorescein) or topically (all others) by using a spraying catheter. The most common dye used to date is fluorescein.

The confocal endoscope can be handled similarly to a standard endoscope. After the application of a contrast dye (e.g. fluorescein, systemically), the distal tip of the endoscope is placed in gentle contact with the mucosa and the position of the focal plane within the specimen adjusted using the buttons on the endoscope control body. In every region of interest images from the surface to deeper parts of the mucosal layer can be obtained and stored digitally in a specific folder associated with the site of collection. Targeted biopsies are possible due to the proximity of the working channel and the endomicroscopic window at the distal tip of the endoscope[18], which allows the position of the confocal scanner on the tissue to be seen via the conventional video endoscopic view.

## CLINICAL DATA

The confocal laser endoscope can be used routinely for screening and surveillance. Suspected lesions can be examined in a targeted fashion by placing the endomicroscopic window onto the lesion. Confocal images can be graduated according to cellular and vascular changes. The images correlated well with conventional histology after targeted biopsies. In the first prospective trial 13 020 confocal images from 390 different locations (256 inconspicuous areas; 134 circumscript lesions) were compared with histological data from 1038 biopsies. Subsurface analysis during confocal laser endoscopy allowed detailed analysis of cellular structures. The presence of neoplastic changes could be predicted by using the new developed confocal pattern (see Figure 4) classification with high accuracy (sensitivity 97.4%, specificity 99.4%, accuracy 99.2%)[18].

In addition, combination of chromoendoscopy and confocal laser endoscopy facilitates surveillance in UC. Chromoendoscopy unmasks circumscript lesions and confocal laser endomicroscopy can be used to predict intraepithelial neoplasias with high accuracy. Thus, targeted biopsies of relevant lesions can be performed and rapid prediction of neoplastic changes by confocal laser endoscopy during colonoscopy may lead to significant improvements in the clinical management of UC patients. Different cellular structures (epithelial and blood cells), capillaries and connective tissue limited to the mucosal layer could be identified by confocal microscopy. Due to the pharmacokinetic properties of fluorescein, nuclei could not be seen. However, the presence of neoplastic changes (sensitivity 94.4%, specificity 95.6%, accuracy 99.3%) and inflammation could be predicted with high accuracy[19] (Figures 4 and 5).

## CONCLUSION

The newly developed high-resolution and magnification endoscopes offer features that allow more and new mucosal details to be seen. They are commonly used in conjunction with chromoendoscopy. The analysis of mucosal surface details is beginning to resemble histological examination. More accurate recognition of small flat and depressed neoplastic lesions is possible. Endoscopic prediction of neoplastic and non-neoplastic tissue is possible by analysis of the surface architecture of the mucosa, which influences endoscopic management. For the diagnosis of flat adenomas chromoendoscopy should belong to the endoscopist's armamentarium. In inflammatory bowel disease chromoendoscopy can be used for patients with long-standing UC to unmask flat intraepithelial neoplasias, and will probably be the new standard method for surveillance colonoscopy in the near future. The new detailed images seen with magnifying chromoendoscopy are the beginning of a new era in which new optical developments such as confocal endomicroscopy allow a unique look at detailed cellular structures.

## References

1.  Gilat T, Fireman Z, Grossman A et al. Colorectal cancer in patients with ulcerative colitis. Gastroenterology. 1988;94:870–7.
2.  Winawer S, Fletcher R, Rex D et al. Colorectal cancer screening and surveillance: clinical guidelines and rationale. Update based on new evidence. Gastroenterology. 2003;124:544–60.
3.  Odze RD, Farraye FA, Hecht JL, Hornick JL. Long-term follow-up after polypectomy treatment for adenoma-like dysplastic lesions in ulcerative colitis. Clin Gastroenterol Hepatol. 2004;2:534–41.
4.  Sinicrope FA, Wang K. Treating polyps in ulcerative colitis: adenoma-like lesions and dysplasia-associated mass lesions. Clin Gastroenterol Hepatol. 2004;2:531–3.
5.  Itzkowitz SH, Harpaz N. Diagnosis and management of dysplasia in patients with inflammatory bowel diseases. Gastroenterology. 2004;126:1634–48.
6.  Suzuki K, Muto T, Shinozaki M, Yokoyama T, Matsuda K, Masaki T. Differential diagnosis of dysplasia-associated lesion or mass and coincidental adenoma in ulcerative colitis. Dis Colon Rectum. 1998;41:322–7.
7.  Jung M, Kiesslich R. Chromoendoscopy and intravital staining techniques. Baillières Best Pract Res Clin Gastroenterol. 1999;13:11–19.
8.  Rutter M, Bernstein C, Matsumoto T, Kiesslich R, Neurath M. Endoscopic appearance of dysplasia in ulcerative colitis and the role of staining. Endoscopy. 2004;36:1109–14.
9.  Kudo S, Tamura S, Nakajima T et al. Diagnosis of colorectal tumorous lesions by magnifying endoscopy. Gastrointest Endosc. 1996;44:814.
10. Kiesslich R, Fritsch J, Holtmann M et al. Methylene blue-aided chromoendoscopy for the detection of intraepithelial neoplasia and colon cancer in ulcerative colitis. Gastroenterology. 2003;124:880–8.
11. Hurlstone DP. Further validation of high-magnification–chromoscopic colonoscopy for the detection of intraepithelial neoplasia and colon cancer in ulcerative colitis. Gastroenterology. 2004;126:376–8.
12. Rutter MD, Saunders BP, Schofield G et al. Pancolonic indigo carmine dye spraying for the detection of dysplasia in ulcerative colitis. Gut. 2004;53:256–60.
13. Kiesslich R, Neurath MF. Chromoendoscopy: an evolving standard in surveillance for ulcerative colitis. Inflamm Bowel Dis. 2004;10:695–6.
14. Rutter M, Saunders B, Wilkinson K et al. Severity of inflammation is a risk factor for colorectal neoplasia in ulcerative colitis. Gastroenterology. 2004;126:451–9.
15. Olliver JR, Wild CP, Sahay P et al. Chromoendoscopy with methylene blue and associated DNA damage in Barrett's oesophagus. Lancet. 2003;362:373–4.
16. Kiesslich R, Burg J, Kaina B et al. Safety andefficacy of methylene blue-aided chromoendoscopy in ulcerative colitis: a prospective pilot study upon previous chromoendoscopies. Gastrointest Endosc. 2004;59:AB97.
17. Dacosta RS, Wilson BC, Marcon NE. New optical technologies for earlier endoscopic diagnosis of premalignant gastrointestinal lesions. J Gastroenterol Hepatol. 2002;17:85–104.
18. Kiesslich R, Burg J, Vieth M et al. Confocal laser endoscopy for diagnosing intraepithelial neoplasias and colorectal cancer *in vivo*. Gastroenterology. 2004;127:706–13.
19. Kiesslich R, Burg J, Vieth M et al. *In vivo* fluorescence confocal laser endoscopy for prediction of neoplasia in patients with ulcerative colitis. Gastrointest Endosc. 2004;59 (Abstract).

# 21
# Can we prevent cancer using current drugs?

E. HERTERVIG

## INTRODUCTION

Patients with ulcerative colitis (UC) are at greater risk of developing colorectal cancer (CRC) than the general population. Both duration and extent of UC are important risk factors for CRC, as is the presence of primary sclerosing cholangitis, family history of CRC, and early age at diagnosis of UC[1]. Perhaps the most important risk factor is the duration of colitis. A recent review representing a meta-analysis of a total of 116 studies revealed that the risk of CRC in UC is approximately 2% at 10 years, 8% at 20 years, and 18% at 30 years. It also highlighted geographical differences in cancer incidence rates, being 5 per 1000 patient-years in the USA and 2 per 1000 patient-years in Scandinavia[2]. The incidence of CRC in a Danish UC population study of 1161 patients was no higher than in the background population, being 0.2% after 10 years, 1.4% after 20 years, and 3.1% by 30 years[3]. Although the reasons for the geographical variations are not fully elucidated, it should be emphasized that a majority of the inflammatory bowel disease (IBD) patients in the Danish cohort (70%) were receiving regular anti-inflammatory therapy with sulphasalazine (SSZ) or 5-aminosalicylic acid (5-ASA). The potential cancer chemopreventive effect of these agents could explain the overall low risk of CRC that was seen in the Danish cohort. In addition to 5-ASA, ursodeoxycholic acid (UDCA) and folate have been in focus as candidate drugs of chemoprevention in IBD. The ultimate proof of a chemopreventive effect of a pharmacological agent on the outcome of neoplastic progression lies in controlled randomized trials. With the exception of one study on UDCA[4] there are no such data. Prospective studies examining rare outcomes such as CRC are not feasible. In addition, withholding medication that treats colitis has ethical complications. Hence, a substantial body of evidence on this issue is based, and will be based, on observational and experimental data.

## 5-ASA

### Epidemiological studies

There are few randomized controlled trials investigating the potential anti-CRC effects of 5-ASA; instead, we have to rely largely on observational data. A number of studies have demonstrated a decrease in occurrence of sporadic CRC among non-steroidal anti-inflammatory drug (NSAID) users[5-7]. The issue of whether NSAID are protective for CRC also in IBD was addressed by a case–control study by Bansal and Sonnenberg[8]. In this study of risk factors for CRC the investigators looked at patients with IBD who had a co-morbid illness that typically requires long-term NSAID therapy (e.g. ischaemic heart disease, peripheral vascular disease, arterial tromboembolism, rheumatoid arthritis, osteoarthritis). Patients with IBD who also had an NSAID-associated diagnosis had a lower rate of CRC (OR 0.84, 95% CI 0.65–1.08) than those without such a diagnosis. Although the difference did not reach statistical significance, the investigators found a significant reduction in mortality among cases who had NSAID-associated diagnoses (OR 0.51, 95% CI 0.28–0.94). Although this study has some limitations – such as lack of data concerning medication use, the absence of information on extent, duration, or colectomy history in IBD – these findings suggest a protective role for NSAID in IBD-associated neoplasia. A recent case–control study by Velayos supports NSAID use as a protective factor. NSAID use was associated with a 90% risk reduction of CRC risk (OR 0.1, 95% CI 0.04–0.5) compared to non-users[9].

Three published studies and three other studies presented as abstracts, have shown that 5-ASA therapy confers significant protection against the development of CRC in IBD patients. The first one was a case–control study from Sweden, comparing 102 UC patients with 196 UC patients without CRC[10]. The study found that a history of having had a minimum 3 months treatment with sulphasalazine (SSZ) was associated with a significant reduction in the risk of CRC development (OR 0.38, 95% CI 0.2–0.69). In 1996 Moody et al. published a study investigating the impact of long-term SSZ therapy on the risk of developing CRC in a 10-year cohort of UC patients[11]. They found that patients who had SSZ therapy for less than 6 months in total (including patients non-compliant with or intolerant of SSZ therapy) had a 10-fold increase in risk of developing CRC (3% in compliers vs 31% in non-compliers).

In 2000 Eaden et al. published a retrospective, matched case–control study, with compelling evidence for a protective effect of 5-ASA use in patients with UC. In total, 102 patients with UC with complicating CRC were matched with 102 UC patients without CRC. The cases were matched for sex, age, extent and duration of disease. Data collected from medical notes were also examined to identify risk factors for developing cancer. The study showed that a history of regular 5-ASA use significantly reduced the risk of CRC by 75% (OR 0.25, 95% CI 0.13–0.48) with a stronger protective effect being observed for mesalazine (MSA) compared with SSZ. When the results were adjusted for other variables, the protective effect of MSA reduced the risk of CRC by 81%, becoming significant at a dose of 1.2 g/day or greater, whereas the protective effect of SSZ was no longer evident. Interestingly, in this study, steroid therapy was also found to confer some protection against the development of CRC. This would imply that anti-inflammatory therapy regardless of drug might reduce the risk of cancer. However, the protective effect of steroids was not significant when multivariate analysis was performed, whereas aminosalicylate therapy remained significant. MSA was the only treatment to be associated with a statistically significant reduction in the risk of developing cancer. Even after adjusting for other variables, MSA at doses >1.2 g /day reduced the risk of cancer by 81% ($p = 0.006$). Frequent visits to the clinician were also associated with a protective effect, reducing the risk by 84% ($p = 0.007$). The authors suggest that MSA has a stronger protective effect than SSZ. A possible explanation for this is the fact that SSZ interferes with folate metabolism and uptake in the gut. Folate deficiency has been shown to be pro-carcinogenic; thus this side-effect of SSZ therapy may antagonize any inherent anticancer properties of the SSZ molecule itself[12].

Another large database study from the UK in 2003 has confirmed the possible preventive effect of 5-ASA in developing CRC in UC patients[13]. A general practice research database was used to identify almost 19 000 patients with UC. In a nested case–control study the investigators looked at a study population consisting of users of various 5-ASA analogues. Each incident CRC case (100 cases) with any exposure to 5-ASA 6 months prior to the CRC diagnosis was matched with six controls also exposed in that period. Patients were classified according to regularity of use. Regular users were found to have a decreased risk of CRC compared to irregular users (OR 0.54, 95% CI 0.35–0.86). Interestingly, MSA conferred protection (OR 0.31, 95% CI 0.11–0.85), while SSZ failed to do so (OR 0.73, 95% CI 0.35–1.50).

Two recent studies, presented at Digestive Disease Week May 2005, give additional knowledge on the question of chemoprotection of 5-ASA. The first, a large database study from the USA, identified 197 CRC cases in a large cohort of IBD patients (119 UC, 78 CD). Patients with at least three 5-ASA prescriptions during the 2-year period prior to CRC diagnosis were 53% less likely to develop CRC compared to patients with only one or two prescriptions (prior to the development of CRC) (OR 0.47, 95% CI 0.24–0.90)[14]. The second is a case–control study from the Mayo Clinic, matching 188 CRC cases in UC patients with 188 controls identifying predictive and protective factors for CRC development[9]. Among protective factors was use of NSAID (OR 0.1, 95% CI 0.04–0.5). Cumulative use of 5-ASA for at least a year was associated with a reduced risk; however, not quite significant (OR 0.6, 95% CI 0.3–1.0, $p = 0.052$). This is in accordance with van Staa et al., who found that 5-ASA use for less than 2 years was not associated with a significant reduced CRC incidence[13].

In contrast three negative studies have been published. Bernstein et al. looked at 25 CRC cases in CD (14 patients) and UC (11 patients) matched with 348 cases of IBD from the same unselected cohort[15]. The cases were selected from the records of Manitoba province and looked at the use of 5-ASA during the last 2 years prior to the development of CRC. A small sample size of incident cases might have biased the results. Lindberg et al. analysed the effect of SSZ in the development of CRC in 143 UC patients in a 20-year surveillance

**Table 1** Summary of studies, published and non-published, investigating the anticarcinogenic effect of 5-ASA therapy on the risk of colorectal cancer

| Reference | | Cases | OR/RR (95% CI) |
|---|---|---|---|
| *Studies showing a protective effect for 5-ASA* | | | |
| Cohort      Moody et al. 1996[11] | UC | 10 | 3% vs 31% S |
| Case–control  Pinczowski et al. 1994[10] | UC | 102 | 0.36 (0.20–0.69) |
| Case–control  Eaden et al. 2000[19] | UC | 102 | 0.25 (0.13–0.48) |
| Case–control  Van Staa et al. 2003[13] | UC | 72 | 0.54 (0.35–0.86) |
| Case–control  Terdiman et al. 2005[14] | UC/CD | 197 | 0.47 (0.24–0.90) |
| Case–control  Velayos et al. 2005[9] | UC | 188 | 0.60 (0.30–1.00) |
| | | | |
| *Studies showing no protective effect for 5-ASA* | | | |
| Cohort      Lindberg et al. 2001[16] | UC | 7 | 32% vs 41% NS |
| Case–control  Bernstein et al. 2001[15] | UC/CD | 25 | 1.46 (0.58–3.73) |
| Case–control  Rutter et al. 2004[17] | UC | 16 | 2.10 (0.52–8.43) |

S, significant; NS nonsignificant.

programme[16]; 51 developed dysplasia or cancer ($n = 3$). SSZ could not prevent the development of dysplasia or cancer. A *post-hoc* analysis revealed that the power of this study was low and that a larger sample size might have yielded significant results. Finally Rutter et al. looked at various risk factors for developing CRC in a case–control study; 68 cases with colorectal neoplasia (14 CRC, 32 adenoma, 8 high-grade dysplasia and 14 low-grade dysplasia) were matched with 134 controls[17]. Neither SSZ nor MSA use was found to be protective regardless of duration of therapy. A summary of all studies on 5-ASA use is presented in Table 1.

In 2004 Velayos and colleagues performed a meta-analysis of six previously published studies containing 251 cases of CRC, 69 cases of dysplasia and a total of 1031 subjects examining the potential chemopreventive effect of any use of 5-ASA for cancer or dysplasia[18]. Three of the studies were case–control studies[10,15,19] and three were cohort studies[11,16,20]. Three studies reported CRC outcome alone. One study reported separate cancer and dysplasia outcome and two studies reported a combined outcome. The pooled odds ratios showed a statistically significant chemopreventive effect for cancer (OR 0.25, 95% CI 0.15–0.40), or combined outcome of cancer/dysplasia (OR 0.47, 95% CI 0.24–0.92). With the added power of a meta-analysis this strongly supports a protective association of 5-ASA and CRC or CRC/dysplasia in patients with UC.

What dose is required? According to Eaden et al. MSA at a dose of $> 1.2$ g/day gave a CRC risk reduction of 81%. In a study by Ullman et al. a daily dose of at least 2.4 g was required to protect against progression to advanced neoplasia. However, the protective effect was not noted in those patients who had already developed low-grade dysplasia[21]. In a case–control study Rubin et al. found that patients taking 5-ASA 1.2 g/day were 76% less likely ($p = 0.024$) to progress to dysplasia or cancer[22]. They conclude that 5-ASA therapy should probably commence early prior to dysplasia development; however, this issue needs further investigation.

Currently 5-ASA is being studied in a non-IBD setting in the German 5-ASA Polyp Prevention Study (GAPPS). In this study the endpoint is new adenomas after 3 years of therapy with MSA 1 g/day vs placebo. So far the results have been discouraging. The study has had a high dropout rate of 30%. Considering other studies the dose may have been too low. The question of whether 5-ASA is chemopreventive in non-inflamed colonic mucosa remains to be answered.

## 5-ASA experimental studies

Two small prospective human studies have investigated the effect of MSA on colonic mucosal growth parameters, which are considered to be surrogate markers of CRC. In a study by Bus et al. 14 patients with rectosigmoid carcinomas were treated with MSA enemas at a dose of 4 g/day, for 14 days, and biopsies were taken from normal mucosa and tumour at the beginning and end of treatment[23]. MSA increased the apoptotic index in the tumour samples, but not in normal colonic mucosa, and had no effect on proliferation in either tumour or normal colonic mucosal samples, suggesting a selective pro-apoptotic effect in tumour cells. A similar study by Reinacher-Schick et al. investigated the effect of oral MSA on apoptosis and proliferation in normal colonic mucosa in patients undergoing colonoscopy for adenoma surveillance[24]. In contrast to the study by Bus et al., MSA at a dose of 1 g/day significantly increased apoptosis and reduced proliferation indices in normal colonic epithelium of patients with a history of sporadic polyps. Although the differences in results found in these two studies are not easily explained, the results suggest that 5-ASA can modulate human colonic epithelial cell turnover *in vivo*. Both studies have a limited number of patients, and the results need to be confirmed in larger controlled trials.

A number of animal studies have been performed to investigate the chemopreventive action of aminosalicylate drugs. The results have been conflicting, contrary to the consistent results of other NSAID. Three studies have been performed using the dimethylhydrazine (DMH) rodent CRC model, all of which showed that aminosalicylates conferred some protection against the development of CRC[25-27]. Brown et al. found that MSA reduced both the number of aberrant crypt foci (ACF) and the number and size of tumours in DMH-treated rodents[25]. Davis et al. found that high-dose MSA(60 mg/kg) was chemopreventive, whereas low-dose MSA (30 mg/kg), olsalazine and SSZ had no beneficial effect[27]. Wargovitz et al. in an azoxymethane (AOM) model, found that SSZ did not confer protection against the development of ACF. A number of studies using models other than the DMH model have also demonstrated anticancer effects of 5-ASA. One such study, in a combined dextran sulphate sodium/azoxymethane murine model of neoplasia in colitis, found that SSZ treatment reduced the number of areas of high-grade dysplasia[28]. The results in APC mutant animal models have also been conflicting. MacGregor et al. found that balsalazide reduced the number of tumours by 80% in the B6 Min/+ mouse model[29]. In another study by Ritland using the APC$^{MIN}$ mouse model, treatment with MSA and SSZ failed to reduce tumour numbers. In contrast control mice, treated with sulindac or piroxicam, showed a significant drop in tumour count. A conclusion in general is that 5-

ASA seems to confer some protection and that it can also do so in non-inflamed mucosa.

Several studies have examined the effects of 5-ASA on cellular proliferation and apoptosis in diverse cell types. SSZ has been shown to induce apoptosis in several cell types and through activation of caspases[30–32]. More recently, MSA at pharmacologically relevant concentrations was shown to time- and dose-dependently induce apoptosis and inhibit proliferation in two colorectal cell lines[33]. It seems that induction of apoptosis both by SSZ and MSA involves activation of the caspase pathway[30,33], but the details of the cellular effects of 5-ASA have not yet been fully elucidated.

## 5-ASA: potential mechanisms

5-ASA are structurally related to NSAID. MSA shares similar molecular targets, interfering with inflammation, proliferation and/or apoptosis, as do aspirin and other NSAID. This can be explained by the close molecular similarity of MSA and aspirin. A large body of experimental evidence shows that NSAID induce apoptosis, inhibit cellular proliferation, and inhibit colorectal tumour formation in a variety of animal models[34,35]. NSAID are thought to have anti-CRC effects through both cyclooxygenase 2 (COX-2)-dependent and -independent mechanisms. COX-independent mechanisms are increasingly recognized to play an important role in mediating the anticancer effects of NSAID.

COX-dependent mechanisms have been shown to be important but do not explain the whole anticarcinogenic effect. Contrary to the irreversible inhibition of aspirin, COX-1 and COX-2 are reversibly inhibited by MSA. An attractive hypothesis for the MSA/NSAID mode of action in this context relates not to COX inhibition itself, but rather to the accumulation of arachidonic acid. Arachidonic acid activates alkaline sphingomyelinase, which leads to increased ceramide production with activation of caspases and other apoptotic reactions. Alkaline sphingomyelinase has been shown to be down-regulated in both sporadic colorectal adenomas and carcinomas, familial adenomatous polyposis and long-standing UC with and without dysplasia[36–38]. In addition 5-ASA has been shown to up-regulate alkaline sphingo-myelinase in normal rat mucosa[39] and in a Caco-2 colon cancer cell line (Duan, personal communication).

A hypothesis linking COX-dependent and COX-independent inhibitory mechanisms together is based on the peroxisome proliferator-activated receptor δ (PPARδ) system as a common pathway for both inflammatory (COX-dependent) and non-inflammatory (COX-independent)-driven carcinogenesis. PPARδ has been identified as a possible downstream target of the APC/B-catenin pathway[40]. NSAID has been shown to inhibit PPARδ from activating pro-proliferative genes, although the exact mechanism is not fully understood. Just recently, PPAR have also been shown to be an important target for 5-ASA. In an animal model of PPARγ, 5-ASA was able to block the inflammatory response in the wild-type animal but not in the heterozygous PPARγ (+/−) animal[41].

Increased nuclear factor kappa beta (NF-κB) expression is a feature described in CRC[42], and this is likely to render the cells more resistant to apoptosis. The antiapoptotic effects of NF-κB have been well described[43]. Thus, inhibition of NF-κB activity by NSAID may contribute to the anticancer effects of these agents[34]. In common with NSAID, SSZ and MSA all inhibit NF-κB activity *in vitro*, mediated by inhibition of I-κB kinase activity, and resulting in reduced nuclear translocation and reduced NF-κB transcriptional activity[44,45].

Other effects of 5-ASA include inhibition of pro-proliferative mitogen-activated protein (MAP) kinase pathways within CRC cells[45], rendering the cells less resistant to apoptosis; 5-ASA may also have antioxidant properties, and scavenging of free radicals may reduce oxidative DNA damage, a potentially mutagenic process[46,47].

A large body of evidence suggests that 5-ASA has selective chemopreventive properties and that the chemopreventive effect is not a result of general anti-inflammatory action in the colonic mucosa. The fact that steroids, more potent as anti-inflammatory therapy than 5-ASA, had a lesser anticancer effect, supports the theory that 5-ASA, like NSAID, may have an inherent protective effect against the development of CRC[19]. The antineoplastic effect seen in non-inflamed mucosa in animal models also speaks in favour of an inherent chemopreventive effect[25, 27].

## URSODEOXYCHOLIC ACID

### Clinical evidence

The background for considering ursodeoxycholic acid (UDCA) as a chemopreventive agent in the UC population has been put forward mainly from two studies of UDCA use in UC patients with primary sclerosing cholangitis (PSC). There is a particularly high risk of CRC in UC patients with PSC, approaching 50% after 25 years of disease[48]. The use of UDCA to treat PSC is associated with improvement in biochemical indices of liver function, although it has not been shown to affect the overall progression of the liver disease.

In a study by Tung et al. the authors investigated the relationship between UDCA use and colonic dysplasia or adenocarcinoma in 59 UC patients with PSC[49]. Colonic dysplasia was established by surveillance colonoscopy. The UDCA group ($n$ = 41) was older at UC onset and had a shorter duration of UC at time of enrollment in this study. There was no difference in Child-Pugh class or duration of liver disease between the two groups. Overall, 26 patients (44%) developed dysplasia, 32% in the UDCA group vs 72% of those not taking UDCA (OR 0.18, 95% CI 0.05–0.61). This difference remained significant after adjusting for all known potential confounders. There was no significant relationship between the dose or duration of UDCA use and the subsequent development of dysplasia. A secondary analysis excluded those patients with indefinite dysplasia as their worst histological lesion and found that UDCA use was still negatively associated with colonic dysplasia (OR 0.21, 95% CI 0.05–

0.99, $p = 0.05$). This association failed to remain significant after adjusting for other variables. When patients with high-grade dysplasia were analysed independently, there was a statistically significant protective effect of UDCA use against development of this advanced neo-plastic lesion (OR 0.17, 95% CI 0.04–0.68, $p = 0.015$). This difference remained significant after adjustment for other variables.

This study indicates that UDCA may have chemopreventive properties in UC patients; however, the study has several limitations. It was not designed as a randomized intervention trial and there may have been biases related to how patients were selected for treatment with UDCA. There were two confounders that characterized the non-UDCA group: earlier age at diagnosis of UC and longer duration of disease, which might act to increase the risk of neoplasia in this group. There was no association between the dose and duration of UDCA treatment. Finally, biomarkers that might confirm patient compliance were not measured.

The study by Pardi et al. adds major impact to the fact that UDCA might be an effective chemopreventive agent[4]. Originally this was a randomized controlled trial to address the efficacy of UDCA in the treatment of PSC. The authors went back and looked at patients with UC and PSC and re-examined histology from surveillance colonoscopies. Fifty-two eligible patients were randomized to UDCA ($n = 29$) or placebo ($n = 23$). Three patients (10%) in the UDCA group compared to eight patients (35%) in the placebo group, developed neoplasia. The authors found a relative risk of 0.26 (95% CI 0.06–0.92; $p < 0.03$) for the development of dysplasia or cancer in the UDCA-treated patients.

The strength of the study is its design, a randomized, placebo-controlled trial performed in a prospective manner. One limitation concerns the number of colonic biopsies. An average of 20 biopsies were taken during the surveillance colonoscopies in this study. Because dysplasia is focal, and the colon is a large organ, it takes 33 biopsies or more to have 90% confidence that dysplasia is not present[50]. Thus, sampling error could play a role in evaluating the results, particularly the patients who were considered negative for dysplasia.

Can these results be applicable to UC patients without PSC, or even to chemoprevention against sporadic colorectal neoplasia? A small randomized study from Sweden on 19 patients with longstanding UC with dysplasia and/or DNA-aneuploidy compared the effect of UDCA vs placebo on dysplasia progression. Two patients in the placebo group progressed to higher grade of dysplasia but none in the UDCA group. The patient number is too low, but indicates that UDCA may be able to prevent the progress of dysplasia in a non-PSC UC population. More randomized trials are needed[51]. Two major multi-centre trials are under way to determine whether UDCA can prevent sporadic adenomas.

## Animal evidence

In 1994 Earnest et al. showed that supplemental UDCA was a chemopreventive agent in the AOM model of experimental carcinogenesis[52]. The chemopreventive action of UDCA was confirmed by Narisawa et al. using a

$N$-methylnitrosurea model[53] and by others, showing reduced numbers of carcinogen-induced adenomas and colon cancers compared with rats fed cholic acid[54,55]. Timing is important in chemoprevention. Neoplastic progression in the colon involves a process of initiation and then promotion. A recent study demonstrated that UDCA could reduce tumour number, but not size, in the initiation and promotion/progression stages[56]. However, UDCA administered late, after the initiation phase, could not inhibit aberrant crypt foci formation. Thus, it is not clear whether UDCA can completely deter formation or growth of the initial precursors of cancer if given after initiation of tumorigenesis is completed.

## Potential mechanisms

How does UDCA exert its protective effect? One potential mechanism for the chemo-preventive effect of UDCA is a reduced concentration within the colon of the secondary bile acid, deoxycholic acid (DCA), a bile acid that has been postulated as a colonic carcinogen. It has previously been shown that patients with UC and colonic dysplasia or carcinoma have higher faecal DCA concentrations than do patients with UC but without colonic neoplasia[57]. DCA has been shown to be cytotoxic to colonic epithelial cells, inducing hyperproliferation. In studies with rats, UDCA has been found to decrease the faecal levels of DCA in the colon[58,59].

Secondly, UDCA blocks two separate neoplastic pathways: modulating protein kinase C and phospholipase $A_2$ expression[54,55,60]. Both of these pathways have been associated with colon cancer formation in rats and humans[61,62]. Khare et al. found that UDCA blocked COX-2 expression[63]. This NSAID-like action could explain why UDCA dose-dependently increases alkaline sphingomyelinase in the normal rat colonic mucosa, together with caspase-3, a marker of apoptosis[64]. Finally, UDCA is an antioxidant that stabilizes the mitochondrial membrane, preventing oxidative injury to DNA[65].

# FOLATE

## Epidemiological studies

Epidemiological studies, including the Nurses' Health Study, suggest that dietary folate can protect against colorectal neoplasia[66,67]. In addition folate deficiency facilitates neoplasia following exposure to chemical carcinogens in animal models and, in humans, results in chromosomal damage. Folate deficiency is known to be a potential consequence of UC. Symptomatic disease may result in inadequate nutritional intake, while active disease may lead to increased intestinal losses of folate. Furthermore, SSZ acts as a competitive inhibitor to folic acid transport across intestinal epithelium. The presence of luminal SSZ can decrease folate absorption by more than 30%. This can result in a decrease in both serum and erythrocyte levels of folate. It could explain why some studies find MSA to be associated with a stronger chemoprotective effect than SSZ[13,19].

Two retrospective studies by Lashner et al. have evaluated the role of folate as a chemopreventive agent in the setting of UC. The first study in 1989 included 99 patients with pancolitis for at least 8 years, with folate daily supplementation doses ranging from 0.4 to 1.0 mg. Thirty-five patients developed a neoplastic lesion in the colon while under surveillance, and folate use was associated with a decreased risk of finding cancer or dysplasia during surveillance; however, this was not statistically significant (OR 0.38, 95% CI 0.12–1.20). There was a lack of information regarding the duration of surveillance, the duration of folate supplementation and measurements of serum or red blood cell folate levels.

A subsequent study by Lashner et al. looked at a cohort of 98 patients with long-standing extensive disease[20]. Only patients with intact colons, and in whom no dysplasia or cancer developed within 2 years of referral, were included. Folate supplementation (0.4 or 1.0 mg/day) was analysed as a dichotomous variable, with use for at least 6 months compared to less than 6 months or no use. The adjusted relative risk of developing dysplasia and cancer for folate use of at least 6 months was 0.72 (95% CI 0.28–1.83). An insignificant trend towards a dose–response effect was observed. Also, in this study the duration of surveillance was recorded, with a mean of 6.7 years for the dysplasia group and 6.1 years for controls. It is possible that most of the patients studied did in fact receive adequate folate in their diets.

Thus, while folate supplementation appears to be protective against sporadic colonic neoplasia, the evidence for a similar effect for folate in IBD patients is less. Folic acid is currently being investigated in prospective trials to evaluate its potential efficacy in sporadic colorectal neoplasia in the Aspirin/Folate Polyp Prevention Study. One milligram of folic acid supplementation daily is being compared with placebo in patients recently having had adenomas removed.

## Experimental studies

Expansion of the proliferation field in colonic mucosa has been shown to be an early event in the chemical induction of adenocarcinoma in mice, and has been demonstrated in the flat mucosa of patients with CRC. It is therefore considered an intermediate biomarker of CRC risk when determining the effectiveness of a therapeutic intervention. Biasco et al. compared the histological effects of folic acid vs placebo in 24 patients with long-standing UC in a double-blinded, randomized trial[68]. After 3 months of once-daily folic acid (15 mg) or placebo, there was a statistically significant decrease in the frequency of proliferating cells in the upper 40% of the crypts from biopsy specimens in the folate group. This was accompanied by an 18-fold increase in serum folate levels and an 8-fold increase in erythrocyte folate levels in the treatment arm ($p < 0.01$ for both), but no such changes in the placebo group. This supports the biological hypothesis for an association for folic acid and colonic dysplasia. In a small study of 12 patients with colorectal carcinoma, 12 with adenomas, and eight healthy controls, pharmacological doses of folic acid were found to modulate genomic DNA hypomethylation in the normal-appearing rectal epithelium of individuals with neoplasms[69]. The usefulness of folate as a chemopreventive agent for colorectal cancer awaits further evaluation.

## Possible mechanisms

Although the mechanism of action of folate as a putative chemopreventive agent against colorectal cancer is not as yet understood, one theory has focused on the role of folate in DNA methylation. Diets that are deficient in folic acid are thought to render individuals at increased risk of malignancy through two mechanisms. First, the requirement of methyl groups for normal cellular metabolism exceeds dietary supply, and insufficiency is prevented by *de-novo* methyl synthesis via one carbon donation from the folate pool[12]. Genes that are methylated at specific locations in the DNA molecule are either not transcribed or are transcribed at a reduced rate; therefore site-specific DNA methylation appears to control gene expression. It is hypothesized, therefore, that folate deficiency can induce DNA hypomethylation and lead to dysregulated activation of proto-oncogenes involved in carcinogenesis. The second hypothesis is that folate deficiency alters nucleotide precursor pools, inducing uracil misincorporation during DNA synthesis, with DNA strand breakage and chromosome damage[12].

## SUMMARY AND CLINICAL IMPLICATIONS

A series of epidemiological, experimental and, in addition, small preliminary clinical trials strongly suggest that 5-ASA is a protective agent against the development of dysplasia and CRC in UC patients. However, randomized trials that ultimately provide evidence for a chemopreventive effect are missing. The mechanisms behind the postulated chemopreventive properties of 5-ASA are not fully elucidated, but the drug may share similar molecular targets as other NSAID, with its close chemical similarity to aspirin. Several lines of evidence suggest that 5-ASA has inherent chemopreventives properties and that protection is not due to a general anti-inflammatory effect, including studies of molecular targets and the absence of a chemopreventive effect of other anti-inflammatory agents used in IBD. The safe side-effect profile with 5-ASA makes it an attractive chemopreventive option. Patients with UC at high risk of CRC (such as those with a family history of sporadic CRC, pancolitis or with PSC) should receive regular 5-ASA, even if the disease has been quiescent. Maintenance therapy in UC patients for disease control is quite often used. However, one particular emerging problem is the diminishing use of 5-ASA in Crohn's colitis, because of the lack of efficacy in maintaining remission. As in UC, the potential cancerpreventive effects should also be considered, when deciding whether to discontinue maintenance 5-ASA therapy in CD.

UDCA therapy should be considered in all patients with UC and PSC. Future studies will shed more light on this issue. At the moment there are no hard data to support UDCA therapy in UC patients without PSC.

Finally, folate therapy seems to be protective against sporadic colorectal neoplasia. Since folate deficiency is associated with UC, it seems logical to treat with folate supplement. The low cost and excellent side-effect profile make it easier to support this view. However, the data to support so far only suggest, but do not prove, a chemopreventive effect for folate in IBD patients.

# References

1. Itzkowitz SH. Inflammatory bowel disease and cancer. Gastroenterol Clin N Am. 1997;26: 129–39.
2. Eaden JA, Abrams KR, Mayberry JF. The risk of colorectal cancer in ulcerative colitis: a meta-analysis. Gut. 2001;48:526–35.
3. Langholz E, Munkholm P, Davidsen M, Binder V. Colorectal cancer risk and mortality in patients with ulcerative colitis. Gastroenterology. 1992;103:1444–51.
4. Pardi DS, Loftus EV Jr, Kremers WK, Keach J, Lindor KD. Ursodeoxycholic acid as a chemopreventive agent in patients with ulcerative colitis and primary sclerosing cholangitis. Gastroenterology. 2003;124:889–93.
5. Kune GA, Kune S, Watson LF. Colorectal cancer risk, chronic illnesses, operations, and medications: case control results from the Melbourne Colorectal Cancer Study. Cancer Res. 1988;48:4399–404.
6. Thun MJ, Namboodiri MM, Heath CW Jr. Aspirin use and reduced risk of fatal colon cancer. N Engl J Med 1991;325:1593–6.
7. Giovannucci E, Rimm EB, Stampfer MJ, Colditz GA, Ascherio A, Willett WC. Aspirin use and the risk for colorectal cancer and adenoma in male health professionals. Ann Intern Med. 1994;121:241–6.
8. Bansal P, Sonnenberg A. Risk factors of colorectal cancer in inflammatory bowel disease. Am J Gastroenterol. 1996;91:44–8.
9. Velayos F, Loftus EV Jr, Jess W et al. A case–control study of predictive factors in 188 patients with colorectal cancer and ulcerativec colitis. Gastroenterology. 2005; DDW, Abstract M1191.
10. Pinczowski D, Ekbom A, Baron J, Yuen J, Adami HO. Risk factors for colorectal cancer in patients with ulcerative colitis: a case–control study. Gastroenterology. 1994;107:117–20.
11. Moody GA, Jayanthi V, Probert CS, MacKay H, Mayberry JF. Long-term therapy with sulphasalazine protects against colorectal cancer in ulcerative colitis: a retrospective study of colorectal cancer risk and compliance with treatment in Leicestershire. Eur J Gastroenterol Hepatol. 1996;8:1179–83.
12. Duthie SJ. Folic acid deficiency and cancer: mechanisms of DNA instability. Br Med Bull. 1999;55:578–92.
13. Van Staa T, Card T, Leufkens H, Logan R. Prior aminosalicylate use and the development of colorectal cancer in inflammatory bowel disease. Am J Gastroenterol. 2003;98:S76–7.
14. Terdiman J, Ullman T, Blumentals W, Rubin D. A case–control study of 5-aminosalicylic acid therapy in the prevention of colitis-related colorectal cancer. DDW, 2005; Abstract M1052.
15. Bernstein CN, Blanchard JF, Kliewer E, Wajda A. Cancer risk in patients with inflammatory bowel disease: a population-based study. Cancer. 2001;91:854–62.
16. Lindberg BU, Broome U, Persson B. Proximal colorectal dysplasia or cancer in ulcerative colitis. The impact of primary sclerosing cholangitis and sulfasalazine: results from a 20-year surveillance study. Dis Colon Rectum. 2001;44:77–85.
17. Rutter M, Saunders B, Wilkinson K et al. Severity of inflammation is a risk factor for colorectal neoplasia in ulcerative colitis. Gastroenterology. 2004;126:451–9.
18. Velayos F, Walsh J, Terdiman J. Effect of 5-aminosalisylic use on colorectal cancer and dysplasia risk in ulcerative colitis: a meta-analysis. Gastroenterology. 2003;126(Suppl. 2): Abstract 136.
19. Eaden J, Abrams K, Ekbom A, Jackson E, Mayberry J. Colorectal cancer prevention in ulcerative colitis: a case–control study. Aliment Pharmacol Ther. 2000;14:145–53.
20. Lashner BA, Provencher KS, Seidner DL, Knesebeck A, Brzezinski A. The effect of folic acid supplementation on the risk for cancer or dysplasia in ulcerative colitis. Gastroenterology. 1997;112:29–32.
21. Ullman T, Croog V, Harpaz N, Itzkovic S, Kornbluth A. Preventing neoplastic progression in ulcerative colitis: role of mesalamine. Gastroenterology. 2003;124:242.
22. Rubin D, Djordevic A, Huo D, Yadron N, Hanauer S. Use of 5-ASA is associated with a decreased risk of dysplasia abd colon cancer (CRC) in ulcerative colitis (UC). Gastroenterology. 2003. DDW, Abstract 279).

23. Bus PJ, Nagtegaal ID, Verspaget HW et al. Mesalazine-induced apoptosis of colorectal cancer: on the verge of a new chemopreventive era? Aliment Pharmacol Ther. 1999;13: 1397–402.

24. Reinacher-Schick A, Seidensticker F, Petrasch S et al. Mesalazine changes apoptosis and proliferation in normal mucosa of patients with sporadic polyps of the large bowel. Endoscopy. 2000;32:245–54.

25. Brown WA, Farmer KC, Skinner SA, Malcontenti-Wilson C, Misajon A, O'Brien PE. 5-aminosalicyclic acid and olsalazine inhibit tumor growth in a rodent model of colorectal cancer. Dig Dis Sci. 2000;45:1578–84.

26. Andrianopoulos GD, Nelson RL, Barch DH, Nyhus LM. Sulfasalazine alters the character of dimethylhydrazine-induced colorectal carcinoma in rats. Anticancer Res. 1989;9:1725–8.

27. Davis AE, Patterson F, Crouch R. The effect of therapeutic drugs used in inflammatory bowel disease on the incidence and growth of colonic cancer in the dimethylhydrazine rat model. Br J Cancer. 1992;66:777–80.

28. Suzuki S, Sakamoto S, Mitamura T, Sassa S, Kudo H, Yamashita Y. Preventive effects of sulphasalazine on colorectal carcinogenesis in mice with ulcerative colitis. In Vivo. 2000;14: 463–6.

29. MacGregor DJ, Kim YS, Sleisenger MH, Johnson LK. Chemoprevention of colon cancer carcinogenesis by balsalazide: inhibition of azoxymethane-induced aberrant crypt formation in the rat colon and intestinal tumor formation in the B6-Min/+ mouse. Int J Oncol. 2000;17:173–9.

30. Rodenburg RJ, Ganga A, van Lent PL, van de Putte LB, van Venrooij WJ. The antiinflammatory drug sulfasalazine inhibits tumor necrosis factor alpha expression in macrophages by inducing apoptosis. Arthritis Rheum. 2000;43:1941–50.

31. Liptay S, Bachem M, Hacker G, Adler G, Debatin KM, Schmid RM. Inhibition of nuclear factor kappa B and induction of apoptosis in T-lymphocytes by sulfasalazine. Br J Pharmacol. 1999;128:1361–9.

32. Akahoshi T, Namai R, Sekiyama N, Tanaka S, Hosaka S, Kondo H. Rapid induction of neutrophil apoptosis by sulfasalazine: implications of reactive oxygen species in the apoptotic process. J Leukoc Biol. 1997;62:817–26.

33. Reinacher-Schick A, Schoeneck A, Graeven U, Schwarte-Waldhoff I, Schmiegel W. Mesalazine causes a mitotic arrest and induces caspase-dependent apoptosis in colon carcinoma cells. Carcinogenesis. 2003;24:443–51.

34. Chan TA. Nonsteroidal anti-inflammatory drugs, apoptosis, and colon-cancer chemoprevention. Lancet Oncol. 2002;3:166–74.

35. Janne PA, Mayer RJ. Chemoprevention of colorectal cancer. N Engl J Med. 2000;342: 1960–8.

36. Hertervig E, Nilsson A, Nyberg L, Duan RD. Alkaline sphingomyelinase activity is decreased in human colorectal carcinoma. Cancer. 1997;79:448–53.

37. Hertervig E, Nilsson A, Bjork J, Hultkrantz R, Duan RD. Familial adenomatous polyposis is associated with a marked decrease in alkaline sphingomyelinase activity: a key factor to the unrestrained cell proliferation? Br J Cancer. 1999;81:232–6.

38. Sjoqvist U, Hertervig E, Nilsson A et al. Chronic colitis is associated with a reduction of mucosal alkaline sphingomyelinase activity. Inflamm Bowel Dis. 2002;8:258–63.

39. Duan RD. Potential link between sphingomyelin metabolism and colonic tumourigenesis. In: Scheppach W, Scheurlen M, editors. Exogenous Factors in Colorectal Carcinogenesis. Dordrecht: Kluwer, 2003:142–56.

40. He TC, Chan TA, Vogelstein B, Kinzler KW. PPARdelta is an APC-regulated target of nonsteroidal anti-inflammatory drugs. Cell. 1999;99:335–45.

41. Rousseaux C, Lefebvre B, Dubuquoy L et al. Intestinal antiinflammatory effect of 5-aminosalicylic acid is dependent on peroxisome proliferator-activated receptor-γ. J Exp Med. 2005;201:1205–15.

42. Lind DS, Hochwald SN, Malaty J et al. Nuclear factor-kappa B is upregulated in colorectal cancer. Surgery. 2001;130:363–9.

43. Schmid RM, Adler G. NF-kappaB/rel/IkappaB: implications in gastrointestinal diseases. Gastroenterology. 2000;118:1208–28.

44. Weber CK, Liptay S, Wirth T, Adler G, Schmid RM. Suppression of NF-kappaB activity by sulfasalazine is mediated by direct inhibition of IkappaB kinases alpha and beta. Gastroenterology. 2000;119:1209–18.

45. Kaiser GC, Yan F, Polk DB. Mesalamine blocks tumor necrosis factor growth inhibition and nuclear factor kappaB activation in mouse colonocytes. Gastroenterology. 1999;116: 602–9.
46. Lewis JG, Adams DO. Inflammation, oxidative DNA damage, and carcinogenesis. Environ Health Perspect. 1987;76:19–27.
47. Ahnfelt-Ronne I, Nielsen OH, Christensen A, Langholz E, Binder V, Riis P. Clinical evidence supporting the radical scavenger mechanism of 5-aminosalicylic acid. Gastroenterology. 1990;98:1162–9.
48. Broome U, Lofberg R, Veress B, Eriksson LS. Primary sclerosing cholangitis and ulcerative colitis: evidence for increased neoplastic potential. Hepatology. 1995;22:1404–8.
49. Tung BY, Emond MJ, Haggitt RC et al. Ursodiol use is associated with lower prevalence of colonic neoplasia in patients with ulcerative colitis and primary sclerosing cholangitis. Ann Intern Med. 2001;134:89–95.
50. Rubin CE, Haggitt RC, Burmer GC et al. DNA aneuploidy in colonic biopsies predicts future development of dysplasia in ulcerative colitis. Gastroenterology. 1992;103:1611–20.
51. Sjoqvist U, Tribukait B, Ost A, Einarsson C, Oxelmark L, Lofberg R. Ursodeoxycholic acid treatment in IBD-patients with colorectal dysplasia and/or DNA-aneuploidy: a prospective, double-blind, randomized controlled pilot study. Anticancer Res. 2004;24: 3121–7.
52. Earnest DL, Holubec H, Wali RK et al. Chemoprevention of azoxymethane-induced colonic carcinogenesis by supplemental dietary ursodeoxycholic acid. Cancer Res. 1994; 54:5071–4.
53. Narisawa T, Fukaura Y, Terada K, Sekiguchi H. Prevention of N-methylnitrosourea-induced colon tumorigenesis by ursodeoxycholic acid in F344 rats. Jpn J Cancer Res. 1998;89:1009–13.
54. Ikegami R, Zheng H, Ong SH, Culotti J. Integration of semaphorin-2A/MAB-20, ephrin-4, and UNC-129 TGF-beta signaling pathways regulates sorting of distinct sensory rays in C. elegans. Dev Cell. 2004;6:383–95.
55. Wali RK, Frawley BP Jr, Hartmann S et al. Mechanism of action of chemoprotective ursodeoxycholate in the azoxymethane model of rat colonic carcinogenesis: potential roles of protein kinase C-alpha, -beta II, and -zeta. Cancer Res. 1995;55:5257–64.
56. Wali RK, Stoiber D, Nguyen L et al. Ursodeoxycholic acid inhibits the initiation and postinitiation phases of azoxymethane-induced colonic tumor development. Cancer Epidemiol Biomarkers Prev. 2002;11:1316–21.
57. Hill MJ, Melville DM, Lennard-Jones JE, Neale K, Ritchie JK. Faecal bile acids, dysplasia, and carcinoma in ulcerative colitis. Lancet. 1987;2:185–6.
58. Rodrigues CM, Kren BT, Steer CJ, Setchell KD. The site-specific delivery of ursodeoxycholic acid to the rat colon by sulfate conjugation. Gastroenterology. 1995;109: 1835–44.
59. Batta AK, Salen G, Holubec H, Brasitus TA, Alberts D, Earnest DL. Enrichment of the more hydrophilic bile acid ursodeoxycholic acid in the fecal water-soluble fraction after feeding to rats with colon polyps. Cancer Res. 1998;58:1684–7.
60. Pongracz J, Clark P, Neoptolemos JP, Lord JM. Expression of protein kinase C isoenzymes in colorectal cancer tissue and their differential activation by different bile acids. Int J Cancer. 1995;61:35–9.
61. Kopp R, Noelke B, Sauter G, Schildberg FW, Paumgartner G, Pfeiffer A. Altered protein kinase C activity in biopsies of human colonic adenomas and carcinomas. Cancer Res. 1991;51:205–10.
62. Minami T, Tojo H, Shinomura Y, Matsuzawa Y, Okamoto M. Increased group II phospholipase A2 in colonic mucosa of patients with Crohn's disease and ulcerative colitis. Gut. 1994;35:1593–8.
63. Khare S, Cerda S, Wali RK et al. Ursodeoxycholic acid inhibits Ras mutations, wild-type Ras activation, and cyclooxygenase-2 expression in colon cancer. Cancer Res. 2003;63: 3517–23.
64. Cheng Y, Tauschel HD, Nilsson A, Duan RD. Ursodeoxycholic acid increases the activities of alkaline sphingomyelinase and caspase-3 in the rat colon. Scand J Gastroenterol. 1999; 34:915–20.

65. Mitsuyoshi H, Nakashima T, Sumida Y et al. Ursodeoxycholic acid protects hepatocytes against oxidative injury via induction of antioxidants. Biochem Biophys Res Commun. 1999;263:537–42.
66. Giovannucci E, Stampfer MJ, Colditz GA et al. Multivitamin use, folate, and colon cancer in women in the Nurses' Health Study. Ann Intern Med. 1998;129:517–24.
67. Giovannucci E, Stampfer MJ, Colditz GA et al. Folate, methionine, and alcohol intake and risk of colorectal adenoma. J Natl Cancer Inst. 1993;85:875–84.
68. Biasco G, Zannoni U, Paganelli GM et al. Folic acid supplementation and cell kinetics of rectal mucosa in patients with ulcerative colitis. Cancer Epidemiol Biomarkers Prev. 1997; 6:469–71.
69. Cravo M, Fidalgo P, Pereira AD et al. DNA methylation as an intermediate biomarker in colorectal cancer: modulation by folic acid supplementation. Eur J Cancer Prev. 1994;3: 473–9.

# 22
# Management of low-grade dysplasia in inflammatory bowel disease

S. ITZKOWITZ

## INTRODUCTION

Essentially all colorectal cancers (CRC) develop from dysplastic precursor lesions. This is true for sporadic cancers arising in the general population, or colitis-associated CRC in the setting of inflammatory bowel diseases (IBD). Indeed, the fact that there is a premalignant phase of CRC offers the opportunity for early detection and cure. In sporadic CRC the dysplastic precursor lesion is the adenomatous polyp; a single, discrete focus of neoplasia that is typically managed by endoscopic polypectomy. In patients with long-standing IBD the dysplasia may be polypoid or flat, localized or diffuse, and marks the entire colon as being at heightened risk of neoplasia. These differences in morphology and biological behaviour make cancer surveillance in IBD more challenging than in the general population. Despite evidence suggesting that overall mortality in patients with ulcerative colitis (UC) is quite similar to patients without UC[1], CRC remains a much-feared long-term complication of IBD, with associated morbidity and mortality.

## RISK OF CRC IN IBD

The prevalence of CRC in patients with UC is approximately 3.7% overall, and 5.4% in those with pancolitis[2]. Cumulative risks for CRC in UC are approximately 8% after 20 years, and 18% after 30 years[2]. While most studies to date have focused mainly on CRC risk and management in patients with UC, patients with long-standing Crohn's colitis involving a substantial extent of colonic mucosa should be considered to have a similar increased risk of CRC[3].

Factors that increase risk for CRC in IBD include long disease duration (with risk beginning at approximately 7–8 years of colitis), greater extent of colitis, presence of primary sclerosing cholangitis, positive family history of CRC, young age of onset (some studies), and higher degrees of inflammation[4]. In an effort to decrease the risk of CRC most patients choose to follow a programme of surveillance rather than undergo a prophylactic total proctocolectomy. Surveillance entails regular visits to the doctor[5] as well as periodic colonoscopy to look for neoplastic transformation of the colonic mucosa. While evidence is lacking from prospective studies as to whether surveillance colonoscopy improves CRC-specific mortality in IBD, population-based case–control data have estimated that surveillance colonoscopy can reduce CRC mortality by almost 80%[6]. Notwithstanding this encouraging observation, there remains considerable controversy as to the efficacy of surveillance, due to a variety of limitations. From a logistical standpoint, patients must be willing and able to comply with regular (typically annual) colonoscopies. Failure to comply with regular surveillance has been associated with adverse consequences[7,8]. Physicians must sample the colonic mucosa adequately during colonoscopy, and they must understand the meaning and implications of finding dysplasia[9,10]. Even if these logistical and technical limitations can be overcome, however, there is no unanimity on what findings should prompt the recommendation for colectomy. In part, gastroenterologists may be reluctant to make such important management decisions in a clinical situation where pathologists may differ among themselves on the presence or severity of dysplasia. However, the matter is further complicated by uncertainty regarding the natural history of dysplasia. This uncertainty is minimal when it comes to managing high-grade dysplasia (HGD). Few would argue with the generally accepted policy of recommending colectomy for HGD, given the over 40% chance that cancer is either already present in the colon or will subsequently arise in this high-risk group[4,11]. The controversy typically centres around the biology and management of low-grade dysplasia (LGD).

## POLYPOID DYSPLASIA – A SEPARATE ENTITY

An important lesson that has been learned only in recent years is that polypoid LGD may indeed behave differently from flat LGD. In the earlier surveillance literature one can find reference to 'adenomas' arising in the setting of UC, with simple endoscopic resection of such lesions being associated with excellent outcomes. However, there was never a clear endoscopic or histological definition of what an adenoma in a colitic colon actually is. Despite the lack of a clear definition, it was subsequently learned that patients in whom polypoid dysplastic lesions could be completely resected endoscopically, and in whom there was no evidence of dysplasia at the polyp base or anywhere else in the colon, such individuals did not develop more advanced degrees of colonic neoplasia when followed for 5–10 years without undergoing colectomy[12–14]. It is worth realizing that such patients still were followed at more frequent intervals (at least initially) than someone without dysplasia, so it is not as if the post-polypectomy patient can simply return for follow-up in 3 or more years as one might do for a sporadic adenoma. When a polypoid dysplastic lesion does not lend itself to complete endoscopic resection, or if it recurs after apparently curative polypectomy, the lesion is then considered a dysplasia-associated lesion or mass (so-called DALM) and colectomy should be strongly considered, assuming co-morbid illnesses or other extenuating circumstances do not dictate otherwise.

## THE BIOLOGY OF LGD

Excluding patients with endoscopically manageable polypoid LGD, a strong argument can be made to consider colectomy in patients who demonstrate flat LGD. This strategy is supported by several lines of evidence. First, at the initial finding of flat LGD, there is an approximate 19–20% risk of an unsuspected cancer already being present in the colon. This estimate is based on a compilation of results from older surveillance studies[15] as well as more recent data from the Mount Sinai Hospital, New York, which took care to only include patients with flat LGD[16]. Curiously, another study found only a 10% rate of HGD and no cancers at resection[17], but whether this is sufficient to offer reassurance to the patient is unclear.

Second, if colectomy is not performed at the first sign of LGD, the actuarial rate of progression can be as high as 54% by 5 years. On the higher end of this statistic are studies from St Mark's Hospital, London[18], the Mayo Clinic[19] and the Mount Sinai Hospital[16] demonstrating 5-year progression to HGD or cancer of 35–54%. Importantly, the St Mark's group demonstrated that when LGD was properly classified according to the modern histological definition of dysplasia established by the International Morphology Study Group in 1983[20], the 5-year rate of progression rose from 16% to 54%, suggesting that lower rates of progression in some studies may be due to the inclusion of samples that are indefinite for dysplasia or reactive atypia. Nonetheless, other studies report rather low 5-year progression. A Swedish study reported no cancers developing after a mean follow-up period of 10 years[17], and the Leeds group found only a 10% rate of progression to HGD or cancer[21]. Whether these differences are due to real geographic differences, different histological interpretation, or other factors, the higher rates of progression must still be taken into account when considering a conservative management plan.

Third, progression to CRC may occur during surveillance. This may be due to a prolonged interval between colonoscopies. Studies suggest that cancers can arise within 2 years of a previous surveillance examination[18]. Thus, most experts support the recommendation that surveillance colonoscopy be performed every 1–2 years[11]. However, despite seemingly adequate surveillance, CRC can still arise. Some have argued that this is due to undersampling of the mucosa (giving the impression that LGD is the worst lesion when in fact cancer is already present)[22], or misinterpretation by the pathologist who might have called a lesion LGD when it was in fact HGD. While these circumstances are certainly possible, there is also evidence that CRC can arise without progressing through an intermediate stage of HGD. Our research group reported that, of seven patients who developed CRC after an initial finding of LGD, only one patient was found to have HGD on colonoscopy prior to the eventual discovery of CRC, and two patients who developed advanced CRC had no dysplasia at all on the last colonoscopy prior to the detection of cancer[16]. More worrisome is the recent realization that a particular type of invasive adenocarcinoma can arise directly from LGD in patients with UC. Harpaz and colleagues have described 'low grade tubular glandular adenocarcinoma', a bona-fide carcinoma which appears cytologically innocent, even in the more invasive portions of the tumour specimen[23]. This histological variant may account for as much as 11% of all CRC in UC, and could explain why some LGD lesions can progess to CRC without an HGD intermediate.

Fourth, following the discovery of LGD, subsequent examinations that are negative for dysplasia offer no reassurance that the risk has been reduced[8], and physicians as well as patients might be lulled into a sense of false security.

Finally, there are no accurate markers of neoplastic progression for patients with LGD. The risk factors cited above have not been shown to separate patients who already have LGD into higher and lower risk categories.

## MANAGING LGD

So how does one manage the patient with LGD? The first step is to confirm that the interpretation of LGD is correct. LGD may be over-interpreted in the setting of a very inflamed biopsy. It is often recommended that two pathologists skilled in gastrointestinal pathology should read the slides before coming to definitive conclusions regarding the presence of LGD. As mentioned above, if LGD occurs in a polyp, and the polyp can be completely resected without any evidence of adjacent or remote dysplasia, those patients can remain under endoscopic surveillance. It has been recommended that such patients be brought back at more frequent intervals of approximately 3–6 months to make sure there is no other focus of dysplasia. With respect to flat LGD, colectomy should be strongly considered, in good operative candidates, for the reasons discussed above. If patients are unwilling to have colectomy, they must be apprised that their risk of cancer will continue despite even the best efforts at surveillance by highly competent physicians and pathologists.

## NEW DEVELOPMENTS IN THE FIELD

Chromoendoscopy holds promise for detecting more LGD lesions than conventional colonoscopy. The dye-spray technique permits the elucidation of otherwise inapparent lesions, with separate studies demonstrating a considerable increase in dysplasia detection[24,25]. It is not yet known, however, whether finding more LGD lesions will change the natural history of LGD in a favourable or unfavourable direction.

Several studies, but not all, have found that regular use of 5-aminosalicylate (5-ASA) compounds can lower the risk of CRC in patients with UC[4]. While this might be considered an important component of long-term management, it is not yet known where in the colitis–dysplasia–carcinoma sequence these compounds might exert their antineoplastic effect. Thus, one cannot yet tell patients with LGD that taking high-dose 5-ASA will cause their dysplasia to regress. Curiously, non-steroidal anti-inflammatory drugs (NSAID) have been shown to regress adenomas in patients with familial polyposis, although it should also be noted that, despite this, CRC can still arise in these patients. Hopefully, in the future, as our understanding of LGD biology improves, our colonoscopic detection becomes sharper, new molecular markers are discovered, and possible pharmaceutical interventions are developed, we will be able to offer a more accurate management plan for IBD patients with LGD and lower the CRC burden in these high-risk patients.

## References

1. Loftus EV, Silverstein MD, Sandborn WJ et al. Ulcerative colitis in Olmstead County, Minnesota, 1940–1993: incidence, prevalence, and survival. Gut. 2000;46:336–43.
2. Eaden J, Abrams KR, Mayberry JF. The risk of colorectal cancer in ulcerative colitis: a meta-analysis. Gut. 2001;48:526–35.
3. Sachar DB. Cancer in Crohn's disease: dispelling the myths. Gut. 1994;35:1507–8.
4. Itzkowitz S, Harpaz N. Diagnosis and management of dysplasia in patients with inflammatory bowel disease. Gastroenterology. 2004;126:1634–48.
5. Eaden J, Abrams K, Ekbom A et al. Colorectal cancer prevention in ulcerative colitis: a case–control study. Aliment Pharmacol Ther. 2000;14:145–53.
6. Karlen P, Kornfeld D, Brostrom O et al. Is colonoscopic surveillance reducing colorectal cancer mortality in ulcerative colitis? A population based case control study. Gut. 1998;42:711–14.
7. Lynch DA, Lobo AJ, Sobala GM et al. Failure of colonoscopic surveillance in ulcerative colitis. Gut. 1993;34:1075–80.
8. Woolrich AJ, DaSilva MD, Korelitz BI. Surveillance in the routine management of ulcerative colitis: the predictive value of low-grade dysplasia. Gastroenterology. 1992;103:431–8.
9. Bernstein CN, Weinstein WM, Levine DS, Shanahan F. Physicians' perceptions of dysplasia and approaches to surveillance colonoscopy in ulcerative colitis. Am J Gastroenterol. 1995;90:2106–14.
10. Eaden JA, Ward BA, Mayberry JF. How gastroenterologists screen for colonic cancer in ulcerative colitis: an analysis of performance. Gastrointest Endosc. 2000;51:123–8.
11. Itzkowitz SH, Present DH, Crohn's and Colitis Foundation of America Colon Cancer in IBD Study Group. Consensus conference: colorectal cancer screening and surveillance in inflammatory bowel disease. Inflamm Bowel Dis. 2005;11:314–21.
12. Rubin PH, Friedman S, Harpaz N et al. Colonoscopic polypectomy in chronic colitis: conservative management after endoscopic resection of dysplastic polyps. Gastroenterology. 1999;117:1295–300.
13. Engelsgjerd M, Farraye FA, Odze RD. Polypectomy may be adequate treatment for adenoma-like dysplastic lesions in chronic ulcerative colitis. Gastroenterology. 1999;117:1288–94.
14. Odze RD, Farraye FA, Hecht JL, Hornick JL. Long-term follow-up after polypectomy treatment for adenoma-like dysplastic lesions in ulcerative colitis. Clin Gastroenterol Hepatol. 2004;2:534–41.
15. Bernstein CN, Shanahan F, Weinstein WM. Are we telling patients the truth about surveillance colonoscopy in ulcerative colitis? Lancet. 1994;343:71–4.
16. Ullman TA, Croog T, Harpaz N et al. Progression of flat low-grade dysplasia to advanced neoplasia in patients with ulcerative colitis. Gastroenterology. 2003;125:1311–19.
17. Befrits R, Ljung T, Jaramillo E, Rubio C. Low-grade dysplasia in extensive, long-standing inflammatory bowel disease; a follow-up study. Dis Colon Rectum. 2002;45:615–20.
18. Connell WR, Lennard-Jones JE, Williams CB et al. Factors affecting the outcome of endoscopic surveillance for cancer in ulcerative colitis. Gastroenterology. 1994;107:934–44.
19. Ullman TA, Loftus EV Jr, Kakar S et al. The fate of low grade dysplasia in ulcerative colitis. Am J Gastroenterol. 2002;97:922–7.
20. Riddell RH, Goldman H, Ransohoff DF et al. Dysplasia in inflammatory bowel disease: standardized classification with provisional clinical applications. Hum Pathol. 1983;14:931–68.
21. Lim CH, Dixon MF, Vail A et al. Ten year follow up of ulcerative colitis patients with and without low grade dysplasia. Gut. 2003;52:1127–32.
22. Rubin CE, Haggitt RC, Burmer GC et al. DNA aneuploidy in colonic biopsies predicts future development of dysplasia in ulcerative colitis. Gastroenterology. 1992;103:1611–20.

23. Levi, G., Harpaz N. Low-grade tubuloglandular adenocarcinoma associated with inflammatory bowel disease: a study of 21 cases. Mod Pathol. 2005;18:110A.
24. Kiesslich R, Fritsch J, Holtmann M et al. Methylene blue-aided chromoendoscopy for the detection of intraepithelial neoplasia and colon cancer in ulcerative colitis. Gastroenterology. 2003;124:880–8.
25. Rutter MD, Saunders BP, Schofield G et al. Pancolonic indigo carmine dye spraying for the detection of dysplasia in ulcerative colitis. Gut. 2004;53:256–60.

# 23
# Low-grade dysplasia in flat mucosa: is it relevant?

A. AXON

## INTRODUCTION

Patients with long-standing, extensive ulcerative colitis are at greater risk of developing colorectal cancer than the normal population. A meta-analysis by Eaden et al.[1] showed that for the first 10 years of colitis an individual has a 2% risk of developing cancer. This is roughly equivalent to the 10-year incidence of colorectal cancer in a normal 60-year-old man. In the second decade, however, the risk rises to 6% and in the third it rises to 10%. In the 1960s and 1970s patients in the at-risk group were advised to undergo total proctocolectomy to protect them from this complication.

A seminal paper by Morsen and Pang in 1967[2] drew attention to the concept of dysplasia. They showed that dysplastic changes in the rectal mucosa of patients with ulcerative colitis predicted adenocarcinoma elsewhere in the colon. With the development of colonoscopy, patients at risk have not been advised to undergo surgery, but to have regular colonoscopic surveillance examinations during which multiple biopsies are taken from the mucosa. These are assessed by pathologists and graded as 'negative for dysplasia', 'indefinite', 'low-grade dysplasia' or 'high-grade dysplasia'.

When high-grade dysplasia is present there is a roughly 30% risk of the patient developing invasive cancer within a relatively short period of time. A similar risk obtains in those patients who have low-grade dysplasia associated with a lesion or mass (DALM). When these premalignant lesions are identified therefore patients are advised to undergo proctocolectomy. Quite frequently, however, low-grade dysplasia is detected in flat mucosa without a macroscopic lesion or mass, the management of these patients is more controversial.

## RECOMMENDATIONS FOR THE MANAGEMENT OF LOW-GRADE DYSPLASIA IN FLAT MUCOSA

In 1994, Bernstein and colleagues published a paper in Lancet[3] which was an analysis of a series of studies that had reported the outcome of colonoscopic surveillance in extensive ulcerative colitis. They showed that the presence of a DALM predicted cancer in 43%, high-grade dysplasia 32%, low-grade dysplasia 8%, indefinite dysplasia 9% and when all patients were considered the risk was 5.5%. On this basis they recommended that not only should patients with DALM and high-grade dysplasia be advised to have surgery, but that those with low-grade dysplasia in flat mucosa should also be recommended for surgery. As a result of this paper and subsequent work, a number of authorities including the British Society of Gastroenterology have recommended that these patients should be advised to undergo surgery[4].

It is difficult to understand why this recommendation has been made because, as indicated earlier, the risk of developing cancer in the third decade of extensive colitis is already 10%, so if it is considered that patients with low-grade dysplasia should be operated on for an 8% risk it follows that those in their third decade of extensive colitis, or even those in their second decade, should be advised to have surgery. In other words, if 8% is taken as the level of risk that warrants surgery we should revert to the system of management that was advised in the 1960s and 1970s before colonoscopic surveillance was introduced.

## MORE RECENT STUDIES

In the years since the Berstein paper was published, a number of studies have been undertaken to assess specifically the risk of flat dysplasia in ulcerative colitis. One of these was from our department in Leeds, by Lim and colleagues[5].

Between 1978 and 1990 consecutive patients with long-standing extensive colitis attending the inflammatory bowel disease service at the General Infirmary were encouraged to enter a prospective colonoscopic screening study. In all 160 patients were recruited and, over the 12-year period, 40 (25%) developed low-grade dysplasia. The results were published in 1990 and Table 1 shows the outcome of the two groups, those with low-grade dysplasia and those without. It can be seen that, over the period of the surveillance, seven in the low-grade dysplasia group had undergone colectomy because of symptoms of ulcerative colitis, two had died for reasons unrelated to the condition and one had developed colorectal cancer. The outcome of the no-dysplasia group was similar, with two patients developing colorectal cancer. At the end of the surveillance period there were 30 patients with low-grade dysplasia and 98 without dysplasia who were alive and had an intact colon. According to current guidelines these 30 patients with low-grade dysplasia would have been advised to have surgery. In 2000 we decided to trace the patients from this cohort in order to determine their outcome, as we felt that this would provide useful information concerning the natural history of low-grade dysplasia, information that would be helpful in determining the true risk of the condition and whether or not surgery was justified.

In 2000 we had contacted directly or indirectly all but two of the cohort that had been alive and with an intact colon in 1990. One patient from each group we were unable to trace. Table 2 shows the outcome. Within the low-grade

**Table 1** Leeds surveillance study: outcome 1990: extensive long-standing ulcerative colitis; 160 entered surveillance, 1978–1990

|                     | LGD | No dysplasia |
| ------------------- | --- | ------------ |
| Total               | 40  | 120          |
| Colectomy           | 7   | 15           |
| Died                | 2   | 5            |
| CRC                 | 1   | 2            |
| Alive + intact colon| 30  | 98           |

**Table 2** What happens to patients with low grade dysplasia? (1999–2000)

|                     | LGD       | No dysplasia |
| ------------------- | --------- | ------------ |
| Total               | 29        | 97           |
| Colectomy           | 0         | 5            |
| Died                | 2         | 11           |
| CRC                 | 3 (10%)   | 4 (4%)       |
| Died from CRC       | 1 (3%)    | 1 (1%)       |
| Alive + intact colon| 24 (83%)  | 77 (79%)     |

dysplasia group patients had generally done well, none had required colectomy for their underlying illness, two had died from unrelated causes, but three (10%) had developed colorectal cancer and, of these, one (3%) had died. In all, 24 (83%) were alive with an intact colon. The no-dysplasia group had not done quite so well in that five had required colectomy because of their disease and 11 had died; however, only four (4%) had developed cancer and only one (1%) had died of this. Seventy-nine percent of the group were alive with an intact colon. In retrospect therefore, had we advised the original 30 to undergo colectomy, one life would have been saved, but 24 unnecessary proctocolectomies would have been performed.

It is interesting that the cancer rate within the low-grade dysplasia group at 10% is identical with that predicted in ordinary patients with colitis in their third decade. Most of our patients with low-grade dysplasia were either in their third decade or entering it in 1990. Their incidence of cancer therefore was no greater than what would have been predicted from an equivalent group of patients without dysplasia.

A number of other papers have been published over the same period (Table 3). it can be seen that the progression from low-grade to high-grade dysplasia or cancer varied widely in the five studies. In the Connell study[6] from St Mark's, London, the rate of progression was estimated at 54% in 5 years (this would be equivalent to around 80% in 10 years). This compares with the results of Befrits et al. from the Karolinska Institute in Stockholm[7] where 60 cases of low-grade dysplasia were found in 207 patients and were followed for 10 years with no progress to high-grade dysplasia or cancer. The Connell paper, however, is unusual because it can be seen that, although 332 patients were screened, only

**Table 3** Outcome of patients with low grade dysplasia

| Reference | No of patients | LGD | Mean follow-up (yrs) | Progression |
|---|---|---|---|---|
| Connell et al. 1994[6] | 332 | 9* | 7.5 | 54% in 5 years |
| Befrits et al. 2002[7] | 207 | 60 | 10 | 0% in 10 years |
| Ullman et al. 2002[8] | ? | 18 | 2.75 | 33% in 5 years[#] |
| Ullman et al. 2003[9] | ? | 46** | 1.25 | 53% in 5 years |
| Lim et al. 2003[5] | 128 | 29 | 17 | 10% in 10 years |

*A total of 51 LGD reclassified to seven.

**125 excluded.

[#]Only 1 cancer.

nine were assessed as having low-grade dysplasia. This, however, was not the first time that this cohort of patients had been reported. In a previous paper low-grade dysplasia had progressed in only 15%. The new paper had been written following re-examination of the pathology using more stringent criteria for the diagnosis of low-grade dysplasia. As a result 51 low-grade dysplasias were re-classified down to seven. Furthermore, the histology of patients with high-grade dysplasia were also re-examined, and two of these were shifted to the low-grade dysplasia group. In all, four patients out of the nine had developed cancer or high-grade dysplasia, and this included the two patients who had been transferred from the high-grade dysplasia group. It is this small group of patients that account for the 54% progression over the 5-year period.

The next two papers shown in Table 3 are the papers by Ullman and co-workers[8,9]. It is not clear how many original patients were screened because the low-grade dysplasia slides were obtained by a retrospective analysis of reports within the pathology department. In both studies, however, the first from the Mayo and the second from the Mount Sinai Hospital, the period of follow-up was surprisingly short, the median lengths being $2\frac{3}{4}$ years and $1\frac{1}{4}$ years respectively. One assumes therefore that the 33% and 53% progression over the 5-year periods were based on an arithmetical/statistical estimation rather than actual follow-up of 5 years.

One possibly important aspect of the Mayo study was that, of the 18 patients shown to have low-grade dysplasia, nine had progressed; however, only one of these had developed colorectal cancer and the rest had advanced only to high-grade dysplasia. The second Ullman et al. paper from the Mount Sinai Hospital included a much larger group of patients with low-grade dysplasia. However, it is interesting that this represented the minority of individuals they had identified with low-grade dysplasia. In all, 171 patients had been found but 125 had been excluded for a variety of reasons, many of them because there had been no endoscopic or surgical follow-up. The danger of excluding such a large number of patients as this is that it implies a degree of selection bias.

One cannot help but draw the conclusion that the results of these studies are, to say the least, most unsatisfactory and have limited scientific value. It certainly does not produce data on which it is appropriate to draw conclusions as to whether or not an individual with low-grade dysplasia should undergo surgery. What, after all, should one tell patients with respect to the risk? Should one go with the St Mark's data and tell them that the risk of cancer over 10 years is 80%, or with the Swedish paper indicating that the likelihood of them developing cancer is remote?

Essentially the problem here is not so much the clinical studies, it is that the diagnosis of low-grade dysplasia is unsafe.

## LACK OF CONSISTENCY IN THE DIAGNOSIS OF LOW-GRADE DYSPLASIA

In the Leeds study the diagnosis made by our pathologists at the time when the biopsy was taken was the gold standard. However, having analysed the data in 2000 we took the precaution of re-staining the slides with this diagnosis together with a further 50 slides taken from the non-dysplasia group. We circulated these to five independent, well-known gastrointestinal pathologists and requested them to grade the biopsies as normal, low-grade dysplasia, or high-grade dysplasia. The results were interesting in that 80% of the 40 low-grade dysplasia slides were agreed to have low-grade dysplasia by at least one pathologist. However, when the diagnosis had to be supported by two pathologists the figure fell to 63%, and when three pathologists (consensus) were involved the proportion agreed fell to 38%.

It occurred to us that this reduced number of diagnoses might have excluded those patients with low-grade dysplasia who were overdiagnosed by our own pathologist. We therefore assessed the outcomes for the 12 patients in whom the consensus view was that they had low-grade dysplasia. The effect of this was that two of the three cancers were lost from the group, including the one who had died; in other words had we used the consensus diagnosis rather than the contemporary one, only 12 patients would have been operated on, but on the other hand we would only have saved one cancer (10%) and we would not have saved any lives.

It is apparent from the above that the ability of pathologists to truly diagnose low-grade dysplasia is limited. We assessed the kappa value between the pathologists and this turned out to be 0.26. Kappa values are the accepted method used for determining the degree of agreement between observers. The scoring extends from −1 (complete disagreement), 0 (random) and 1 (complete agreement). −0.2 to +0.2 is tantamount to chance agreement, 0.2–0.4 is fair agreement, 0.4–0.6 moderate agreement and 0.6–1.0 good agreement. It is clear that the diagnosis of low-grade dysplasia by specialized pathologists is little better than by chance. It is failure of the diagnostic technique that is responsible for the disparate results in the studies; a diagnosis of low-grade dysplasia is of little, if any, value.

## LIKELIHOOD OF DEVELOPING LOW-GRADE DYSPLASIA

A further concern with respect to low-grade dysplasia is the frequency with which the diagnosis is made. If a patient undergoes colonoscopy every year, and has 30 biopsies taken, there is a likelihood that over time one or other of these biopsies will be assessed as low-grade dysplasia. It was shown by Lashner et al.[10], and in our own service, that within the lifetime of a cohort nearly all will eventually develop low-grade dysplasia. The insistence on more frequent colonoscopy and larger numbers of biopsies is likely to accelerate the speed with which members of the cohort will receive this diagnosis. This is not a new observation; similar data were used by Provenzale and co-workers in 1995[11] when creating a model to assess the cost effectiveness of colonoscopic surveillance. These workers made the assumption that by the end of the surveillance period virtually everyone would have received a diagnosis of low-grade dysplasia and would have undergone colectomy.

## DRAWBACKS OF SURGERY

The introduction of restorative proctocolectomy with the creation of an ileal pouch was an important step forward. Patients with ulcerative colitis no longer had to assume that if they underwent surgery they would require an ileostomy for the rest of their lives. As a result of this our threshold for advising surgery has fallen; however, restorative proctocolectomy is not without its problems. Roughly 10% of pouches have to be removed because of failure. Two recent surgical series have shown that pouchitis may occur in up to 50% of individuals and can be severe in 19–37%, intestinal obstruction in 8–16%, re-operation required in 17–20%. At the same time stool frequency in 24 h is usually around six or seven, and incontinence occurs in 38–48%. Mortality for this operation is low, but morbidity is significant. These drawbacks must be considered when advising patients whether to continue with colonoscopic surveillance or to opt for surgery[12,13].

Low-grade dysplasia is a poor predictor of cancer. The diagnosis of low-grade dysplasia is unsafe and most patients will eventually receive that diagnosis. Had we followed current advice on the management of our patients we would have saved one life in the 20–30 patients who originally developed low-grade dysplasia. This, however, would have been at the cost of unnecessary surgery in 23 patients.

## CONCLUSIONS

What conclusion should we draw from these data? In today's era of patient empowerment it is only right and proper that patients be allowed to decide for themselves whether they should undergo surgery or continue on surveillance. They should therefore be provided with the information, but it should be emphasized that the evidence base is poor, that a diagnosis of low-grade dysplasia is unsafe. In my view it is reasonable to tell them that their risk of developing cancer over the subsequent 10 years is roughly 10% and the risk of death around 3%. When asked by the patient for my own opinion (as is usually the case) I advise them that a conservative approach seems to me their best option.

The British Society of Gastroenterology Guidelines with respect to low-grade dysplasia are didactic. This approach is, in my view, misconceived. First it exerts pressure on doctors to abandon their own judgement. Secondly they are unhelpful from a medicolegal perspective. We know that patients with ulcerative colitis in this age group have a 10% risk of developing cancer whether or not they have low-grade dysplasia. Some of them will therefore develop cancer, and we run a risk of litigation if we do not offer advice that is consistent with the society's guidelines. This may lead to the practice of defensive medicine which, in this case, may not be in the interest of the patient.

## References

1.   Eaden J, Abrams K, McKay H et al. Inter-observer variation between general and specialist gastrointestinal pathologist when grading dysplasia in ulcerative colitis. J Pathol. 2001;194:152-7.
2.   Morson BC, Pang LS. Rectal biopsy as an aid to cancer control in ulcerative colitis. Gut. 1967;8:423-34.
3.   Bernstein CN, Shanahan F, Weinstein WM. Are we telling patients the truth about surveillance colonoscopy in ulcerative colitis? Lancet. 1994;343:71-4.
4.   Eaden JA, Mayberry JF. Guidelines for screening and surveillance of asymptomatic colorectal cancer in patients with inflammatory bowel disease. Gut. 2002;51(Suppl. V):10-12.
5.   Lim CH, Dixon MF, Vail A, Forman D, Lynch DAF, Axon ATR. Ten year follow up of ulcerative colitis patients with and without low grade dysplasia. Gut. 2003;52:1127-32.
6.   Connell WR, Lennard-Jones JE, Williams CB, Talbot IC, Price AB, Wilkinson KH. Factors affecting the outcome of endoscopic surveillance for cancer in ulcerative colitis. Gastroenterology. 1994;107:934-44.
7.   Befrits R, Ljung T, Jaramillow E, Rubio C. Low-grade dysplasia in extensive, long-standing inflammatory bowel disease: a follow-up study. Dis Colon Rectum. 2002;45:615-20.
8.   Ullman TA, Loftus EV, Kakar S, Burgart LJ, Sandborn WJ, Tremaine WJ. The fate of low grade dysplasia in ulcerative colitis. Am J Gastroenterol. 2002;97:922-7.
9.   Ullman T, Croog V, Harpaz N, Sachar D, Itzkowtiz S. Progression of flat low-grade dysplasia to advanced neoplasia in patients with ulcerative colitis. Gastroenterology. 2003;125:1311-19.
10.  Lashner BA, Silverstein MD, Hanauer SB. Hazard rates for dysplasia and cancer in ulcerative colitis. Results from a surveillance program. Dig Dis Sci. 1989;34:1536-41.
11.  Provenzale D, Kowdley KV, Arora S et al. Prophylactic colectomy or surveillance for chronic ulcerative colitis? A decision analysis. Gastroenterology. 1995;109:1188-96.
12.  Johnson E, Carlsen E, Nazir M et al. Morbidity and functional outcome after restorative proctocolectomy for ulcerative colitis. Eur J Surg. 2001;167:40-5.
13.  Tiainen J, Matikainen M. Long-term clinical outcome and anemia after restorative proctocolectomy for ulcerative colitis. Scand J Gastroenterol. 2000;35:1170-3.

# Section VIII
# New therapeutic approaches

Chair: F. PALLONE and E.F. STANGE

# 24
# Leucocytapheresis

## J. EMMRICH

Recently published studies have suggested that leucocytapheresis is a useful adjunct to therapy of rheumatoid arthritis and the inflammatory bowel diseases ulcerative colitis (UC) and Crohn's disease (CD) after failure of conventional treatment[1-8]. Leucocytapheresis involves extracorporeal removal of leucocytes either by adsorptive systems or by centrifugation. There are two commonly used adsorptive systems; one contains cellulose acetate beads (Adacolumn, Otsuka, Japan) and the other a polyester fibre filter (Cellsorba, Asahi-Kasei, Japan). Neutrophils and monocytes bind to cellulose acetate beads of the Adacolumn system, whereas the polyester fibre system removes neutrophils, monocytes and lymphocytes[9-13].

Since 2001 both Cellsorba and Adacolumn have been listed as medical devices reimbursed by the Japanese national health insurance system to be used in the therapy of active ulcerative colitis. Several clinical studies could demonstrate the efficacy of leucocytapheresis treatment in ulcerative colitis, as well as the safety of this therapy[2,12-16].

The procedure of leucocytapheresis is similar to dialysis therapy in nephrology. Vascular access for apheresis requires peripheral venepuncture in both arms. Venous blood is drawn from one arm and passed through the adsorptive system, driven by a blood pump, before being returned to the contralateral arm. For this process a flow rate of 30–50 ml/h is used. This flow rate for leucocytapheresis is much more lower than in dialysis procedures for removal of toxic substances. Sessions usually last for 60 to 90 min allowing 2–4.5 L of blood to pass through the adsorptive apparatus. A course of treatment typically comprises five to 10 sessions twice weekly or at weekly intervals. Moreover, all systems require the use of anticoagulation with heparin or citrate.

An overshooting reaction of the mucosal immune system against luminal antigens is one of the key pathogenic processes in IBD. This immune reaction is mediated by lymphocytes, monocytes, and neutrophils. These cells communicate with a cytokine network. Removal of activated circulating leucocytes, and their replacement with bone marrow-derived unactivated leucocytes, should reduce inflammatory cellular infiltration in the gut. However, the overall number of circulating leucocytes may not be decreased by leucocytapheresis. Other mechanisms are suggested to induce the

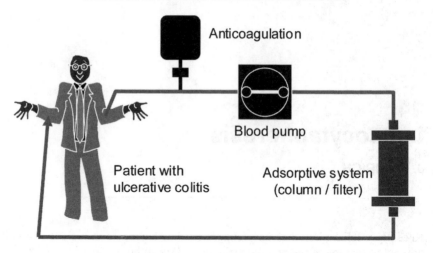

**Figure 1**  Extracorporeal circulation in leucocytapheresis

therapeutic effects[2,11,17–19]. The mechanisms and consequences of leucocyte removal differ between the adsorptive systems used in leucocytapheresis.

Interaction between blood and cellulose acetate beads of the Adacolumn system causes complement activation and the production of active fragments such as C3a and C5a[11]. These fragments bind to the beads together with immunoglobulins. Activated leucocytes expressing Fc receptors or complement receptors can be adsorbed by the beads[9]. In addition, plasma cytokines and the cytokine-producing capacity of immunocompetent cells were decreased regarding IL-1, TNF-$\alpha$, IL-6 and IL-8[9]. The down-regulation of L-selectin is also induced by the cellulose acetate beads, resulting in a decrease in neutrophil adhesion to endothelial cells[11,19]. Neutrophil apoptosis should also be induced[9]. The system removes about 65% of neutrophils, 55% of monocytes and 2% of lymphocytes[20].

The polyester fibre filter system also removes leucocytes by adsorption. This results in the removal of almost 100% of neutrophils and monocytes, and 20–60% of leucocytes[21]. Leucocytes filtered through the Cellsorba system contained a decreased percentage of CD4$^+$DR$^+$ cells and an increased percentage of CD4$^+$DR$^-$ cells compared to the peripheral blood[12]. IL-4 production of the filter-passed lymphocytes was increased significantly[18]. Based on these results redistribution of the T lymphocytes producing IL-4 locally at the inflamed site may be one of the mechanisms in leucocytapheresis.

However, the effective mechanisms of leucocytapheresis have not yet been exactly defined. Leucocyte removal could mobilize cells from the bone marrow to have an impact on the immunological imbalance in the peripheral blood. In addition there is a quantitative change of leucocytes over a short period of time. After the completion of apheresis the peripheral leucocyte levels increased transiently. The general redistribution of leucocytes may be an important factor for the efficacy of leucocytapheresis.

Leucocytapheresis is able to remove 20–40% of platelets. Activated platelets are not only prothrombotic but also proinflammatory, and may be important in the pathogenesis of IBD.

In several open and controlled trials using both systems for adsorptive apheresis in UC and CD, remission rates with a wide variation were observed (Tables 1 and 2). In these studies 40–80% of patients came into remission after therapy. Indications for leucocytapheresis with adsorptive systems were steroid-refractory or steroid-dependent IBD. Unfortunately, several aspects of the published studies, including the heterogeneous clinical characteristics of the patients, the outcome measures used, and variations in steroid dosages, make its interpretation difficult.

**Table 1**  Clinical studies with the Adacolumn system

| Authors | Patients (n) | Remission (%) | Improvement (%) |
|---|---|---|---|
| *Ulcerative colitis* | | | |
| Shimoyama et al., 2001[16] | 53 | 21 | 38 |
| Hanai et al., 2003[14] | 39 | 82 | 8 |
| Suzuki et al., 2004[22] | 20 | 85 | 0 |
| Sawada et al., 2003[20] | 39 | 23 | 51 |
| Hanai et al., 2004[15] | 46 | 83 | n.a. |
| Kruis et al., 2004[23] | 34 | 38 | 12 |
| Emmrich et al., 2005[24] | 31 | 52 | 9 |
| | | | |
| *Crohn's disease* | | | |
| Fukuda et al., 2004[25] | 29 | 34 | 10 |
| Emmrich et al., 2005[26] | 18 | 45 | 7 |

**Table 2**  Clinical studies with the Cellsorba system

| Authors | Patients (n) | Remission (%) | Improvement (%) |
|---|---|---|---|
| *Ulcerative colitis* | | | |
| Sawada et al., 1995[13] | 8 | 50 | 25 |
| Amano et al., 1998[17] | 37 | 48 | 43 |
| Sasaki et al., 1998[27] | 9 | 33 | 33 |
| Yajima et al., 1998[28] | 8 | 38 | 25 |
| Kawamura et al., 1999[10] | 12 | 92 | 0 |
| Sakata et al., 2003[29] | 51 | 65 | 18 |
| Emmrich et al., 2003[30] | 20 | 70 | 0 |

Kanke et al.[5] treated 60 patients with active UC with up to 10 apheresis sessions using the Adacolumn system. Fifty patients improved, of whom 14 went into remission, and the courses of treatment allowed reduction in steroid intake by the steroid-dependent patients. In another study, 78 patients were randomly assigned to receive either an increase in their dosage of prednisolone, the magnitude of which varied according to the severity of the disease, or to leucocytapheresis. Leucocytapheresis was apparently twice as effective in improving UC as was increasing the dose of prednisolone[20]. Recently, an uncontrolled study has suggested that leucocytapheresis may be effective as a first-line alternative to steroids in steroid-naive patients[22].

In a pilot study we evaluated the potential of leucocytapheresis with Cellsorba filter in UC (LCAP). Twenty patients suffering from chronic active steroid-dependent UC (CAI according to Rachmilewitz: 6–10) were recruited. Azathioprine was not effective in these patients or induced side-effects. LCAP was performed weekly for 5 weeks (intensive therapy). After this treatment patients in remission were randomized into two groups followed by tapering the steroids. In one group LCAP was continued monthly for 5 months (maintenance therapy), whereas patients in the second group were not treated with LCAP. Remission of diseases was achieved in 14 of 20 patients after intensive therapy with LCAP. After the maintenance therapy five of eight patients had no disease activity without steroids. Only one of five patients treated with intensive therapy but without following maintenance therapy was still in remission without steroids after 5 months[30].

There are only a few studies using leucocytapheresis in CD. We performed an open trial to treat CD with granulocyte and monocyte adsorption apheresis (GMCAP, Adacolumn system). Eighteen steroid-dependent patients with chronic active CD (CDAI 200–400) were involved in this trial. All patients failed to respond to azathioprine. GMCAP was performed twice a week for 3 weeks and weekly for an additional 3 weeks. Remission of CD was achieved in eight of 18 patients[26].

Apheresis treatment is a safe therapeutic option. In the published studies common symptoms such as nausea, vomiting, fever, chills and nasal obstruction, respiratory distress, palpitations and chest tightness were described. Among the patients 1–5% had these side-effects. No severe adverse events were observed[31,32].

Summarizing the results of published clinical studies leucocytapheresis could be established as a new therapeutic strategy in IBD. The results seem to be more promising in UC than in CD. Further well-designed randomized controlled trials are needed to confirm the results of the preliminary studies. In patients refractory to aminosalicylates and immunosuppressive drugs leucocytapheresis might be a suitable therapy.

## References

1.  Hanai H, Watanabe F, Saniabadi A, Matsushita I, Takeuchi K, Iida T. Therapeutic efficacy of granulocyte and monocyte adsorption apheresis in severe active ulcerative colitis. Dig Dis Sci. 2002;47:2349–53.

2.  Hidaka T, Suzuki K, Matsuki Y et al. Changes in CD* T lymphocyte subsets in circulating blood and synovial fluid following filtration leukocytapheresis therapy in patients with rheumatoid arthritis. Ther Apher. 1999;2:178–85.
3.  Hidaka T, Suzuki K, Kawakami M et al. Dynamic changes in cytokine levels in serum and synovial fluid following filtration leukocytapheresis therapy in patients with rheumatoid arthritis. J Clin Apheresis. 2001;16:74–81.
4.  Ishida H, Ohara M, Watanabe S, Takase Y, Kasukawa R. Treatment of rheumatoid arthritis by granulo-monocytapheresis. Jpn J Rheumatol. 1996;6:113–24.
5.  Kanke K, Nakano M, Hiraishi H, Terano A. Clinical evaluation of granulocyte/monocyte apheresis therapy for active ulcerative colitis. Dig Liver Dis. 2004;36:811–17.
6.  Kashiwagi N, Hirata I, Kasukawa R. A role for granulocyte and monocyte apheresis in the treatment of rheumatoid arthritis. Ther Apher. 1998;2:134–41.
7.  Kondo K, Shinoda T, Yoshimoto H, Takazoe M, Hamada T. Effective maintenance leukocytapheresis for patients with steroid dependent or resistant ulcerative colitis. Ther Apher. 2001;5:462–5.
8.  Saniabadi AR, Hanai H, Takeuchi K et al. Adacolumn, an adsorptive carrier based granulocyte and monocyte apheresis device for the treatment of inflammatory and refractory diseases associated with leukocytes. Ther Apher Dial. 2003;7:45–59.
9.  Kashiwagi N, Sugimura K, Koiwai H et al. Immunomodulatory effects of granulocyte and monocyte adsorption apheresis as a treatment for patients with ulcerative colitis. Dig Dis Sci. 2002;47:1334–41.
10. Kawamura A, Saitoh M, Yonekawa M et al. New technique of leukocytapheresis by the use of nonwoven polyester fiber filter for inflammatory bowel disease. Ther Apher. 1999;3:334–7.
11. Ramlow W, Emmrich J, Ahrenholz P et al. In vitro and in vivo evaluation of adacolumn® cytapheresis in healthy subjects. J Clin Apher. 2005;19:1–9.
12. Sawada K, Ohnishi K, Fukui S et al. Leukocytapheresis therapy, perfomed with leukocyte removal filter, for inflammatory bowel disease. J Gastroenterol. 1995;30:322–9.
13. Sawada K, Ohnishi K, Kosaka T et al. Leukocytapheresis therapy with leukocyte removal filter for inflammatory bowel disease. J Gastroenterol. 1995;30:124–7.
14. Hanai H, Watanabe F, Takeuchi K et al. Leukocyte adsorptive apheresis for the treatment of active ulcerative colitis: a prospective, uncontrolled, pilot study. Clin Gastroenterol Hepatol. 2003;1:28–35.
15. Hanai H, Watanabe F, Yamada M et al. Adsorptive granulocyte and monocyte apheresis versus prednisolone in patients with corticosteroid-dependent moderately severe ulcerative colitis. Digestion. 2004;70:36–44.
16. Shimoyama T, Sawada K, Hiwatashi N et al. Safety and efficacy of granulocyte and monocyte adsorption apheresis in patients with active ulcerative colitis: a multicenter study. J Clin Apher. 2001;16:1–9.
17. Amano K, Amano K. Filter leukapheresis for patients with ulcerative colitis: clinical results and the possible mechanism. Ther Apher. 1998;2:97–100.
18. Noguchi M, Hiwatishi N, Hayakawa T, Toyota T. Leukocyte removal filter-passed lymphocytes produce large amounts of interleukin-4 in immunotherapy for inflammatory bowel disease: role of bystander suppression. Ther Apher. 1998;2:109–14.
19. Rembacken BJ, Newbould HE, Richards SJ et al. Granulocyte apheresis in inflammatory bowel disease: possible mechanisms of effect. Ther Apher. 1998;2:93–6.
20. Sawada K, Muto T, Shimoyama T et al. Multicenter randomized controlled trial for the treatment of ulcerative colitis with a leukocytapheresis column. Curr Pharm design. 2003;9:307–21.
21. Shirokaze J. Leukocytapheresis using a leukocyte removal filter. Ther Apher. 2002;6:261–6.
22. Suzuki Y, Yoshimura N, Saniabadi AR, Saito Y. Selective granulocyte and monocyte adsorptive apheresis as a first-line treatment for steroid naœve patients with active ulcerative colitis: a prospective uncontrolled study. Dig Dis Sci. 2004;49:565–71.
23. Kruis W, Morgenstern J, Loefberg R et al. Successful apheresis in active steroid refractory ulcerative colitis. Gastroenterology. 2004;1216:A628.
24. Emmrich J, Rieckeheer K, Petermann S, Franz M, Liebe S, Ramlow W. Leukocyte removal in steroid-dependent ulcerative colitis using granulocyte and monocyte adsorption apheresis. Gastroenterology. 2005;128:A577.

25. Fukuda Y, Matsui T, Suzuki Y et al. Adsorptive granulocyte and monocyte apheresis for refractory Crohn's disease: an open multicenter prospective study. J Gastroenterol. 2004;39:1158–64.
26. Emmrich J, Rieckeheer K, Liebe S, Franz M, Ramlow W. Granulocyte and monocyte adsorption apheresis in chronic active Crohn's disease. Gastroenterology. 2005;128:A577.
27. Sasaki M, Tsujikawa T, Fujiyama Y, Bamba T. Leukocytapheresis therapy for severe ulcerative colitis. Ther Apher. 1998;2:101–4.
28. Yajima T, Takaishi H, Kanai T et al. Predictive factors of response to leukocytapheresis therapy for ulcerative colitis. Ther Apher. 1998;2:115–19.
29. Sakata H, Kawamura N, Horie T et al. Successful treatment of ulcerative colitis with leukocytapheresis using non-woven polyester filter. Ther Apher Dial. 2003;7:536–9.
30. Emmrich J, Brock P, Nowak D et al. Leucocytapheresis in patients with steroid dependent ulcerative colitis. Z Gastroenterol. 2003;41:A775.
31. Nagase K, Sawada K, Ohnishi K, Egashira A, Ohkusu K, Shimoyama T. Complications of leukocytapheresis. Ther Apher. 1998;2:120–4.
32. Takazoe M, Tanaka T, Kondo K, Ichimori T, Shinoda T. The present status and the recent development of the treatment for inflammatory bowel diseases: desirable effect of extracorporeal immunomodulation. Ther Apher. 2002;6:305–11.

# 25
# Helminths and immune modulation of inflammatory bowel disease

**J. V. WEINSTOCK and D. E. ELLIOTT**

---

Inflammatory bowel disease (IBD) may result from loss of immune tolerance to the normal enteric bacteria that reside in the intestine. Expression of disease in mouse models of IBD requires normal intestinal flora[1]. Ulcerative colitis (UC) and Crohn's disease (CD) develop mostly in regions of the intestine with the highest concentration of bacteria. Diversion of the faecal stream also improves CD in bowel segments distal to the diversion[2]. These observations suggest that interaction between intestinal flora and the immune system are important in disease pathogenesis.

UC and CD are unlikely to be two distinct diseases resulting from single causes. Each is more apt to be several conditions sharing similar clinical and histological phenotypes. No single genetic defect is the cause of either UC or CD. Twin pairs separated at birth show a higher concordance rate for CD and to a lesser degree UC among monozygotic as opposed to dizygotic twins[3,4] suggesting that genes play a role.

CARD15 (NOD2) is a susceptibility gene associated with CD. People with one of several variants of CARD15 that renders this molecule dysfunctional are 2–3-fold more at risk for CD[5–7]. However, CARD15 mutations are absent in most patients with CD and most persons with such defects never get CD. CARD15 and other genetic traits only influence the frequency of IBD, but are not the primary cause of these diseases.

Geographic variations in IBD frequency suggest that environmental factors affect the risk of disease[8]. The prevalence of CD has increased steadily in North American and Western Europe in the last half of the 20th century[9]. The frequency of other immunological diseases such as asthma and multiple sclerosis has also increased[10]. Europe and the USA have an uneven distribution in IBD frequency, with disease being more common in the north than in the south[11,12]. The ethnic and racial prevalences of IBD have changed over time and are influenced by undefined geographic factor[13]. Children acquire greater risk for disease if they move from regions of low IBD prevalence to locations of high disease frequency[14–16].

Hygiene is a risk factor for IBD. IBD is less common in people whose work exposes them to dirt[17]. Patients with CD live in more hygienic environments with hot water and indoor plumbing[18,19]. The disease is more common in urban versus rural areas[20]. Helminth infection could be a protective factor against the development of immunological diseases.

Helminths are complex multicellular, worm-like parasitic animals. Various annelids (the leeches), nematodes (the roundworms) and platyhelminths (the tapeworms and flukes) can parasitize humans.

More than one in every three people have helminths. These organisms are spread through contact with contaminated soil, water or food. Ten thousand-year-old petrified human waste discovered in caves contains helminth ova, suggesting that humans and helminths have coexisted for thousands of years[21]. Many children and adults in the USA carried helminths before the 1940s. Helminth colonization has steadily declined except in indigenous populations living in underserved regions[22] and in recent immigrants from less developed countries[23].

Eating dirt (geophagia) is a common practice of humans and other animals that may be an evolutionary adaptation to allow enteric interactions with soil organisms[24]. Intentional geophagia is nearly a universal practice of children less than 2 years of age. Both children and adults have inadvertent exposure to dirt through inhalation of dust in the air, contaminants in food and water, and exposure to soiled hands. This may have immunological consequences. Topsoil can harbour many of the infective forms of animal and human helminthic parasites. Geophagy of soil containing dog or cat faeces leads to exposure to *Toxocara canis*[25,26]; its seroprevalence is 4–8%, rising to 16–30% among some groups of Afro-Americans and Hispanics. Children living on farms may readily encounter animal helminths whose ova are in the faeces of farm animals (e.g. *Trichuris suis*, the pig whipworm).

Various helminthic species have different life cycles and occupy different niches within their human host, e.g. the intestinal lumen, blood stream or lymphatics. For instance, some are ingested orally and have a strict intestinal existence (e.g. *Trichuris trichiura* – whipworm, *Enterobius vermicularis* – pinworm). Other helminths migrate through the body to reach the gut (e.g. *Ascaris lumbricoides* – roundworm, *Necator americanus* and *Ancylostoma duodenale* – hookworm, *Strongyloides* – threadworm). Some reside in the human blood stream after migrating through the skin and the lungs (*Schistosoma* species). Still others enter through the skin to live in the lymphatics (e.g. *Wuchereria bancrofti* and *Brugia malayi* – filarial worms). The overall incidence of severe morbidity related to worm carriage is relatively low considering the prevalence of these organisms.

There are some epidemiological data suggesting that helminth infection protects from immunological diseases. The prevalence of IBD is highest in industrialized nations where helminth infection is rare, while the frequency of IBD is low in developing countries where helminthic colonization is common[27]. Helminth infections associate with a lower risk of allergic disorders. Infection with *Schistosoma hematobium* correlates with suppression of atopic reactivity[28]. Repeated anti-helminthic treatment of chronically helminth-infected children results in increased allergic sensitivity to house dust mites[29]. There is a lower frequency of asthma in people infected with hookworm[30].

Animal models of IBD support this concept of protection. Rodents treated with non-viable schistosome ova[31] or infected with the vascular fluke *Schistosoma mansoni*[32], or with various intestinal worms like *Trichiura muris, Trichinella spiralis*[33], *Heligmosomoides polygyrus* or *Hymenolepis diminuta* are protected from trinitrobenzene sulfonic acid (TNBS)-induced colitis. Mice deficient in IL-10 production develop a chronic Th1-type colitis that is prevented or reversed by colonization with *T. muris* or *H. polygyrus*[9,34], or by exposure to non-viable schistosome ova.

Favourable clinical trials using helminths to treat human IBD also support the concept that lack of exposure to worms is leading to a rise in the prevalence of IBD and other immunological disorders. In clinical trials, patients received live ova from the porcine whipworm *Trichuris suis*, which is genetically related to the human whipworm *Trichuris trichiura*[35]. Individuals acquire *T. trichiura* by ingesting mature ova located in contaminated soil, food or water. The ova hatch in the small bowel to release larvae that eventually mature into adult helminthic worms, which settle mostly on the right side of the colon. Both the larvae and adults worms remain confined to the intestines. Adult worms lay immature ova that pass with the stool. In warm moist soil the ova require 4–6 weeks of incubation to mature. The worms cannot multiply in the host or be easily transmitted to others because of this requirement for soil incubation. There is no readily available source of human whipworm, since it cannot colonize other animal species. The porcine whipworm (*T. suis*) can colonize people only briefly[36]. About 20% of the pig herds in Iowa carry this worm, and there are no reported human diseases resulting from farm exposure to this organism. *T. suis* can be grown in pigs maintained in a pathogen-free environment. The worms can be harvested and grown *in vitro* to produce ova for therapeutic use.

Two studies provide evidence that *T. suis* ova therapy is effective in both ulcerative colitis and Crohn's disease. In patients with active ulcerative colitis, *T. suis* ova were tested in a 24-week crossover, double-blind controlled clinical trial. Patients consumed 2500 ova orally once every 2 weeks. The agent induced an overall response rate of about 50%, while the rate of improvement with placebo was only about 15%. The therapeutic response required about 6 weeks from the time of initial helminthic exposure. Also completed was an open trial in Crohn's disease. A total of 29 patients were enrolled for 24 weeks. Patients ingested 2500 *T. suis* ova every 3 weeks. At week 24, 72.4% were in remission. No adverse clinical effects were detected as a result of therapy in either study. Long-term maintenance treatment suggests that the agent will afford prolonged benefit (unpublished observation). Human hookworm currently is being tested for clinical efficacy in asthma

There is a strong immunological basis to suspect that helminths can protect from IBD. Helminths exert a strong influence on the host immune system. They usually stimulate production of Th2 cytokines (IL-4, IL-5, IL-9, IL-13)[37-41] and can alter host immune reactivity to immunological stimuli unrelated to the parasite. Studies in humans suggest that exposure to various helminths results in decreased host T cell reactivity[42] and raised level of the important immune modulatory cytokine IL-10[43]. In mice the Th2 response to helminths can deviate Th1 antigenic immunity towards Th2[44-46]. People carrying helminths can show immune bias away from the Th1 response normally elicited with tetanus vaccination[47] or *in-vitro* mitogen stimulation[43].

Induction of Th2 pathways (IL-4 and/or IL-13 and their *Stat6* signalling pathway) also may contribute to protection from IBD. TNBS is a murine model of IBD driven by Th1 cytokines. In rats, concurrent infection with *S. mansoni* decreases the inflammatory response to TNBS and shortens the duration of the colitis[32]. Mice given non-viable eggs of the helminthic parasite *S. mansoni* are resistant to TNBS-induced colitis[31]. The resistance to TNBS colitis requires IL-4 and intact *Stat6* circuitry[31].

However, with worm exposure there can be concomitant dampening of Th2-type reactivity[29,48,49] and reduced lymphocyte responsiveness to various antigens and mitogens. Helminths may induce production of regulatory T cells in their host, which may explain why helminths affect both Th1 and Th2 responses.

Regulatory T cells can induce peripheral tolerance and constrain mucosal reactivity[50–52]. Such regulatory cells can control self-reactive T cells and are functionally important in limiting inflammation in various animal models of IBD[53] and other immunological diseases. There are several regulatory T cell phenotypes. For instance, some express CD4; others express CD8[54]. There are naturally occurring $CD4^+$ $CD25^+$ regulatory T cells that develop in the thymus. Also described are $CD4^+$ regulatory T cells that produce high levels of IL-10 and/or TGF-β (Tr1, Th3)[55]. These are secondary suppressor cells that develop from $CD4^+$ $CD25^-$ T cells in the periphery.

T cells from the mesenteric lymph node (MLN) of *H. polygyrus*-colonized IL-10-deficient mice, unlike MLN cells from their worm-free IL-10 littermates, abrogate established colitis when transferred into IL-10-deficient recipient[34]. Lamina propria (LP) T cells from distal bowel segments of healthy wild-type (WT) mice also acquire the capacity to make large amounts of IL-10 and TGF-β after *H. polygyrus* infection, which is an indicator of regulatory activity.

It was recently shown that *H. polygyrus*, a mouse helminth, enhances expression of a class I-dependent, $CD8^+$ regulatory T cell in the murine intestine that blocks proliferation of other types of T cell in a class I-dependent fashion. This could prove important, since failure to limit expansion of overly reactive T cells in the gut could be one of the mechanisms leading to IBD. The function of this regulatory cell requires cell contact. This is akin to the natural regulatory T cells that mediate much of their suppressor activity through direct cell–cell contact[56].

Natural regulatory cells either secrete TGF-β or express on their surface latency-associated peptide, which is the amino-terminal domain of the TGF-β precursor peptide[57]. Expression of TGF-β is an important mechanism through which these cells exercise suppression both *in vitro* and *in vivo*[58]. It also may have an important role in the function of acquired T regulatory cells (e.g. Th3). However, the worm-induced, CD8 regulatory T cells differ from natural regulatory cells in that they do not need TGF-β signalling through the T cell to limit responder T cell proliferation.

IL-10 also is a strong modulator of immune functions[59]. IL-10 inhibits production of various important proinflammatory cytokines such as IL-12 and TNF-α, and blocks dendritic and macrophage cell function. Transgenic mice lacking IL-10 develop a severe Th1-type colitis showing the importance of IL-10 for mucosal protection. Without IL-10, *H. polygyrus* induces CD8$^+$ regulatory T cells normally. This suggests that IL-10 is not essential for their regulatory activity either.

T cell suppression mediated by CD8$^+$ T cells has been characterized in several animal models of inflammation. They participate in resistance to the autoimmune disease model of experimental allergic encephalomyelitis[60]. CD8$^+$ T cells are also involved in the down-regulation of the CD4$^+$ T cell response to superantigen staphylococcal enterotoxin B[61]. CD8 T cells can kill activated T cells[61] and B cells[62] through recognition of specific TCR-derived peptides associated with the non-classical MHC molecule Qa-1 on these cells. They require priming by activated CD4$^+$ T cells during the primary immune response to regulate the secondary immune response. This is in contrast to the CD4$^+$CD25$^+$ regulatory T cells that occur naturally and function during the primary phases of an immune reaction.

It remains unknown how the CD8 regulatory T cell limits responder T cell proliferation. It has also not yet been shown that these cells can prevent or limit colitis in an animal model.

Helminths also may induce production of other types of regulatory-type immune cells (T and non-T cell) in their host. Infection of mice with *H. polygyrus* induces some of the T cells in distal regions of the intestine to make large amounts of IL-10 and TGF-β, and to express high levels of *FoxP3*. These cells may prove important for limiting IFN-γ and IL-12 production, and for blunting Th1 responses. In humans, T cells that produce IL-10 and/or TGF-β have been cloned from the blood of patients who have the filarial nematode *O. volvulus* and peripheral T cell hyporesponsiveness[63,64]. Mice having the filarial parasite *Brugia pahangi* or *B. malayi* exhibit regulatory macrophages that suppress Th1 cell function[65] and lymphocyte proliferation[66].

Lipopolysaccharide (LPS), a product of Gram-negative bacteria, interacts with LPS receptors (TLR4) on various cell types to stimulate production of proinflammatory molecules. However, intestinal lamina propria mononuclear cells are anergic to LPS because of their close proximity to LPS-producing luminal flora.

*H. polygyrus* infection induces TLR4 expression on mucosal T cells. Once inducd, LPS engagement of TLR4 stimulates production of TGF-β rather than synthesis of the usual proinflammatory cytokines (manuscript in preparation). CD4$^+$CD25$^+$ regulatory T cells express TLR4 and respond to LPS with enhanced proliferation and increased suppressor activity[67]. This once more suggests that helminths induce expression of regulatory T cells in the mucosa.

## SUMMARY

Loss of immune tolerance to the normal enteric bacteria is a leading hypothesis regarding the aetiology of IBD. Genetic traits influence the frequency and clinical course of IBD, but are not the central cause of these diseases. Environmental factors greatly affect the chance for disease, as suggested by the geographic variations in IBD frequency, and may prove more influential than genetic predisposition. Good hygiene is a risk factor for IBD. Helminths are worm-like organisms that can live within the host. People acquire helminths through exposure to contaminated food, water and soil. Epidemiological data suggest that helminth infection protects from immunological diseases. Favourable clinical trials using helminths to treat human IBD support this concept. Live enteric helminthic parasites, helminths with a systemic distribution and even non-viable schistosome ova can shield animals from IBD. The protection coincides with induction in the lamina propria of Th2 and regulatory cytokines such as IL-10, TGF-β and PgE2, and local development of regulatory-type T cells. These regulatory factors (e.g. IL-10, TGF-β) and regulatory cells suppress pro-inflammatory cytokine production (e.g. IFN-γ and IL-12 P40) in the LPMC and inhibit expansion of T cells that drive inflammation. Future studies will determine if helminths or derivatives from these animals will prove highly effective for prevention or treatment of IBD and other immunological diseases.

## References

1.  Sartor RB. Review article: Role of the enteric microflora in the pathogenesis of intestinal inflammation and arthritis. Aliment Pharmacol Ther. 1997;11(Suppl):22.
2.  Rutgeerts P, Goboes K, Peeters M et al. Effect of faecal stream diversion on recurrence of Crohn's disease in the neoterminal ileum [comment]. Lancet. 1991;338:771–4.
3.  Tysk C, Lindberg E, Jarnerot G, Floderus-Myrhed B. Ulcerative colitis and Crohn's disease in an unselected population of monozygotic and dizygotic twins. A study of heritability and the influence of smoking. Gut. 1988;29:990–6.
4.  Halfvarson J, Bodin L, Tysk C, Lindberg E, Jarnerot G. Inflammatory bowel disease in a Swedish twin cohort: a long-term follow-up of concordance and clinical characteristics. Gastroenterology. 2003;124:1767–73.
5.  Cuthbert AP, Fisher SA, Mirza MM et al. The contribution of NOD2 gene mutations to the risk and site of disease in inflammatory bowel disease [comment]. Gastroenterology. 2002; 122:867–74.
6.  Abreu MT, Taylor KD, Lin YC et al. Mutations in NOD2 are associated with fibrostenosing disease in patients with Crohn's disease. Gastroenterology. 2002;123:679–88.
7.  Radlmayr M, Torok HP, Martin K, Folwaczny C. The c-insertion mutation of the NOD2 gene is associated with fistulizing and fibrostenotic phenotypes in Crohn's disease. Gastroenterology. 2002;122:2091–2.
8.  Loftus EV Jr, Sandborn WJ. Epidemiology of inflammatory bowel disease. Gastroenterol Clin N Am. 2002;31:1–20.
9.  Elliott DE, Urban JF, Jr., Argo CK, Weinstock JV. Does the failure to acquire helminthic parasites predispose to Crohn's disease? FASEB J. 2000;14:1848–55.
10. Bach JF. The effect of infections on susceptibility to autoimmune and allergic diseases [see comment]. New Engl J Med 2002;347:911–20.
11. Sonnenberg A, McCarty DJ, Jacobsen SJ. Geographic variation of inflammatory bowel disease within the United States [see comment.]. Gastroenterology. 1991;100:143–9.
12. Shivananda S, Lennard-Jones J, Logan R et al. Incidence of inflammatory bowel disease across Europe: is there a difference between north and south? Results of the European Collaborative Study on Inflammatory Bowel Disease (EC-IBD). Gut. 1996;39:690–7.
13. Odes HS, Fraser D, Krawiec J. Inflammatory bowel disease in migrant and native Jewish populations of southern Israel. Scand J Gastroenterol (Supplement). 1989;170:36–8.
14. Carr I, Mayberry JF. The effects of migration on ulcerative colitis: a three-year prospective study among Europeans and first- and second-generation South Asians in Leicester (1991–1994). Am J Gastroenterol. 1999;94:2918–22.
15. Jayanthi V, Probert CS, Pinder D, Wicks AC, Mayberry JF. Epidemiology of Crohn's disease in Indian migrants and the indigenous population in Leicestershire. Q J Med. 1992; 82:125–38.

16. Probert CS, Jayanthi V, Hughes AO, Thompson JR, Wicks AC, Mayberry JF. Prevalence and family risk of ulcerative colitis and Crohn's disease: an epidemiological study among Europeans and south Asians in Leicestershire. Gut. 1993;34:1547–51.

17. Sonnenberg A. Occupational distribution of inflammatory bowel disease among German employees. Gut. 1990;31:1037–40.

18. Duggan AE, Usmani I, Neal KR, Logan RF. Appendicectomy, childhood hygiene, Helicobacter pylori status, and risk of inflammatory bowel disease: a case–control study [see comments]. Gut. 1998;43:494–8.

19. Gent AE, Hellier MD, Grace RH, Swarbrick ET, Coggon D. Inflammatory bowel disease and domestic hygiene in infancy [comment]. Lancet. 1994;343:766–7.

20. Ekbom A, Helmick C, Zack M, Adami HO. The epidemiology of inflammatory bowel disease: a large, population-based study in Sweden. Gastroenterology. 1991;100:350–8.

21. Goncalves ML, Araujo A, Ferreira LF. Human intestinal parasites in the past: new findings and a review. Memorias do Instituto Oswaldo Cruz. 2003;98(Suppl. 1):103–18.

22. Healy GR, Gleason NN, Bokat R, Pond H, Roper M. Prevalence of ascariasis and amebiasis in Cherokee Indian school children. Publ Health Rep. 1969;84:907–14.

23. Salas SD, Heifetz R, Barrett-Connor E. Intestinal parasites in Central American immigrants in the United States. Arch Intern Med. 1990;150:1514–16.

24. Callahan GN. Eating dirt. Emerging Infect Dis. 2003;9:1016–21.

25. Overgaauw PA. Aspects of Toxocara epidemiology: toxocarosis in dogs and cats. Crit Rev Microbiol. 1997;23:233–51.

26. Overgaauw PA. Aspects of Toxocara epidemiology: human toxocarosis. Crit Rev Microbiol. 1997;23:215–31.

27. Weinstock JV, Summers R, Elliott DE. Helminths and harmony [comment]. Gut. 2004;53:7–9.

28. van den Biggelaar AH, Lopuhaa C, van Ree R et al. The prevalence of parasite infestation and house dust mite sensitization in Gabonese schoolchildren. Int Arch Allergy Immunol. 2001;126:231–8.

29. van den Biggelaar AH, Rodrigues LC, van Ree R et al. Long-term treatment of intestinal helminths increases mite skin-test reactivity in Gabonese schoolchildren. J Infect Dis. 2004;189:892–900.

30. Scrivener S, Yemaneberhan H, Zebenigus M et al. Independent effects of intestinal parasite infection and domestic allergen exposure on risk of wheeze in Ethiopia: a nested case–control study [see comment]. Lancet. 2001;358:1493–9.

31. Elliott DE, Li J, Blum A et al. Exposure to schistosome eggs protects mice from TNBS-induced colitis. Am J Physiol Gastrointest Liver Physiol. 2003;284:G385–91.

32. Moreels TG, Nieuwendijk RJ, De Man JG et al. Concurrent infection with Schistosoma mansoni attenuates inflammation induced changes in colonic morphology, cytokine levels, and smooth muscle contractility of trinitrobenzene sulphonic acid induced colitis in rats [see comment]. Gut. 2004;53:99–107.

33. Khan WI, Blennerhasset PA, Varghese AK et al. Intestinal nematode infection ameliorates experimental colitis in mice. Infect Immun. 2002;70:5931–7.

34. Elliott DE, Setiawan T, Metwali A, Blum A, Urban JF Jr, Weinstock JV. Heligmosomoides polygyrus inhibits established colitis in IL-10-deficient mice. Eur J Immunol. 2004;34:2690–8.

35. Ooi HK, Tenora F, Itoh K, Kamiya M. Comparative study of Trichuris trichiura from non-human primates and from man, and their difference with T. suis. J Vet Med Sci. 1993;55:363–6.

36. Beer RJ. The relationship between Trichuris trichiura (Linnaeus 1758) of man and Trichuris suis (Schrank 1788) of the pig. Res Vet Sci. 1976;20:47–54.

37. Maxwell C, Hussain R, Nutman TB et al. The clinical and immunologic responses of normal human volunteers to low dose hookworm (Necator americanus) infection. Am J Trop Med Hygiene 1987;37:126–34.

38. Loukas A, Prociv P. Immune responses in hookworm infections. Clin Microbiol Rev. 2001;14:689–703.

39. Turner JD, Faulkner H, Kamgno J et al. Th2 cytokines are associated with reduced worm burdens in a human intestinal helminth infection. J Infect Dis. 2003;188:1768–75.

40. Dunne DW, Pearce EJ. Immunology of hepatosplenic schistosomiasis mansoni: a human perspective. Microbes Infect. 1999;1:553–60.

41. Gause WC, Urban JF Jr, Stadecker MJ. The immune response to parasitic helminths: insights from murine models. Trends Immunol. 2003;24:269–77.
42. Borkow G, Leng Q, Weisman Z et al. Chronic immune activation associated with intestinal helminth infections results in impaired signal transduction and anergy. J Clin Invest. 2000; 106:1053–60.
43. Bentwich Z, Weisman Z, Moroz C, Bar-Yehuda S, Kalinkovich A. Immune dysregulation in Ethiopian immigrants in Israel: relevance to helminth infections? Clin Exp Immunol. 1996; 103:239–43.
44. Kullberg MC, Pearce EJ, Hieny SE, Sher A, Berzofsky JA. Infection with *Schistosoma mansoni* alters Th1/Th2 cytokine responses to a non-parasite antigen. J Immunol. 1992; 148:3264–70.
45. Pearlman E, Kazura JW, Hazlett FE Jr, Boom WH. Modulation of murine cytokine responses to mycobacterial antigens by helminth-induced T helper 2 cell responses. J Immunol. 1993;151:4857–64.
46. Sacco R, Hagen M, Sandor M, Weinstock JV, Lynch RG. Established T(H1) granulomatous responses induced by active *Mycobacterium avium* infection switch to T (H2) following challenge with *Schistosoma mansoni*. Clin Immunol. 2002;104:274–81.
47. Sabin EA, Araujo MI, Carvalho EM, Pearce EJ. Impairment of tetanus toxoid-specific Th1-like immune responses in humans infected with *Schistosoma mansoni*. J Infect Dis. 1996;173:269–72.
48. Bashir ME, Andersen P, Fuss IJ, Shi HN, Nagler-Anderson C. An enteric helminth infection protects against an allergic response to dietary antigen. J Immunol. 2002;169: 3284–92.
49. Lynch NR, Hagel I, Perez M, Di Prisco MC, Lopez R, Alvarez N. Effect of anthelmintic treatment on the allergic reactivity of children in a tropical slum. J Allergy Clin Immunol. 1993;92:404–11.
50. Jonuleit H, Schmitt E. The regulatory T cell family: distinct subsets and their interrelations. J Immunol. 2003;171:6323–7.
51. Uraushihara K, Kanai T, Ko K et al. Regulation of murine inflammatory bowel disease by CD25$^+$ and CD25$^-$ CD4$^+$ glucocorticoid-induced TNF receptor family-related gene+ regulatory T cells. J Immunol. 2003;171:708–16.
52. Liu H, Hu B, Xu D, Liew FY. CD4$^+$CD25$^+$ regulatory T cells cure murine colitis: the role of IL-10, TGF-β and CTLA4. J Immunol. 2003;171:5012–17.
53. Mottet C, Uhlig HH, Powrie F. Cutting edge: cure of colitis by CD4$^+$CD25$^+$ regulatory T cells. J Immunol. 2003;170:3939–43.
54. Field AC, Caccavelli L, Bloch MF, Bellon B. Regulatory CD8$^+$ T cells control neonatal tolerance to a Th2-mediated autoimmunity. J Immunol. 2003;170:2508–15.
55. McGuirk P, Mills KH. Pathogen-specific regulatory T cells provoke a shift in the Th1/Th2 paradigm in immunity to infectious diseases. Trends Immunol. 2002;23:450–5.
56. Fehervari Z, Sakaguchi S. Development and function of CD25$^+$CD4$^+$ regulatory T cells. Curr Opin Immunol. 2004;16:203–8.
57. Oida T, Zhang X, Goto M et al. CD4$^+$CD25$^-$ T cells that express latency-associated peptide on the surface suppress CD4$^+$CD45RBhigh-induced colitis by a TGF-beta-dependent mechanism. J Immunol. 2003;170:2516–22.
58. Nakamura K, Kitani A, Fuss I et al. TGF-beta 1 plays an important role in the mechanism of CD4$^+$CD25$^+$ regulatory T cell activity in both humans and mice. J Immunol. 2004;172: 834–42.
59. Moore KW, de Waal MR, Coffman RL, O'Garra A. Interleukin-10 and the interleukin-10 receptor. Ann Rev Immunol. 2001;19:683–765.
60. Jiang H, Zhang SI, Pernis B. Role of CD8$^+$ T cells in murine experimental allergic encephalomyelitis. Science. 1992;256:1213–15.
61. Jiang H, Ware R, Stall A, Flaherty L, Chess L, Pernis B. Murine CD8$^+$ T cells that specifically delete autologous CD4$^+$ T cells expressing V beta 8 TCR: a role of the Qa-1 molecule. Immunity. 1995;2:185–94.
62. Noble A, Zhao ZS, Cantor H. Suppression of immune responses by CD8 cells. II. Qa-1 on activated B cells stimulates CD8 cell suppression of T helper 2 responses. J Immunol. 1998; 160:566–71.
63. Doetze A, Satoguina J, Burchard G et al. Antigen-specific cellular hyporesponsiveness in a chronic human helminth infection is mediated by T(h)3/T(r)1-type cytokines IL-10 and

transforming growth factor-beta but not by a T(h)1 to T(h)2 shift. Int Immunol. 2000;12: 623–30.

64. Satoguina J, Mempel M, Larbi J et al. Antigen-specific T regulatory-1 cells are associated with immunosuppression in a chronic helminth infection (onchocerciasis). Microbes Infect. 2002;4:1291–300.

65. Osborne J, Devaney E. Interleukin-10 and antigen-presenting cells actively suppress Th1 cells in BALB/c mice infected with the filarial parasite *Brugia pahangi*. Infect Immun. 1999; 67:1599–605.

66. Loke P, MacDonald AS, Robb A, Maizels RM, Allen JE. Alternatively activated macrophages induced by nematode infection inhibit proliferation via cell-to-cell contact. Eur J Immunol. 2000;30:2669–78.

67. Caramalho I, Lopes-Carvalho T, Ostler D, Zelenay S, Haury M, Demengeot J. Regulatory T cells selectively express toll-like receptors and are activated by lipopolysaccharide [see comment]. J Exp Med. 2003;197:403–11.

# 26
# Probiotics for inflammatory bowel disease

**P. MARTEAU**

---

## INTRODUCTION

The pathogenesis of inflammatory bowel disease (IBD) involves an interaction between genetically determined host susceptibility, dysregulated immune response and the resident enteric bacterial flora[1]. The deleterious role of some intestinal microorganisms is well established in experimental models and in humans[1]. On the other hand some other microorganisms seem to be protective and may contain or produce molecules of potential therapeutic interest[2]. This led to the concept of using ingested living microorganisms to produce and transport these molecules to targets in the intestine, and try some of them in IBD. Probiotics are defined as living non-pathogenic microorganisms which, when ingested, exert a positive influence on host health or physiology[3]. The originalities of this pharmacological approach include the potential for *in-vivo* production of active molecules, targeting immune cells, and presenting immunogenic molecules in a microbial context. This review summarizes facts and ideas about the use of probiotics in IBD considering the results of randomized controlled trials (RCT), elements of pharmacokinetics, mechanisms of action, and safety.

## CURRENT EVIDENCE FOR EFFICACY: CLINICAL TRIALS IN HUMANS WITH IBD

The best evidence for the efficacy of probiotics relies on double-blind RCT. Meta-analysis of trials testing probiotics in antibiotic-associated diarrhoea and gastroenteritis have been performed[4-7]. However, as the active components may differ between probiotics, one should be very cautious when considering meta-analyses of results with different probiotics.

## Pouchitis

Pouchitis is associated with an imbalance of the endogenous flora including reduced counts of bifidobacteria and lactobacilli[8]. Antibiotics such as metronidazole or ciprofloxacin constitute its usual treatment. Two double-blind placebo-controlled trials showed that the probiotic mixture VSL#3 was effective to prevent recurrence of chronic relapsing pouchitis[9,10]. VSL#3 (CSL, Milan, Italy) contains 300 billion viable lyophilized bacteria per gram, including four strains of lactobacilli (*L. casei, L. plantarum, L. acidophilus, L. delbrueckii* subsp. *bulgaricus*), three strains of bifidobacteria (*B. longum, B. breve, B. infantis*), and one strain *of Streptococcus salivarius* subsp. *thermophilus*. The rationale for the selection of these strains and the composition of this product has not been presented. The first study included 40 patients with chronic relapsing pouchitis. They were treated for an acute pouchitis episode by ciprofloxacin and rifabutin, and then received the probiotic or a placebo for 9 months[9]. A relapse occurred in 15% of the subjects in the probiotic group vs 100% in the placebo group (*p* < 0.001). This result was confirmed in the second RCT which included 36 subjects[10]. At 12 months the remission was maintained in 85% of the patients receiving the probiotic vs 6% in the placebo group (*p* < 0.0001). A third RCT showed that VSL#3 could prevent the first episode of pouchitis after ileopouch–anal anastomosis for ulcerative colitis (UC)[11]. Forty patients who had colectomy and ileopouch–anal anastomosis for UC were randomized to receive either VSL#3 (3 g/day) or placebo immediately after ileostomy closure and for 1 year. Pouchitis occurred in 10% of the patients in the VSL#3 group vs 40% of those in the placebo group (*p* < 0.01). Other probiotics were tried in this setting but the evidence of their efficacy is presently low. In an open trial with historical control, Gosselink et al. suggested that daily administration of *L. rhamnosus* GG decreased the risk of pouchitis (at 3 years the risk was 7% vs 29% in the historical controls (*p* = 0.01)[12].

## Ulcerative colitis

Three double-blind RCT compared the efficacy of living *E. coli* Nissle 1917 to that of mesalazine to prevent relapse of UC, but no trial compared it to placebo[13–15]. Kruis et al.[13] included 120 patients with inactive UC in a double-blind RCT. Half of them received 1.5 g/day of mesalazine, and the other half received 200 mg/day of mutaflor (Ardeypharm GmbH, Herdecke, Germany) i.e. $5 \times 10^{10}$ colony-forming units (cfu)/day of *E. coli* Nissle 1917. After 12 weeks, 11.3% of the subjects receiving mesalazine and 16% of those receiving the *E. coli* had relapsed (difference not significant, n.s.). Rembacken et al. performed a second trial comparing *E. coli* strain Nissle 1917 to mesalazine in 116 patients[14]. Patients with active UC were randomized to receive 2.4 g/day of mesalazine or 200 mg/day of mutaflor. All patients were also initially given a course of oral gentamycin and steroids. Remission was attained in 75% of the patients in the mesalazine group vs 68% in the *E. coli* group (n.s.). When remission was reached, the steroids were tapered and stopped over 4 months, and the dose of mesalazine was reduced to 1.2 g/day. Relapse occurred in 73% of the patients in the mesalazine group vs 67% in the *E. coli* group (n.s.). These first two trials were criticized because of the too-low statistical power to test for the equivalence of the treatments. A third RCT has been more convincing as it included an appropriate number of patients and had the longer follow-up period[15]. In this study, 327 patients with quiescent UC received either the probiotic or mesalazine (1.5 g/day) for 1 year. The relapse rate was 36.4% in the probiotic group vs 33.9% in the mesalazine group (per-protocol analysis) and the statistical tests disclosed equivalence of the two drugs. The evidence for efficacy of other probiotics in UC is lower, although some interesting trials have been published. Ishikawa et al.[16] treated 21 subjects suffering from UC, giving them 100 ml/day of fermented milk for 1 year. Eleven received *B. bifidum* YIT 4007, *B. breve* YIT 4065, and *L. acidophilus* YIT 0168 in the milk and the other 10 did not. This probiotic mixture was well tolerated and there were fewer relapses in the group receiving the probiotic (27%) than in the control group (90%).

The majority of the studies using probiotics in patients with UC aimed at decreasing the risk of relapse. A recent randomized double-blind pilot trial suggested for the first time that an ecological treatment combining *B. longum* with fructo-oligosaccharides could have therapeutic benefits in patients with acute UC[17]. A significant decrease of endoscopic lesions in the distal colon was observed only in the 'symbiotic' group and the biological markers of inflammation in the mucosa TNF-$\alpha$, interleukin 1$\alpha$ and the human-$\beta$-defensins 2, 3 and 4 were ameliorated. However, this study is still too preliminary to convince clinicians of using this synbiotic as a treatment because of the low number of subjects (18 only), the use of additional treatments, and the lack of histological inflammation score. Studies like this one will hopefully help selecting products for powered RCT.

## Crohn's disease

The evidence for efficacy of probiotics in Crohn's disease (CD) is still low. The RCT were all performed to try to prevent recurrence. Malchow tested *E. coli* Nissle 1917[18] in a pilot double-blind, placebo-controlled study enrolling 28 patients. At 1 year there was a non-significant trend of lower relapse rate in the probiotic group (30% vs 63.6%, n.s.). This pilot study has not been reproduced. Guslandi et al.[19] examined the effect of *S. boulardii*. Thirty-two patients received either 1 g/day of *S. boulardii* plus mesalamine 2 g/day or 3 g/day of mesalamine, and were followed for 6 months. A clinical relapse occurred in 6.25% of the probiotic group vs 37.5% in the control group ($p = 0.04$). This pilot study was not blinded and a confirmation double-blind study is ongoing. *L. rhamnosus* GG has been studied in small series of patients[20] but the results of a large controlled trial performed a few years ago are still not presented.

Postoperative recurrence is an attractive target for probiotics; indeed, there is strong evidence that luminal bacteria are involved in the occurrence of new lesions, and nitroimidazole antibiotics have proven efficacy[21,22]. Prantera et al. compared *L. rhamnosus* GG to placebo in 45 patients[23]; this was a double-blind, placebo-controlled study. At 1 year the percentages of endoscopic or clinical relapse did not differ between the two groups. Endoscopic relapse was 60% in the probiotic group vs 35.3% with the placebo ($p = 0.297$). Campieri et al. carried out a single-blind study to evaluate the efficacy of a combined treatment consisting in the administration of rifaximin (a non-absorbed broad-spectrum antibiotic) for 3 months followed by VSL#3 (two packets/day for 9 months) vs mesalazine (4 g/day for 12 months)[24]. Forty patients were randomized and their clinical situation and endoscopic lesions were assessed 3 and 12 months after surgery. The authors reported a lower rate of severe endoscopic recurrence both at 3 and 12 months in patients of the antibiotic–probiotic group (10% and 20% vs 40% and 40% respectively, $p < 0.01$). We performed a double-blind, randomized placebo-controlled study in 98 patients who had just been operated for CD and who received for 6 months either *L. johnsonii* LA1 ($4 \times 10^9$ cfu/day) or a placebo. At 6 months an endoscopic recurrence was observed in 49% of patients in the LA1 group, and 64% of patients in the placebo group (n.s.). The endoscopic recurrence rate did not differ significantly between the LA1 and placebo groups for any given endoscopic grade. There were four clinical recurrences in the LA1 group and three in the placebo group[25].

## PHARMACOLOGY

Probotics are living microorganisms and their pharmacokinetics is thus very original. Probiotic properties have been demonstrated among bacteria such as lactobacilli, bifidobacteria, and *E. coli*, but also yeast such as *Saccharomyces*[26]. The effects can be either direct effects due to the expression *in vivo* of intrinsic metabolic properties of the microorganism or to some part of its architecture, or indirect effects due to modifications of the endogenous flora or of the immune system[26]. The survival of the strain in the gastrointestinal tract, and for some researchers its adhesion to the mucosa (especially the mucus), seem to be relevant pharmacokinetic characteristics[26].

### Mechanisms of action

Microbial signals in the intestinal lumen are detected by pattern-recognition receptors, especially the toll-like receptors (TLR) expressed on immune and epithelial cells. TLR2 recognizes bacterial peptidoglycan, TLR4 recognizes lipopolysaccharide, and TLR9 recognizes special sequences of bacterial DNA (unmethylated CpG motifs). Interestingly, the positive effect of the probiotic mixture VSL#3 on dextran sulphate-induced colitis in mice was also observed after oral administration of its extracted CpG DNA and suppressed in TLR9-deficient animals[27]. This does not mean that all effects of probiotics are due to their CpG DNA, but shows that at least some immunomodulatory effects may be due to this bacterial component. Endogenous bacteria and probiotics have variable influence on the NF-κB and MAP kinase transduction signalling pathways[28]. This explains why immunocompetent cells do not secrete the same inflammatory or immunoregulatory cytokines when challenged with various microorganisms or probiotics[29]. Some probiotics can significantly stimulate the innate immunity, including the phagocytosis capacity of polymorphonuclear leucocytes and the expression of defensins by epithelial cells[30,31]. They may also enhance immunoglobulin-A (IgA) secretion. For example, in a RCT performed in children suffering from rotavirus gastroenteritis[32], the children receiving *L. rhamnosus* GG had significantly higher numbers of circulating antibody-secreting cells than those receiving a placebo. A higher proportion of children in the probiotic group exhibited rotavirus-specific IgA antibody-secreting cell response (90% vs 46% in the placebo group), and this may explain the significant shortening of diarrhoea in this group. Wehkamp et al. recently observed that several probiotic bacteria including *E. coli* Nissle 1917 strongly induced the expression of the human-β-defensin-2 in Caco2 cells in contrast to (or much more than) a large series of non-probiotic bacteria[30]. Some trials have shown that probiotics can protect from pathological leakage of tight junctions observed in infectious or inflammatory conditions. For example, *S. boulardii* maintained the tight-junction structure of T84 cells during enteropathogenic *E. coli* (EPEC) infection[33]. This yeast and its culture supernatant also prevented chloride secretion induced by *E. coli* heat-labile toxin and cholera toxin[33]. Other studies showed that *S. thermophilus* ATCC19258 and *L. acidophilus* ATCC4356 blocked the effect of enteroinvasive *E. coli* (EIEC) on chloride secretion[34]. Probiotics may also modulate mucin gene secretion. *L. plantarum* 299v increased the expression of mucins MUC-2 and MUC-3 mRNA in HT-29 cells[35] and *L. rhamnosus* GG up-regulated MUC-2 mRNA and protein in CaCo-2 cells. Two RCT showed that *B. animalis* DN-173010 shortened the transit time in the sigmoid colon in healthy women[36,37], but the mechanism for this effect remains unknown[37]. The effects of probiotics on the endogenous ecosystem are difficult to assess because of inter-individual variability in the composition of the intestinal flora. Probiotics may interact with endogenous microorganisms by competition for essential nutrients, production of antimicrobial factors, modifications of ecological conditions (pH, for example), and competition for adhesion sites. Some probiotics decreased the faecal concentrations of Bacteroides, clostridia, and *E. coli*[38] and sometimes also increased the endogenous bifidobacteria and lactobacilli[39].

## Pharmacokinetics

Probiotics act as vectors which deliver their active constituents at various target sites in the gastrointestinal tract. The majority of the effects occur only (or mainly) when the microorganisms are ingested alive, and this suggested that the survival of the probiotic until its target could be a desirable property[2]. The survival of probiotics in the gastrointestinal tract varies greatly not only between genera but between species and even strains[18]. Some strains are destroyed in the stomach while others have a high survival until faeces. *L. bulgaricus*, *S. thermophilus* and *L. lactis* have a poor intrinsic resistance to acid and bile and are rapidly lysed in the stomach and duodenum. On the contrary, strains of *L. acidophilus, L. reuteri, L. rhamnosus, L. plantarum, L. salivarius, L. casei* and *L. johnsonii* have a higher survival and may reach the distal parts of the intestine. For example, about 1–10% of *L. acidophilus* were found to survive until the ileum in human studies using intestinal intubation techniques[18]. *L. plantarum* NCIB 8826 and some *Bifidobacterium* spp. demonstrated a very high survival capacity, i.e. 25–30% of the ingested bacteria were recovered in the terminal ileum and in faeces[2,40–43]. The ability to adhere to the intestinal mucosa and/or to intestinal mucus is also a characteristic which varies between strains[44]. It is believed (but not proven) that this property may favour competitive exclusion of pathogens and immunomodulation. Even the best surviving and adhering probiotics usually do not colonize the intestine for long periods[18]. However, it was observed that *L. rhamnosus* GG or *L. plantarum* 299 could colonize the intestinal mucus of some subjects for several days or weeks[45,46]. Another originality is that probiotics may reach the inductive mucosal immune system through M cells or dendritic cells[47,48]. This has not been studied until now in humans.

## Genetically modified probiotics

Selection of probiotic strains or combinations for clinical trials is presently a challenge. One strategy is to search for microorganisms with potentially interesting intrinsic properties. A recent trial has shown that a nitric oxide-producing strain of *L. farciminis* improved TNBS-induced colitis in rats via the nitric oxide delivery[49]. Another strategy is to select candidate microorganisms on their pharmacokinetics and engineer them to make them produce therapeutic molecules *in vivo*. The majority of studies on genetically modified probiotics used lactococci (especially *L. lactis* MG1363) as vector for the transgene[50–52] as these bacteria are easy to manipulate. However, lactococci (including *L. lactis* MG1363) have a low survival capacity in the human gastrointestinal tract[43] and may therefore not be the best vector for ileal or colonic diseases in humans. Steidler et al. pioneered the field when they reported that lactococci which had been genetically manipulated to produce interleukin-10 had a therapeutic effect in murine models of colitis[50]. Clinical studies are now ongoing using this 'biologically contained *L. lactis* secreting IL-10' in patients with CD. In a recent trial Vandenbroucke et al. used the same principle for *in-situ* delivery of trefoil factors[52]. These molecules play important roles in the protection and healing of the intestinal epithelium. They have a significant therapeutic efficacy on histological lesions of dextran sulphate-induced colitis when administered rectally, but not when given orally because they stick to the mucus of the small bowel and are removed from the lumen at the caecum[52]. In the series of experiments, gastric administration of this 'trefoil factor secreting probiotic' led to active delivery of trefoil factors in the colon and to prevention and healing of dextran sulphate-induced colitis in mice, while the vector without the transgene and the trefoil peptides alone were ineffective. These studies open a large field of potential applications for preclinical and clinical research and hopefully will lead to new treatments of IBD.

## Safety

Currently used probiotic products are safe. However, they may theoretically be responsible for four types of side-effects in susceptible individuals: infections, deleterious metabolic activities, excessive immune stimulation, and gene transfer. Probiotics are not selected among pathogens, and the theoretical risk of infections is thus very low. A few cases of infections have been traced back to *S. boulardii* and *L. rhamnosus* GG[53–57]. Noticeably, the majority of the cases occurred in hospitalized patients (adults or infants) who had a central venous catheter. The probiotic capsules or packets were often opened in the patient room and catheter contamination through hand-related transmission is likely. Hennequin et al.[53] showed that opening a packet of *S. boulardii* induced contamination of the surrounding surfaces, the arm of a simulated patient, and the hands of the nurse. Nosocomial transmission is further suggested by demonstration of clusters of isolates among patients concurrently hospitalized in the same unit[56], and by a case of nosocomial fungaemia in a patient who had not been treated with the probiotic[57]. Translocation of a probiotic from the patient's intestine has not been observed until now, even in patients with intestinal ulceration[58], but one case of endocarditis was reported in a man with mitral valve regurgitation who had chewed *L. rhamnosus* after dental extraction[59]. The risk for immunosuppressed patients is not established. One case of liver abscess due to *L. rhamnosus* GG was observed in a 74-year-old woman with diabetes[54]. Genetically modified probiotics should not contaminate the environment. In order to 'contain' genetically modified IL-10 producing lactococci, and avoid their survival in the external environment, Steidler et al. replaced the *Lactococcus* gene for thymidilate synthase by the IL-10 transgene so that the microorganism becomes dependent on the presence of thymidine and does not survive in the environment[60].

## CONCLUSIONS

RCT have demonstrated the efficacy of some probiotics to treat or prevent specific situations of IBD, especially pouchitis and UC. Probiotics differ greatly from one another even at the strain level; therefore results obtained with one strain cannot be extrapolated to another one. Dose–response studies are too few to establish the dose needed or the optimal number of administrations per day. It is often quoted that only living microorganisms had therapeutic value, that probiotics had to be of human origin and that they had to survive in the gastrointestinal tract in order to be efficient. However, there are now examples showing that these characteristics are in fact not needed in every case[2]. Other statements or hypotheses such as 'probiotic mixtures should be preferred to single strains', 'probiotics should only used in prevention' or 'probiotics should always be used in combination with antibiotics or with prebiotics' are also presently unproven, although they may contain some truth. One will certainly learn from probiotic studies and develop drugs containing only their active component (without risk of infection). However, the originality of the *in-vivo* pharmacokinetics of probiotics is such that this method of vectoring activities in the intestine and especially to the immune cells has to be studied further.

# References

1. Sartor RB. Therapeutic manipulation of the enteric microflora in inflammatory bowel diseases: antibiotics, probiotics, and prebiotics. Gastroenterology. 2004;126:1620–33.
2. Marteau P, Shanahan F. Basic aspects and pharmacology of probiotics: an overview of pharmacokinetics, mechanisms of action and side-effects. Best Pract Res Clin Gastroenterol. 2003;17:725–40.
3. Schrezenmeir J, de Vrese M. Probiotics, prebiotics and synbiotics – approaching a definition. Am J Clin Nutr. 2001;73(Suppl. 2):361s–4s.
4. Cremonini F, Di Caro S, Nista EC et al. Meta-analysis: the effect of probiotic administration on antibiotic-associated diarrhoea. Aliment Pharmacol Ther. 2002;16: 1461–7.
5. D'Souza AL, Rajkumar C, Cooke J, Bulpitt CJ. Probiotics in prevention of antibiotic associated diarrhoea: meta-analysis. Br Med J. 2002;324:1361–5.
6. Huang JS, Bousvaros A, Lee JW, Diaz A, Davidson EJ. Efficacy of probiotic use in acute diarrhea in children: a meta-analysis. Dig Dis Sci. 2002;47:2625–34.
7. Van Niel CW, Feudtner C, Garrison MN, Christakis DA. *Lactobacillus* therapy for acute infectious diarrhoea in children: a meta analysis. Pediatrics. 2002;109:678–84.
8. Ruseler van Embden JGH, Schouten WR, van Lieshout LMC. Pouchitis: result of microbial imbalance? Gut. 1994;35:658–64.
9. Gionchetti P, Rizzello F, Venturi A et al. Oral bacteriotherapy as maintenance treatment in patients with chronic pouchitis: a double-blind, placebo-controlled trial. Gastroenterology. 2000;119:305–9.
10. Mimura T, Rizzello F, Helwig U et al. Once daily high dose probiotic therapy (VSL#3) for maintaining remission in recurrent or refractory pouchitis. Gut. 2004;53:108–14.
11. Gionchetti P, Rizzello F, Helwig U et al. Prophylaxis of pouchitis onset with probiotic therapy: a double-blind, placebo-controlled trial. Gastroenterology. 2003;124:1202–9.
12. Gosselink MP, Schouten WR, van Lieshout LM et al. Delay of the first onset of pouchitis by oral intake of the probiotic strain *Lactobacillus rhamnosus* GG. Dis Colon Rectum. 2004; 47:876–84.
13. Kruis W, Schutz E, Fric P, Fixa B, Judmaier G, Stolte M. Double-blind comparison of an oral *Escherichia coli* preparation and mesalazine in maintaining remission of ulcerative colitis. Aliment Pharmacol Ther. 1997;11:853–8.
14. Rembacken BJ, Snelling AM, Hawkey PM, Chalmers DM, Axon AT. Non-pathogenic *Escherichia coli* versus mesalazine for the treatment of ulcerative colitis: a randomised trial. Lancet. 1999;354:635–9.
15. Kruis W, Fric P, Pokrotnieks J et al. Maintaining remission of ulcerative colitis with the probiotic *Escherichia coli* Nissle 1917 is as effective as with standard mesalazine. Gut. 2004; 53:1617–23.
16. Ishikawa H, Akedo I, Umesaki Y, Tanaka R, Imaoka A, Otani T. Randomized controlled trial of the effect of bifidobacteria-fermented milk on ulcerative colitis. J Am Coll Nutr. 2003;22:56–63.
17. Furrie E, Macfarlane S, Kennedy A et al. Synbiotic therapy (*Bifidobacterium longum*/ SynergyITM) initiates resolution of inflammation in patients with active ulcerative colitis: a randomised controlled pilot trial. Gut. 2005;54:242–9.
18. Malchow HA. Crohn's disease and *Escherichia coli*. A new approach in therapy to maintain remission of colonic Crohn's disease? J Clin Gastroenterol. 1997;25:653–8.
19. Guslandi M, Mezzi G, Sorghi M, Testoni PA. *Saccharomyces boulardii* in maintenance treatment of Crohn's disease. Dig Dis Sci. 2000;45:1462–4.
20. Schultz M, Timmer A, Herfarth HH, Sartor RB, Vanderhoof JA, Rath HC. *Lactobacillus* GG in inducing and maintaining remission of Crohn's disease. BMC Gastroenterol. 2004;4:5.
21. Rutgeerts P, Hiele M, Geboes K et al. Controlled trial of metronidazole treatment for prevention of Crohn's recurrence after ileal resection. Gastroenterology. 1995;108:1617–21.
22. Rutgeerts P, Van Assche G, Vermeire S et al. Ornidazole for prophylaxis of postoperative Crohn's disease recurrence: a randomized, double-blind, placebo-controlled trial. Gastroenterology. 2005;128:856–61.

23. Prantera C, Scribano ML, Falasco G, Andreoli A, Luzi C. Ineffectiveness of probiotics in preventing recurrence after curative resection for Crohn's disease: a randomised controlled trial with *Lactobacillus* GG. Gut. 2002;51:405–9.
24. Campieri M, Rizzello F, Venturi A et al. Combination of antibiotic and probiotic treatment is efficacious in prophylaxis of post-operative recurrence of Crohn's disease: a randomized controlled study vs mesalamine. Gastroenterology. 2000;118:G4179.
25. Marteau P, Lémann M, Seksik P et al. Ineffectiveness of the probiotic strain *Lactobacillus johnsonii* LA1 in preventing recurrence after curative resection for Crohn's disease – a randomized double-blind, placebo controlled trial. Gastroenterology. 2005;128:47541 (abstract).
26. Marteau P, Seksik P, Lepage P, Doré J. Cellular and physiological effects of probiotics and prebiotics. Mini-rev Med Chem. 2004;4:889–96.
27. Rachmilewitz D, Katakura K, Karmeli F et al. Toll-like receptor 9 signaling mediates the anti-inflammatory effects of probiotics in murine experimental colitis. Gastroenterology. 2004;126:520–8.
28. Dahan S, Dalmasso G, Imbert V, Peyron JF, Rampal P, Czerucka D. *Saccharomyces boulardii* interferes with enterohemorrhagic *Escherichia coli*-induced signaling pathways in T84 cells. Infect Immun. 2003;71:766–73.
29. Haller D, Bode C, Hammes WP, Pfeifer AM, Schiffrin EJ, Blum S. Non-pathogenic bacteria elicit a differential cytokine response by intestinal epithelial cell/leucocyte co-cultures. Gut. 2000;47:79–87.
30. Schiffrin EJ, Rochat F, Link-Amster H, Aeschlimann JM, Donnet-Hughes A. Immunomodulation of human blood cells following the ingestion of lactic acid bacteria. J Dairy Sci. 1995;78:491–7.
31. Wehkamp J, Harder J, Wehkamp K et al. NF-kB- and AP-1-mediated induction of human beta defensin-2 in epithelial cells by *Escherichia coli* Nissle 1917: a novel effect of a probiotic bacterium. Infect Immun. 2004;72:5750–8.
32. Kaila M, Isolauri E, Soppi E, Virtanen E, Laine S, Arvilommi H. Enhancement of the circulating antibody secreting cell response in human diarrhea by a human *Lactobacillus* strain. Pediatr Res. 1992;32:141–4.
33. Czerucka D, Dahan S, Mograbi B, Rossi B, Rampal P. *Saccharomyces boulardii* preserves the barrier function and modulates the signal transduction pathway induced in enteropathogenic *Escherichia coli*-infected T84 cells. Infect Immun. 2000;68:5998–6004.
34. Resta-Lenert S, Barrett KE. Live probiotics protect intestinal epithelial cells from the effects of infection with enteroinvasive *Escherichia coli* (EIEC). Gut. 2003;52:988–97.
35. Mack DR, Michail S, Wei S, McDougall L, Hollingsworth MA. Probiotics inhibit enteropathogenic *E. coli* adherence *in vitro* by inducing intestinal mucin gene expression. Am J Physiol. 1999;276:G941–50.
36. Bouvier M, Méance S, Bouley C, Berta JL, Grimaud JC. Effects of consumption of a milk fermented with the probiotic strain *Bifidobacterium animalis* DN-173 010 on colonic transit times in healthy humans. Biosci Microflor. 2001;20:43–8.
37. Marteau P, Cuillerier E, Meance S et al. *Bifidobacterium animalis* strain DN-173 010 shortens the colonic transit time in healthy women: a double-blind, randomized, controlled study. Aliment Pharmacol Ther. 2002;16:587–93.
38. Fooks LJ, Gibson GR. Probiotics as modulators of the gut flora. Br J Nutr. 2002;88(Suppl. 1):S39–49.
39. Spanhaak S, Havenaar R, Schaafsma G. The effect of consumption of milk fermented by *Lactobacillus casei* strain Shirota on the intestinal microflora and immune parameters in humans. Eur J Clin Nutr. 1998;52:899–907.
40. Marteau P, Pochart P, Bouhnik Y, Zidi S, Goderel I, Rambaud JC. Survie dans l'intestin grêle de *Lactobacillus acidophilus* et *Bifidobacterium* sp. *Ingérés* dans unlait fermenté: une base rationnele pouir l'utilisation des probiotiques chez l'homme. Gastroenterol Clin Biol. 1992;16:25–8 (in French).
41. Bouhnik Y, Pochart P, Marteau P, Arlet G, Goderel I, Rambaud JC. Fecal recovery in humans of viable *Bifidobacterium* sp. ingested in fermented milk. Gastroenterology. 1992; 102:875–8.
42. Pochart P, Marteau P, Bouhnik Y, Goderel I, Bourlioux P, Rambaud JC. Survival of *Bifidobacteria* ingested via fermented milk during their passage through the human small intestine: an *in vivo* study using intestinal perfusion. Am J Clin Nutr. 1992;55:78–80.

43. Vesa T, Pochart P, Marteau P. Pharmacokinetics of *Lactobacillus plantarum* NCIMB 8826, *Lactobacillus fermentum* KLD, and *Lactococcus lactis* MG 1363 in the human gastrointestinal tract. Aliment Pharmacol Ther. 2000;14:823–8.

44. Servin AL, Coconnier MH. Adhesion of probiotic strains to the intestinal mucosa and interaction with pathogens. Best Pract Res Clin Gastroenterol. 2003;17:741–54.

45. Johansson ML, Molin G, Jeppsson B, Nobaek S, Ahrne S, Bengmark S. Administration of different *Lactobacillus* strains in fermented oatmeal soup: *in vivo* colonization of human intestinal mucosa and effect on the indigenous flora. Appl Environ Microbiol. 1993;59:15–20.

46. Alander M, Satokari R, Korpela R et al. Persistence of colonization of human colonic mucosa by a probiotic strain, *Lactobacillus rhamnosus* GG, after oral consumption. Appl Environ Microbiol. 1999;65:351–4.

47. Mavris M, Sansonetti P. Microbial–gut interactions in health and disease. Epithelial cell responses. Best Pract Res Clin Gastroenterol. 2004;18:373–86.

48. Drakes M, Blanchard T, Czinn S. Bacterial probiotic modulation of dendritic cells. Infect Immun. 2004;72:3299–309.

49. Lamine F, Fioramonti J, Bueno L et al. Nitric oxide released by *Lactobacillus farciminis* improves TNBS-induced colitis in rats. Scand J Gastroenterol. 2004;39:37–45.

50. Steidler L, Hans W, Schotte L et al. Treatment of murine colitis by *Lactococcus lactis* secreting interleukin-10. Science. 2000 25;289:1352–5.

51. Pavan S. Evaluation des capacités probitioques de *Lactobacillus plantarum* et *Lactococcus lactis* pour le traitement des maladies inflammatoires chroniques de l'intestin. Thèse de l'Université de Lille I. 2002.

52. Vandenbroucke K, Hans W, Van Huysse J et al. Active delivery of trefoil factors by genetically modified *Lactococcus lactis* prevents and heals acute colitis in mice. Gastroenterology. 2004;127:502–13.

53. Hennequin C, Kauffmann-Lacroix C, Jobert A et al. Possible role of catheters in *Saccharomyces boulardii* fungemia. Eur J Clin Microbiol Infect Dis. 2000;19:16–20.

54. Rautio M, Jousimies-Somer H, Kauma H et al. Liver abscess due to a *Lactobacillus rhamnosus* strain indistinguishable from *L. rhamnosus* strain GG. Clin Infect Dis. 1999;28:1159–60.

55. Land MH, Rouster-Stevens K, Wood CR, Cannon ML, Cnota J, Shetty AK. *Lactobacillus* sepsis associated with probiotic therapy. Pediatrics. 2005;115:178–81.

56. Lherm T, Monet C, Nougiere B et al. Seven cases of fungemia with *Saccharomyces boulardii* in critically ill patients. Intens Care Med. 2002;28:797–801.

57. Cassone M, Serra P, Mondello F et al. Outbreak of *Saccharomyces cerevisiae* subtype *boulardii* fungemia in patients neighboring those treated with a probiotic preparation of the organism. J Clin Microbiol. 2003;41:5340–53.

58. Borriello SP, Hammes WP, Holzapfel W et al. Safety of probiotics that contain lactobacilli or bifidobacteria. Clin Infect Dis. 2003;36:775–8.

59. MacKay A, Taylor M, Kibbler C, Hamilton Miller J. *Lactobacillus* endocarditis caused by a probiotic microorganism. Clin Microbiol Infect. 1999;5:290–2.

60. Steidler L. Genetically engineered probiotics. Best Pract Res Clin Gastroenterol. 2003;17:861–76.

# Index

# Falk Symposium Series

*These titles were published under the MTP Press imprint.

# Falk Symposium Series

# Falk Symposium Series

83. Dobrilla G, Felder M, de Pretis G, eds.: *Advances in Hepatobiliary and Pancreatic Diseases: Special Clinical Topics.* Falk Symposium 83. 1995.    ISBN 0-7923-8892-5
84. Fromm H, Leuschner U, eds.: *Bile Acids – Cholestasis – Gallstones: Advances in Basic and Clinical Bile Acid Research.* Falk Symposium 84. 1995    ISBN 0-7923-8893-3
85. Tytgat GNJ, Bartelsman JFWM, van Deventer SJH, eds.: *Inflammatory Bowel Diseases.* Falk Symposium 85. 1995    ISBN 0-7923-8894-1
86. Berg PA, Leuschner U, eds.: *Bile Acids and Immunology.* Falk Symposium 86. 1996
ISBN 0-7923-8700-7
87. Schmid R, Bianchi L, Blum HE, Gerok W, Maier KP, Stalder GA, eds.: *Acute and Chronic Liver Diseases: Molecular Biology and Clinics.* Falk Symposium 87. 1996
ISBN 0-7923-8701-5
88. Blum HE, Wu GY, Wu CH, eds.: *Molecular Diagnosis and Gene Therapy.* Falk Symposium 88. 1996    ISBN 0-7923-8702-3
88B. Poupon RE, Reichen J, eds.: *Surrogate Markers to Assess Efficacy of TReatment in Chronic Liver Diseases.* International Falk Workshop. 1996    ISBN 0-7923-8705-8
89. Reyes HB, Leuschner U, Arias IM, eds.: *Pregnancy, Sex Hormones and the Liver.* Falk Symposium 89. 1996    ISBN 0-7923-8704-X
89B. Broelsch CE, Burdelski M, Rogiers X, eds.: *Cholestatic Liver Diseases in Children and Adults.* International Falk Workshop. 1996    ISBN 0-7923-8710-4
90. Lam S-K, Paumgartner P, Wang B, eds.: *Update on Hepatobiliary Diseases 1996.* Falk Symposium 90. 1996    ISBN 0-7923-8715-5
91. Hadziselimovic F, Herzog B, eds.: *Inflammatory Bowel Diseases and Chronic Recurrent Abdominal Pain.* Falk Symposium 91. 1996    ISBN 0-7923-8722-8
91B. Alvaro D, Benedetti A, Strazzabosco M, eds.: *Vanishing Bile Duct Syndrome – Pathophysiology and Treatment.* International Falk Workshop. 1996
ISBN 0-7923-8721-X
92. Gerok W, Loginov AS, Pokrowskij VI, eds.: *New Trends in Hepatology 1996.* Falk Symposium 92. 1997    ISBN 0-7923-8723-6
93. Paumgartner G, Stiehl A, Gerok W, eds.: *Bile Acids in Hepatobiliary Diseases – Basic Research and Clinical Application.* Falk Symposium 93. 1997    ISBN 0-7923-8725-2
94. Halter F, Winton D, Wright NA, eds.: *The Gut as a Model in Cell and Molecular Biology.* Falk Symposium 94. 1997    ISBN 0-7923-8726-0
94B. Kruse-Jarres JD, Schölmerich J, eds.: *Zinc and Diseases of the Digestive Tract.* International Falk Workshop. 1997    ISBN 0-7923-8724-4
95. Ewe K, Eckardt VF, Enck P, eds.: *Constipation and Anorectal Insufficiency.* Falk Symposium 95. 1997    ISBN 0-7923-8727-9
96. Andus T, Goebell H, Layer P, Schölmerich J, eds.: *Inflammatory Bowel Disease – from Bench to Bedside.* Falk Symposium 96. 1997    ISBN 0-7923-8728-7
97. Campieri M, Bianchi-Porro G, Fiocchi C, Schölmerich J, eds. *Clinical Challenges in Inflammatory Bowel Diseases: Diagnosis, Prognosis and Treatment.* Falk Symposium 97. 1998    ISBN 0-7923-8733-3
98. Lembcke B, Kruis W, Sartor RB, eds. *Systemic Manifestations of IBD: The Pending Challenge for Subtle Diagnosis and Treatment.* Falk Symposium 98. 1998
ISBN 0-7923-8734-1
99. Goebell H, Holtmann G, Talley NJ, eds. *Functional Dyspepsia and Irritable Bowel Syndrome: Concepts and Controversies.* Falk Symposium 99. 1998
ISBN 0-7923-8735-X
100. Blum HE, Bode Ch, Bode JCh, Sartor RB, eds. *Gut and the Liver.* Falk Symposium 100. 1998    ISBN 0-7923-8736-8

# Falk Symposium Series

101. Rachmilewitz D, ed. *V International Symposium on Inflammatory Bowel Diseases.* Falk Symposium 101. 1998                                    ISBN 0-7923-8743-0
102. Manns MP, Boyer JL, Jansen PLM, Reichen J, eds. *Cholestatic Liver Diseases.* Falk Symposium 102. 1998                                    ISBN 0-7923-8746-5
102B. Manns MP, Chapman RW, Stiehl A, Wiesner R, eds. *Primary Sclerosing Cholangitis.* International Falk Workshop. 1998.       ISBN 0-7923-8745-7
103. Häussinger D, Jungermann K, eds. *Liver and Nervous System.* Falk Symposium 102. 1998                                    ISBN 0-7924-8742-2
103B. Häussinger D, Heinrich PC, eds. *Signalling in the Liver.* International Falk Workshop. 1998                                    ISBN 0-7923-8744-9
103C. Fleig W, ed. *Normal and Malignant Liver Cell Growth.* International Falk Workshop. 1998                                    ISBN 0-7923-8748-1
104. Stallmach A, Zeitz M, Strober W, MacDonald TT, Lochs H, eds. *Induction and Modulation of Gastrointestinal Inflammation.* Falk Symposium 104. 1998
                                                                  ISBN 0-7923-8747-3
105. Emmrich J, Liebe S, Stange EF, eds. *Innovative Concepts in Inflammatory Bowel Diseases.* Falk Symposium 105. 1999            ISBN 0-7923-8749-X
106. Rutgeerts P, Colombel J-F, Hanauer SB, Schölmerich J, Tytgat GNJ, van Gossum A, eds. *Advances in Inflammatory Bowel Diseases.* Falk Symposium 106. 1999
                                                                  ISBN 0-7923-8750-3
107. Špičák J, Boyer J, Gilat T, Kotrlik K, Mareček Z, Paumgartner G, eds. *Diseases of the Liver and the Bile Ducts – New Aspects and Clinical Implications.* Falk Symposium 107. 1999                                    ISBN 0-7923-8751-1
108. Paumgartner G, Stiehl A, Gerok W, Keppler D, Leuschner U, eds. *Bile Acids and Cholestasis.* Falk Symposium 108. 1999             ISBN 0-7923-8752-X
109. Schmiegel W, Schölmerich J, eds. *Colorectal Cancer – Molecular Mechanisms, Premalignant State and its Prevention.* Falk Symposium 109. 1999
                                                                  ISBN 0-7923-8753-8
110. Domschke W, Stoll R, Brasitus TA, Kagnoff MF, eds. *Intestinal Mucosa and its Diseases – Pathophysiology and Clinics.* Falk Symposium 110. 1999
                                                                  ISBN 0-7923-8754-6
110B. Northfield TC, Ahmed HA, Jazwari RP, Zentler-Munro PL, eds. *Bile Acids in Hepatobiliary Disease.* Falk Workshop. 2000            ISBN 0-7923-8755-4
111. Rogler G, Kullmann F, Rutgeerts P, Sartor RB, Schölmerich J, eds. *IBD at the End of its First Century.* Falk Symposium 111. 2000       ISBN 0-7923-8756-2
112. Krammer HJ, Singer MV, eds. *Neurogastroenterology: From the Basics to the Clinics.* Falk Symposium 112. 2000                ISBN 0-7923-8757-0
113. Andus T, Rogler G, Schlottmann K, Frick E, Adler G, Schmiegel W, Zeitz M, Schölmerich J, eds. *Cytokines and Cell Homeostasis in the Gastrointestinal Tract.* Falk Symposium 113. 2000                                ISBN 0-7923-8758-9
114. Manns MP, Paumgartner G, Leuschner U, eds. *Immunology and Liver.* Falk Symposium 114. 2000                                    ISBN 0-7923-8759-7
115. Boyer JL, Blum HE, Maier K-P, Sauerbruch T, Stalder GA, eds. *Liver Cirrhosis and its Development.* Falk Symposium 115. 2000            ISBN 0-7923-8760-0
116. Riemann JF, Neuhaus H, eds. *Interventional Endoscopy in Hepatology.* Falk Symposium 116. 2000                                    ISBN 0-7923-8761-9
116A. Dienes HP, Schirmacher P, Brechot C, Okuda K, eds. *Chronic Hepatitis: New Concepts of Pathogenesis, Diagnosis and Treatment.* Falk Workshop. 2000
                                                                  ISBN 0-7923-8763-5

# Falk Symposium Series

117. Gerbes AL, Beuers U, Jüngst D, Pape GR, Sackmann M, Sauerbruch T, eds. *Hepatology 2000 – Symposium in Honour of Gustav Paumgartner.* Falk Symposium 117. 2000                                                      ISBN 0-7923-8765-1
117A. Acalovschi M, Paumgartner G, eds. *Hepatobiliary Diseases: Cholestasis and Gallstones.* Falk Workshop. 2000                                ISBN 0-7923-8770-8
118. Frühmorgen P, Bruch H-P, eds. *Non-Neoplastic Diseases of the Anorectum.* Falk Symposium 118. 2001                                            ISBN 0-7923-8766-X
119. Fellermann K, Jewell DP, Sandborn WJ, Schölmerich J, Stange EF, eds. *Immunosuppression in Inflammatory Bowel Diseases – Standards, New Developments, Future Trends.* Falk Symposium 119. 2001                                ISBN 0-7923-8767-8
120. van Berge Henegouwen GP, Keppler D, Leuschner U, Paumgartner G, Stiehl A, eds. *Biology of Bile Acids in Health and Disease.* Falk Symposium 120. 2001
                                                                ISBN 0-7923-8768-6
121. Leuschner U, James OFW, Dancygier H, eds. *Steatohepatitis (NASH and ASH).* Falk Symposium 121. 2001                                            ISBN 0-7923-8769-4
121A. Matern S, Boyer JL, Keppler D, Meier-Abt PJ, eds. *Hepatobiliary Transport: From Bench to Bedside.* Falk Workshop. 2001                        ISBN 0-7923-8771-6
122. Campieri M, Fiocchi C, Hanauer SB, Jewell DP, Rachmilewitz R, Schölmerich J, eds. *Inflammatory Bowel Disease – A Clinical Case Approach to Pathophysiology, Diagnosis, and Treatment.* Falk Symposium 122. 2002        ISBN 0-7923-8772-4
123. Rachmilewitz D, Modigliani R, Podolsky DK, Sachar DB, Tozun N, eds. *VI International Symposium on Inflammatory Bowel Diseases.* Falk Symposium 123. 2002                                                                    ISBN 0-7923-8773-2
124. Hagenmüller F, Manns MP, Musmann H-G, Riemann JF, eds. *Medical Imaging in Gastroenterology and Hepatology.* Falk Symposium 124. 2002 ISBN 0-7923-8774-0
125. Gressner AM, Heinrich PC, Matern S, eds. *Cytokines in Liver Injury and Repair.* Falk Symposium 125. 2002                                        ISBN 0-7923-8775-9
126. Gupta S, Jansen PLM, Klempnauer J, Manns MP, eds. *Hepatocyte Transplantation.* Falk Symposium 126. 2002                                          ISBN 0-7923-8776-7
127. Hadziselimovic F, ed. *Autoimmune Diseases in Paediatric Gastroenterology.* Falk Symposium 127. 2002                                            ISBN 0-7923-8778-3
127A. Berr F, Bruix J, Hauss J, Wands J, Wittekind Ch, eds. *Malignant Liver Tumours: Basic Concepts and Clinical Management.* Falk Workshop. 2002
                                                                ISBN 0-7923-8779-1
128. Scheppach W, Scheurlen M, eds. *Exogenous Factors in Colonic Carcinogenesis.* Falk Symposium 128. 2002                                          ISBN 0-7923-8780-5
129. Paumgartner G, Keppler D, Leuschner U, Stiehl A, eds. *Bile Acids: From Genomics to Disease and Therapy.* Falk Symposium 129. 2002              ISBN 0-7923-8781-3
129A. Leuschner U, Berg PA, Holtmeier J, eds. *Bile Acids and Pregnancy.* Falk Workshop. 2002                                                          ISBN 0-7923-8782-1
130. Holtmann G, Talley NJ, eds. *Gastrointestinal Inflammation and Disturbed Gut Function: The Challenge of New Concepts.* Falk Symposium 130. 2003
                                                                ISBN 0-7923-8783-X
131. Herfarth H, Feagan BJ, Folsch UR, Schölmerich J, Vatn MH, Zeitz M, eds. *Targets of Treatment in Chronic Inflammatory Bowel Diseases.* Falk Symposium 131. 2003
                                                                ISBN 0-7923-8784-8
132. Galle PR, Gerken G, Schmidt WE, Wiedenmann B, eds. *Disease Progression and Carcinogenesis in the Gastrointestinal Tract.* Falk Symposium 132. 2003
                                                                ISBN 0-7923-8785-6

# Falk Symposium Series